Pyridostigmine Bromide

A Review of the Scientific Literature As It Pertains to Gulf War Illnesses

VOLUME 2

PYRIDOSTIGMINE BROMIDE

Beatrice Alexandra Golomb

Prepared for the Office of the Secretary of Defense

National Defense Research Institute

RAND

This literature review, one of eight commissioned by the Special Assistant to the Deputy Secretary of Defense for Gulf War Illnesses, summarizes the existing scientific literature on the health effects of pyridostigmine bromide that may have affected service members who served in Operations Desert Shield and Desert Storm. The eight RAND reviews are intended to complement efforts by the Defense Department and other federal agencies as they attempt to understand the full range of health implications of service in that conflict.

While many veterans have reported an array of physical and mental health complaints since the war, it is not yet clear the extent to which veterans are experiencing either higher-than-expected rates of identifiable illnesses with known etiologies or any other illnesses from as yet unidentified origins.

The other seven RAND literature reviews deal with chemical and biological warfare agents, depleted uranium, pesticides, oil well fires, immunizations, infectious diseases, and stress. The topics of these reviews all represent plausible causes of some of the illnesses Gulf War veterans have reported.

These reviews are intended principally to summarize the scientific literature on the known health effects of given exposures to these risk factors. Where available evidence permits, the reviews also summarize what is known about the range of actual exposures in the Gulf and assess the plausibility of the risk factor at hand as a cause of illnesses. Statements related to the Gulf War experience should be regarded as suggestive rather than definitive, for much more research both on health effects and exposures remains to be completed before more definitive statements are made. Recommendations for additional research where appropriate are also made.

These reviews are limited to literature published or accepted for publication in peer-reviewed journals, books, government publications, and conference proceedings. Unpublished information was occasionally used, but only to develop hypotheses.

This work is sponsored by the Office of the Special Assistant and was carried out jointly by RAND Health's Center for Military Health Policy Research and the Forces and Resources Policy Center of the National Defense Research Institute. The latter is a federally funded research and development center sponsored by the Office of the Secretary of Defense, the Joint Staff, the unified commands, and the defense agencies.

CONTENTS

FIGURES

TABLES

Pyridostigmine bromide (PB) is a drug, often given as a tablet, that has been approved since 1955 by the U.S. Food and Drug Administration for treatment of myasthenia gravis, a disease characterized by weakness and fatigability of the muscles. During the Persian Gulf War (PGW), PB was used as an "investigational new drug" (IND) by the U.S. military and some other allied forces as a pretreatment adjunct to protect military personnel from death in event of attack with the nerve agent soman. (IND status conferred by the FDA does not permit unrestricted use but may, as in this case, have conditions attached.) PB is called a pretreatment adjunct because it must be given before exposure to be effective. Also, it is not effective alone but only confers benefit if postexposure treatments are given as well.

PB is used primarily to protect troops against attack by one particular nerve agent, soman. During the PGW, Iraq was known to have nerve agents, including sarin, and had weaponized them by putting them into rockets, bombs, and missile warheads. While it was not known whether Iraq had militarized the nerve agent soman, it was known that the former Soviet Union had soman, and there were concerns, particularly since the fragmentation of the former Soviet Union, that Iraq may have purchased soman. Iraq used chemical weapons against Iran and the Kurds. Because of the possibility that Iraq had soman, coalition troops were provided with PB, to be used for protection when the threat of chemical warfare was deemed high. Evidence from that time and subsequent to the PGW suggests that Iraq had weaponized the nerve agents sarin, cyclosarin, and perhaps tabun and VX, but no evidence uncovered suggests they had soman or had weaponized it.

This report examines issues surrounding the safety and to a lesser degree the effectiveness of PB. The sections on safety consider seven hypotheses of how PB might lead to negative health effects. Each hypothesis is investigated to determine if it can be rejected as a possible causal factor. If sufficient evidence cannot be marshaled to rule out a hypothesis, this does not imply that it is necessarily a causal factor, only that the possibility cannot be dismissed.

HOW PB PROTECTS AGAINST SOMAN EXPOSURE

To understand how PB protects against soman requires understanding the action of nerve agents. Nerve agents act by irreversibly binding to, and inhibiting, the normal action of acetylcholinesterase (AChE), an enzyme. Acetylcholine (ACh) is a major neurotransmitter, or nerve-signaling chemical, and acts as a signaling chemical both in the brain and elsewhere in the body; for example, it is the main signaling chemical used by nerves to tell muscles to contract. AChE breaks down ACh in the synapse, the area where a nerve sends signals to another nerve, or to a muscle (see Figure S.1). Thus, AChE serves a critical role in regulating nerve signaling to other nerve cells or to muscle cells. When AChE is inhibited by a nerve agent, an excessive accumulation of ACh occurs in the synapse, followed by excessive binding of ACh to the receptors on the receiving cell (see Figure S.2). Consequently, cells are overstimulated. This condition leads to an array of possible symptoms based on ACh binding to different types of receptors.

For most nerve agents, postexposure treatment confers adequate protection from death with amounts of nerve agent that are presumed likely in warfare. The postexposure treatments in use by the military are atropine and pralidoxime (also called "2PAM"). Atropine antagonizes (blocks) the effects of ACh at one type of receptor, and pralidoxime pulls the nerve agent off the AChE, restoring the action of AChE to normal. In addition to PB, troops were given three "Mark I" kits containing injections of both atropine and pralidoxime for use after a nerve agent attack (Army and possibly Marines) or were given individual injectors of these agents (Air Force and Navy).

RAND*MR1018/2-(1)*

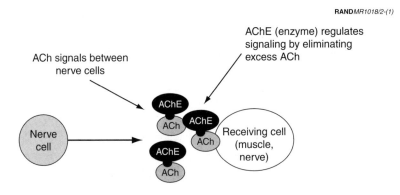

ACh is important in: Muscle action, pain, memory, and sleep.

Figure S.1—How Normal Neurotransmission Works

RAND*MR1018/2-(2)*

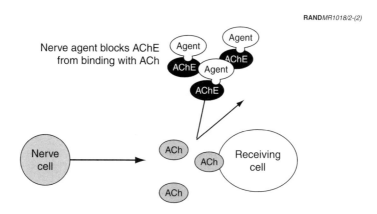

Excess ACh accumulates, signals occur when they should not.
Results may include muscle twitching, paralysis, seizures.

Figure S.2—Nerve Agent Blocks AChE Enzyme

Unfortunately, in the case of soman, a reaction termed "aging" takes place in the nerve agent–AChE complex within only minutes of exposure. Once this reaction has taken place, pralidoxime can no longer pull the nerve agent off the AChE molecule. Thus, troops would not have enough time to administer pralidoxime before AChE is permanently inactivated, which could ultimately result in death. Aging also happens with other nerve agents, but it takes hours to occur after sarin, cyclosarin, tabun, or VX exposure, which allows troops adequate time to administer pralidoxime before aging has taken place, helping to restore AChE action. Animal evidence suggests that to ensure adequate protection against death in the event of a soman attack, PB pretreatment must be employed.[1]

PB acts—it is thought—by reversibly binding to (and, incidentally, inhibiting) the AChE on the site where the nerve agent would bind, thus blocking soman from permanently inactivating the AChE (see Figure S.3). As soman is cleared from the body, PB spontaneously leaves the AChE and restores functional

---

[1]PB may also slightly raise the protection against the nerve agent tabun in rodents, although good primate data are not available, and the increase in protection against tabun is substantially more modest. This is important because any potential side effects of use of the agent must be weighed against the far smaller number of personnel who could be exposed in a realistic battle scenario to more LD_{50}s (lethal doses for 50 percent of subjects) of tabun than after-exposure treatment alone could protect against, but fewer than PB plus after-exposure treatments could protect against. Moreover, this assumes that people will respond as rodents do. But extrapolation of oxime effects from guinea pigs to primates is problematic; primates may be more oxime-sensitive than guinea pigs so that PB may confer no advantages or possibly reduce protection efficacy.

RAND*MR1018/2-(3)*

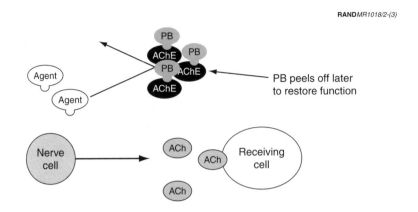

Figure S.3—PB Prevents Nerve Agent from Binding to AChE Enzyme

AChE. The dose of PB used by troops, 30 mg each eight hours, is chosen to inhibit 20 to 40 percent of the AChE. The goal is to ensure that at least this proportion of AChE is relatively safe from permanent inactivation in case of exposure to soman, while allowing enough residual AChE activity (60–80 percent) to prevent significant side effects and to allow personnel to adequately carry out their functions. It is believed that to protect most troops from death by amounts of soman that might realistically occur in a combat setting, a person must be able to withstand approximately five times the normal lethal dose. This level of protection has not been achieved with postexposure treatments alone (that is, with atropine and pralidoxime) but requires use of PB as a pretreatment adjunct in tests in nonhuman primates.

HOW EFFECTIVE IS PB?

The dose of PB needed to protect humans against the effects of soman is not clear and may be higher than previously thought. Tests done in primates to determine the protection by PB against soman have used higher doses of PB (three to 50 times as high on a mg/kg basis), as well as higher doses of atropine (four times as high on a mg/kg basis) than those actually used in humans for nerve agent protection. In addition, these tests commonly have given the equivalent of all three atropine-pralidoxime postexposure treatments at once. Higher doses of PB are given to achieve a similar percentage of AChE inhibition, while the higher doses of atropine are given on the grounds that the nonhuman primates tested are this much "less sensitive" to the effects of atropine. The extrapolation of these data to humans then rests on the assumption that the percentage of AChE inhibition is the exclusive relevant "measure" of the "pharmacologically equivalent" dose of PB (with an analogous argument for atropine), which may or may not be so. According to the only identified study (Smith, 1981)[2] that directly compared the ability of PB to protect against the effects of soman in human and primate muscle tissue, 10 times as high an in vitro dose of PB was needed in humans as in monkeys to provide comparable protection (whereas we give only one-tenth the oral dose to achieve a comparable AChE percentage inhibition). These data arouse concerns about the validity of extrapolation from primate data to humans. It is known that the protective ability of PB, atropine, and oximes vary widely from one species to another.

In monkeys and to a lesser extent in other animals, PB protects against the lethal effects of the nerve agent soman; but it does not prevent severe incapacitation of the animals from high doses of the nerve agent. So even if data signifying protection in primates at higher doses of PB do extrapolate to humans at lower doses, troops are likely to be incapacitated in the presence of a soman attack. Moreover, in animal studies, PB appears to reduce somewhat the protection (conferred by postexposure atropine and pralidoxime) against lethal effects of some other nerve agents, such as sarin and cyclosarin. This apparent reduction in protection still provides for high protection in some animals (with "protective ratios," characterizing protection against lethal effects, that are still several times higher than the fivefold protection that has been designated as desirable). However, no direct evidence ensures that the increased vulnerability to death (*reduced* protection) that PB may bring for such nerve agents as sarin leaves high or "adequate" (fivefold) protection intact in humans. Again, substantial interspecies differences have been seen, with changes not only in magnitude but also in the sign (direction) of the effect of PB, and testing of protection by PB against lethal effects of nerve agents in humans cannot, of course, be done.

IS PB SAFE? SAFETY CONSIDERATIONS OF USING PB

The short-term side effects of taking PB—which also may occur with exposure to any nerve agent—are those of AChE inhibition and the resulting excess of ACh action. These effects may include muscle twitching, muscle spasms, weakness or paralysis, and secretions from glands. Consequences may include difficulty in breathing, cramping, feeling of urge to urinate or frequent urination, tearing, runny nose, salivation, increased bronchial secretions, diarrhea, and sweating.

---

[2]Source citations for other references in the "Summary" can be found in the corresponding chapters of the main body of this report.

PB is normally largely excluded from entry to the brain by the "blood-brain barrier," which bars access to the brain of many chemicals and organisms that circulate in the blood. If PB gains entry to the brain, adverse effects can result from the binding of PB to ACh receptors in the brain. These effects may include confusion, emotional changes such as depression, sleep alterations, and difficulties with concentration and memory.

This report explores whether PB—with this panoply of *acute* effects—could plausibly have contributed to *chronic* symptoms reported by ill PGW veterans. Far higher doses of PB, used for far longer times (typically lifelong) have been employed for decades to treat patients with myasthenia gravis, and this has been assumed by many to indicate that lower-dose, briefer use in nerve agent pretreatment will be safe. However, data from patients with myasthenia might not extrapolate completely to those taking PB for other purposes. For one thing, PB is used in patients with myasthenia gravis to restore nicotinic cholinergic function (at least in the muscles) *toward* normal. In those without myasthenia gravis, PB raises ACh function *away* from normal. Thus, extrapolating evidence of safety from patients with myasthenia gravis is somewhat analogous to assuming that, since high doses of insulin are tolerated—or even necessary— in some patients with diabetes (to bring their blood sugar toward normal), therefore a smaller dose of insulin should surely be safe in those without diabetes. We know this is not the case and that smaller doses of insulin given to normal individuals can cause adverse effects and even death. There are other important reasons PB may not be safe for nonmyasthenic individuals, which are discussed later.

HYPOTHESES RELATING PB USE TO ILLNESSES IN PGW VETERANS

A literature review was performed to identify hypotheses or theories that might link PB to illnesses in PGW veterans and to evaluate evidence pertaining to these hypotheses. Hypotheses are divided into two categories: those that may explain how some individuals may have had heightened susceptibility to PB and those that purport to link exposure to PB—perhaps enabled by such heightened susceptibility—to development of chronic illnesses.

Hypotheses regarding heightened susceptibility to effects of PB include the following:

- Stressful or other special conditions may allow PB to breach the blood-brain barrier and penetrate the brain, producing effects that would not "normally" occur.

- Individual differences in physiology may lead to widely different levels of and susceptibility to PB.

- Interactions between PB and other chemicals may produce toxicity greater than that produced by either alone.

Hypotheses that propose mechanisms by which PB exposure could produce subsequent chronic symptoms include the following:

- The bromide in PB may accumulate in the body, leading to development of a condition termed bromism, which can produce many neuropsychiatric symptoms.

- Exposure to AChE-inhibiting agents, such as PB, may promote a "syndrome" termed "multiple chemical sensitivity" with symptoms similar to those reported by PGW veterans.

- PB may lead to chronic effects on the neuromuscular junction.

- PB may lead to abnormal regulation of the ACh neurotransmitter system.

Several other considerations, including possible effects of PB on sleep and serotonin, are also discussed. The evidence appears to be adequate to dismiss one hypothesis of PB as a significant contributor to illness—that of bromism—but is insufficient to rule out the other hypotheses as possible explanations of how PB might have contributed to PGW illnesses.

HYPOTHESES REGARDING HEIGHTENED EFFECTS OF PB

Blood-Brain Barrier: Does PB Cross the Blood-Brain Barrier During Conditions of Stress?

The permeability of the "blood-brain barrier" in PGW veterans may have been enhanced due to stress and other conditions of war, permitting increased access of PB to the brain. Moreover, PB itself may increase the access of other agents to the brain. Data demonstrating breach of the blood-brain barrier, consequently allowing increased access of PB to the brain in conditions of stress, comes from recent limited research conducted on rodents. However, human data suggest a possible increase in central nervous system (CNS) side effects of PB during the war compared to peacetime, which could also reflect increased access of PB to the brain during stressful circumstances.

The degree to which the blood-brain barrier may have been compromised in conditions of stress may influence the possible contribution of several other hypotheses. For example, dysregulation of the brain's cholinergic system is less likely to result from PB use unless PB gains access to the brain—or other AChE inhibitors do so, perhaps facilitated by PB. (In fact, however, changes in cholinergic function occurring in the periphery could have central consequences).

Individual Differences: Do Physiologic Differences Influence Susceptibility to PB?

Individual differences in susceptibility may also contribute to a connection between PB and chronic illnesses. How is it, if PB is a contributor to chronic illnesses in PGW veterans, that some PGW veterans who took PB became ill, while others who took a similar amount did not? Individual differences of many kinds play a role in the effect of PB on the body. First, differences occurred in the dose of PB actually taken by troops. Moreover, different absorption of PB pills from the gut into the blood; differences in chemical structure, in efficiency of action, and in available amounts of enzymes that clear PB from the blood; and differences in other factors all may lead to different PB blood levels. Furthermore, differences in AChE inhibition occur even for the same blood level of PB. Finally, differences in toxic effects may occur even if individuals experience the same degree of AChE inhibition, perhaps reflecting individual differences at baseline in elements of the complex ACh system.

Altogether, these factors provide substantial opportunity for differences in effect from the "same" oral dose of PB from one individual to another. From a clinical standpoint, individual differences in *acute* susceptibility to PB obviously occur and are reflected in differences in side effects individuals experienced in response to PB. There is limited evidence that the acute susceptibility differences may arise from mechanisms relevant to differences in chronic symptoms in PGW veterans—one study finds a relation between certain chronic illness "syndromes" in ill PGW veterans and self-reported adverse acute response to administration of PB. If PB is a contributor to chronic illnesses in some PGW veterans, then individual differences in susceptibility could play a role in determining which individuals are affected.

Interactions with Other Exposures: Do Interactions Between PB and Other Exposures Enhance the Toxicity of Effects?

Another factor that may play a role in the connection between PB and illnesses in PGW veterans involves possible interactions between PB and other exposures. Animal studies indicate that additive or even synergistic toxicity—that is, toxic effects from a group of chemicals that are more than the sum of the toxic effects from the individual chemicals—may occur with PB and other exposures that some veterans may have experienced. These may include pesticides and insect repellents, as well as caffeine, perhaps nerve agents, and chemicals released by the body itself in conditions of stress.

The degree to which these interactions between PB and other exposures may play a role in PGW veterans is unclear for several reasons. First, we do not have good data regarding who received which exposures, complicating any epidemiological studies to determine the effect of these interactions. Second, the data from animal studies are difficult to extrapolate to PGW veterans because extremely high doses of both PB and the interactants have been used in studies in animals—doses many times higher than those experienced by PGW veterans.

Addressing the question of whether important synergistic effects would occur with lower doses of interactants—more comparable to those administered to PGW veterans—is not simple. There is no good way to assess whether low doses in animals produce effects comparable to those reported by ill veterans. In the existing animal studies, relatively crude measures, such as gross incoordination in walking, or death, are often employed because it is difficult to test animals for more-subtle effects. If lower doses are studied, more-sensitive measures will need to be found. Nonetheless, because evidence of synergistic toxicity exists, interactions between PB and other agents or exposures remain a possible avenue by which increased effect or toxicity of PB may have occurred in some veterans.

HYPOTHESES PROPOSING A LINK BETWEEN PB AND DEVELOPMENT OF CHRONIC SYMPTOMS

Bromism: Does Accumulation of the Bromide from PB Produce Bromism?

Bromism is a condition characterized by neurological and psychiatric symptoms and caused by the accumulation of bromide in the body. It has been suggested that PB administration during the PGW may have led to this condition. However, bromism emerges as an unlikely cause of chronic illness, because the cumulative doses of bromide ingested in PB pills by most PGW veterans were too small to cause bromism, and the time-course of illness in many ill PGW veterans is too long to be typical of this condition, which usually abates within days to months of discontinuing exposure to bromide. Although it is conceivable that bromism could have contributed to illnesses for some rare veterans with special circumstances, bromism is highly unlikely as a significant contributor to illnesses in most ill veterans.

Multiple Chemical Sensitivity (MCS): Does PB Lead to MCS?

MCS is a putative symptom complex involving multiple self-reported "sensitivities" or adverse subjective responses to low levels of a host of apparently unrelated foods and chemicals. Symptoms may include headaches, difficulty concentrating, memory impairment, and musculoskeletal and abdominal complaints. MCS is not universally accepted as a syndrome by scientists or clinicians. It lacks a widely accepted case definition, and no objective technique has been identified to distinguish those who report symptoms from those who do not. Since MCS itself is not universally accepted or well understood, it is poorly positioned to explain illnesses in PGW veterans.

Still, there are several intriguing similarities. First, symptoms reported by patients with MCS are not confined to chemical sensitivities; and other symptoms, such as musculoskeletal symptoms and headaches, are reportedly similar to those described by ill PGW veterans. Second, some ill PGW veterans report that they have developed new chemical sensitivities since their return from the PGW. Third, many or most ill PGW veterans and MCS patients experienced exposures to AChE-inhibiting drugs or chemicals prior to developing their symptoms. Moreover, the genesis of MCS has been proposed to relate to excessive ACh activity, or reduced AChE activity, which may presumably have been experienced by PGW veterans exposed to PB. At present, because of limitations noted above, MCS cannot serve as an explanation for illnesses in any PGW veterans. However, it can be hoped that ongoing research into each condition (MCS and illnesses in PGW veterans) will advance understanding of possible cholinergic mechanisms for both, whether or not these conditions are found to converge.

Neuromuscular Junction (NMJ) Effects: Does PB Produce NMJ Changes?

Nerves signal to muscles using ACh at the neuromuscular junction (NMJ), and this signaling causes the muscles to contract. Administration of high doses of AChE-inhibiting drugs, such as PB, has been shown in animals to produce destructive changes to the muscle tissue and to produce pre- and postsynaptic changes in the NMJ—that is, changes that occur both at the side of the signal-sending nerve cell and at the side of the signal-receiving muscle cell. These changes begin after a single dose of PB. Though some destructive effects begin to recede even if use of PB is continued, partially restoring the appearance of the muscle and of the NMJ, this restoration has not been complete in all cases, even long after administration of PB has been stopped. Thus, chronic—and perhaps permanent—changes take place.

Findings at the NMJ are important for two reasons. First, some of the symptoms reported by PGW veterans include musculoskeletal problems and fatigue, to which the effects of PB at the NMJ might contribute. Second, the NMJ is the most accessible cholinergic synapse, and it is therefore the easiest one to study. Researchers have hoped that effects evident at the NMJ will accurately reflect effects at acetylcholinergic synapses in the brain. In some instances, but not others, this hope has been borne out. Additional and different processes play important roles in brain synapses.

Neurotransmitter Dysregulation: Does PB Alter Regulation of Neurotransmitters, Particularly ACh?

Abnormal regulation of neurotransmitter systems may occur following the administration of drugs that act on these systems. "Downregulation," in this case the (hypothesized) attenuation or suppression of the acetylcholinergic system following use of such AChE-inhibiting drugs as PB, is an instance of dysregulation. That is, during and after PB use, effects may occur that counteract the abnormally high activity of ACh induced by PB. Changes consistent with downregulation have been demonstrated in the NMJ with drugs like PB. Moreover, some evidence suggests that dysregulation changes may also occur in the brain, when AChE-inhibiting chemicals gain access to it. These changes have been demonstrated in animals, using AChE inhibitors that readily gain access to the CNS, and typically at doses that achieve higher levels of AChE inhibition than expected for doses to which veterans were exposed. These may include both changes that enhance and that depress ACh action, with different effects occurring for different components of the ACh system and in different parts of the brain. Different effects may also occur with widely differing time-scales, from very brief to long-term or perhaps permanent. They may involve changes in production, packaging, and release of the neurotransmitter; changes in the number of receptors for ACh, in the "affinity" of these receptors for ACh (the avidity with which ACh attaches), and in their response to ACh; and changes in production and degradation of the enzymes that regulate breakdown of ACh.

By hypothesis, symptoms described by PGW veterans could be manifestations of a prolonged dysregulation effect from PB use. But this hypothesis has not been directly substantiated by data. *If* PB gains access to the brain, discontinuing PB exposure might lead to symptoms of low (or altered) ACh activity. However, little basic science has been done to characterize the time-course of dysregulation changes, and more needs to be understood about the doses and the durations of use that might produce it—recalling that individual differences are surely at play. Clinically, ACh is known to play an important role in memory, sleep, and pain, as well as muscle action, and the most prominent symptoms reported by PGW veterans include problems with memory, sleep, pain, and fatigue. Moreover, studies have been done in which drugs that boost ACh function, particularly nicotinic function, have specifically benefited memory, pain, fatigue, diarrhea, and sleep apnea. (Sleep apnea is a specific sleep abnormality that has been reported among ill PGW veterans). These findings, indicating the selective benefit of ACh-enhancing drugs for problems that figure prominently in complaints of ill PGW veterans, are consistent with the possibility that these symptoms in PGW veterans could derive from ACh downregulation (or, more generally, dysregulation) resulting from use of PB.

However, they are not proof of this hypothesis. In addition, these studies showing benefit to these symptoms from ACh-enhancing drugs have not been done in ill PGW veterans, and it is unknown whether ill veterans would derive similar benefit. At present, the idea of neurotransmitter dysregulation as an explanation for illnesses in some PGW veterans is speculative. Research is needed to clarify what role, if any, such dysregulation might have in the development of chronic symptoms.

Chronic Effects

Some literature suggests the possibility of chronic effects by AChE inhibitors generally, including PB. Data regarding chronic effects, particularly from low-dose exposures that do not produce acute symptoms, are meager and studies are frequently of poor quality. Some studies fail to demonstrate such abnormalities on neuropsychological or other tests in persons with prior AChE exposures. Other studies report chronic changes in nerve and muscle function, EEGs, regional cerebral blood flow, or neuropsychological tests, typically following exposure to AChE-inhibiting pesticides or to nerve agents.

Still other studies have evaluated whether ill PGW veterans indeed have chronic neurological abnormalities. The findings of these studies have been mixed. Differences in findings may reflect both the strategy for selecting ill veterans and the character of the tests performed. If chronic effects are present, they could be missed by failing to properly identify cases and controls or by performing tests that are not sensitive to the specific deficits that ill veterans may have. Of course, if chronic neuropsychological effects are not present in PGW veterans more often than in others, then neither PB nor any other exposure will need to be invoked as an explanation.

A few small studies of chronic neuropsychological findings in ill PGW veterans suggest that selected ill veterans have statistically lower scores on neuropsychological tests than do healthy controls. Although it appears that *some* ill veterans do have mildly diminished neurocognitive function, the extent to which an excess number of veterans do so remains to be clarified. The reductions in function that have been observed do not appear to relate to one or a small number of neurocognitive abilities. However, since the acetylcholinergic system plays a prominent role in many functions of the brain, abnormalities resulting from the disruption of the ACh system might be expected to span many functions. An additional important issue is whether such impairment, if present, is related to use of—or an adverse response to—PB. One study suggested a connection between adverse acute response to PB and current neuropsychological syndromes in Gulf War veterans. Moreover, a recent study from Britain found that self-report of exposure to PB was strongly and significantly linked to current CDC-defined Gulf War illness among British veterans. These and other completed works are limited by the use of self-reporting to determine exposure to PB. Individuals who are ill may remember use of PB differently from individuals who are not ill. (Self-report appears to be the best gauge of use available because records of who received PB, who took PB, and how much they took, were not maintained. Moreover, in the British study, risk ratios were not materially different for troops for whom records were available to confirm risk-factor status, compared to the group as a whole, suggesting against a major role for recall bias.) In short, there is suggestive evidence that some AChE inhibitors may cause chronic neurological changes. There is some objective evidence that chronic neurological changes exist in some ill PGW veterans compared with healthy controls. There is limited evidence that development of some types of chronic neuropsychological changes may be linked to acute response to administration of PB. Consequently, one cannot rule out the possibility that long-term effects of PB might occur and might participate in the production of neuropsychological and other deficits reported by some PGW veterans.

Other Effects

PB's effects on hormones, sleep, the serotonergic and other neurotransmitter systems, and the observation of increased deaths from accidents in PGW veterans after the war may merit additional study. Many PGW veterans report difficulties with sleep. Sleep is prominently regulated by the ACh and serotonin/melatonin systems, both of which might be influenced by PB. Sleep apnea may be particularly common in ill PGW veterans, and some studies outside the PGW population suggest that sleep apnea may respond to nicotine (a "nicotinic" acetylcholinergic agent), consistent with proposed dysregulation of the ACh system in ill PGW veterans. PB may mimic serotonin, providing another avenue for association between PB use and sleep difficulties in PGW veterans. Disruption of sleep, in turn, has been shown to have a role in some pain syndromes. Moreover, sleep disruption is strongly linked to susceptibility to motor vehicle accidents, and epidemiologic studies show an increase in death by motor vehicle accidents in PGW veterans. (Other neurological characteristics that some researchers are investigating in subsets of ill PGW veterans may also dispose them to increased risk of accidental death, perhaps independent of sleep difficulties. For instance, abnormalities in eye movement coordination if confirmed could retard reaction times, which could translate to increased risk when at the wheel.)

LIMITATIONS OF THIS REVIEW AND FUTURE DIRECTIONS

The combined literature related to PB, to PGW illnesses, and particularly to acetylcholinergic function is quite extensive. Although this document is far from being a complete evaluation of each of these areas, it does present a much more thorough discussion of the acetylcholinergic system and its relation to possible mechanisms of illness than have previous discussions of PB as a contributor to illnesses in PGW veterans. Certainly, all possible issues have not been addressed, and it is hoped that future efforts can build on the foundation laid here.

Several issues important to military use of PB were reviewed but are not discussed in detail in this report, including data regarding the efficacy of PB as a nerve agent pretreatment adjunct, data on acute physiological and performance effects of PB, and information about acute side effects outside the warfare setting. (Limited information on the acute effects of PB is included in Appendix B.) While important to the future military use of PB, these data do not directly address the development of chronic illnesses in PGW veterans.

Concern regarding PB as a possible source of chronic symptoms is relatively new, and research in this area is in its infancy. Human data regarding chronic effects are mostly observational, and these epidemiological studies are complicated by lack of a consistent clinical case definition distinguishing which PGW veterans should be counted as ill or as neurologically symptomatic as a result of their involvement in the PGW. The lack of good data regarding who received which exposures hinders study as well. When both the exposure and the outcome are not well characterized, it is doubly difficult to evaluate clearly the connection between PB exposure and an adverse outcome. While some experimental data related to short-term PB effects are available from studies using non-war volunteers, such studies have not looked at long-term effects and have not entailed conditions of high stress and interactions with other exposures that may have conditioned susceptibility to PB in the PGW. Most experimental studies relating to toxic effects, and involving stress and drug interactions, are done in animals at relatively high doses, and the degree to which this evidence extrapolates to humans is unknown.

The findings reported here, in which it is concluded that PB cannot be excluded as a contributor to illness in PGW veterans, differ from conclusions of some prior investigating bodies, such as the Presidential Advisory Committee and the Institute of Medicine. Three significant factors contribute to these differences. First, a more extensive literature review, and particularly a more in-depth examination of the ACh system, has been performed. Second, the approach to evaluation of evidence differs. Some prior reports appear to have interpreted the evidence as though absence of proof that PB contributed to illness constitutes proof that it did not. Finally, new evidence has become available that provides additional rationale for concern regarding PB—evidence not available to previous groups. Similarly, our own findings are provisional and subject to change as new evidence emerges.

CONCLUSIONS

Two major conclusions emerge from this review of the scientific literature, one pertaining to the safety and one to the effectiveness of PB. First, PB cannot be ruled out as a possible contributor to the development of unexplained or undiagnosed illness in some PGW veterans. Of the hypotheses considered, the evidence permits the rejection of only one—bromism. The others remain scientifically viable. By their nature, these hypotheses are not mutually incompatible.

Second, uncertainties remain concerning the effectiveness of PB in protection of humans against nerve agents. Most data on effectiveness of PB in primates derive from studies using higher doses, and how well these extrapolate to lower dose use in humans remains ambiguous. Finally, some literature, again mostly based on animal studies, indicates that use of PB may reduce somewhat the effectiveness of postexposure treatment for some nonsoman nerve agents. The extent and importance this reduction would have in humans is unknown.

These findings based on the scientific literature raise many questions and have important implications relating to the use of PB in military deployments. Clearly, substantially more research into the effectiveness of PB for humans is needed—and quickly. Meanwhile, the issue is a complex one, involving trading off uncertain health risks—but risks now shown to be biologically plausible—against uncertain gains from use of PB in the warfare setting.

ACKNOWLEDGMENTS

Many individuals assisted in the present effort. I thank the principal investigators, Ross Anthony and Mike Hix, for their effective leadership. I thank Dr. Caren Kamberg and Dr. Roberta Shanman for their invaluable assistance identifying, aggregating, and keeping track of literally thousands of references. I thank Beth Giddens for her efforts to make the document more reader-friendly. I thank Dr. Terrence Sejnowski for his ever-available neuroscience expertise. I thank Dr. Hermona Soreq for providing very helpful feedback on Chapter Eight. I thank the reviewers for their advice, expertise, and assistance with this difficult document.

I am indebted to many individuals for discussions or assistance, including (but not confined to) the following: Muhammed Abou-Donia, Edson Albuquerque, Walter Allan, William Augerson, Mike Boyle, Barbara Brake, Clarence Broom-field, Kelley Brix, William Baumsweiger, Ronald Clawson, Bhupendra Doctor, Albert Donnay, William Doyle, Edward Elson, Marge Filbert, Timothy Finnegan, Ari Friedman, Lunette Friend, Clem Furlong, Tim Gerrity, Arnold Gass, Mary Gentry, Chris Gillin, Robert Haley, Arlene Hudson, Randy Hudspeth, David Janowsky, William Kane, Michael Kilpatrick, Katherine Murray Leisure, Oksana Lockridge, Brian Malkin, William McCain, Robert McPhail, Charles Millard, Claudia Miller, Edward Moldenhauer, Dee Morris, James Moss, John Otten-weller, Stephanie Padilla, James Patrick, Carey Pope, Joan Porter, Douglas Reichard, Richard Rettig, David Rhine, Elihu Richter, Kenneth Robinson, Thomas Tiedt, David Trump, and Dale Vesser. These individuals, however, bear no responsibility for any errors herein. We are also particularly indebted to the British, who declassified a host of documents and provided us access to them; this occurred late in the process of developing this document, and many more findings from these studies could have been included than were. Nonetheless, the studies led to important insights, some of which are reflected in the current pages.

ACh	Acetylcholine
AChE	Acetylcholinesterase
BChE	Butyrylcholinesterase
CCEP	Comprehensive Clinical Evaluation Program
CNS	Central nervous system
COPD	Chronic obstruction pulmonary disease
CW	Chemical warfare
DFP	Diisopropyl fluorophosphate
DoD	Department of Defense
EEG	Electroencephalogram, a measure of brain activity
EMG	Electromyography
FDA	Food and Drug Administration
GABA	Gamma amino butyric acid
GI	Gastrointestinal
IND	Investigational new drug
IOM	Institute of Medicine
LD_{50}	Lethal dose for 50 percent of subjects
MCS	Multiple chemical sensitivity
NAPP	Nerve Agent Pretreatment Pack
NAPS	Nerve Agent Pretreatment System
NMJ	Neuromuscular junction
NTE	Neurotoxic esterase
OP	Organophosphate
OPIDN	Organophosphate induced delayed neurotoxicity
PAC	Presidential Advisory Commission
2PAM	Pralidoxime, a postexposure treatment for nerve agent protection
PB	Pyridostigmine bromide
PGW	Persian Gulf War
PNS	Peripheral nervous system
PON	Paraoxonase

PR   Protective ratio; LD_{50} with treatment divided by LD_{50}
                      without treatment
PTSD   Posttraumatic stress disorder
RBC   Red blood cell
REM   Rapid eye movement
SPECT imaging   Single Photon Emission Computer Tomography, a
                      method of evaluating regional (brain) blood flow at a
                      cross section in time
SVN   Sindbis virus strain

Chapter One

INTRODUCTION

BACKGROUND

An estimated 250,000 to 300,000 U.S. veterans of Operation Desert Storm/Operation Desert Shield, also called the Persian Gulf War (PGW) took pyridostigmine bromide (PB), used as a pretreatment adjunct to protect troops in the event of chemical warfare using the nerve agent soman (Brake, 1997). This report examines the evidence regarding whether PB may be linked to illnesses in Persian Gulf War veterans.

Veterans of the Persian Gulf War have reported such symptoms as joint pains, sleep disorder, memory loss, and fatigue more frequently than those who were not deployed (Joseph, 1997) (Table 1.1). The exact number of veterans reporting symptoms that they attribute to involvement in the PGW is difficult to characterize; about 100,000 have enrolled in VA (Veterans Affairs) and DoD (Department of Defense) registries. However, some of those enrolled do not report symptoms (although most do). Some who report symptoms—perhaps as many as 80 percent—have been given a "diagnosis." This has been presumed by some to imply that their symptoms have been "explained" and were thus unrelated to Gulf War involvement, but this does not necessarily follow. First, some "diagnoses," such as "tension headache," are little more than descriptors of symptoms, which may have any of a host of root "causes" or contributing factors. (For instance, headaches may result from drug or chemical exposures—e.g., nitrates or monosodium glutamate, insecticides, or caffeine withdrawal; from COPD or other factors producing reduced oxygen to the brain; from high or low blood pressure, from muscular injury or inappropriate muscular contraction; from conditions of the eyes, ears, teeth, or throat; from systemic infectious illness; from collagen vascular disease; from tumor; from cerebrovascular accident; or from endocrine conditions, such as hyperthyroidism, hypo- or hyperglycemia, among many other causes (Adler, Lam, et al., 1994)). Second, a "diagnosis" may be correct and may be unrelated to Gulf War

1

Table 1.1

Most Frequent Symptoms Among 3,558 Registry Participants with a Primary Diagnosis of "Symptoms, Signs, and Ill-Defined Conditions"

Symptom	As Chief Complaint (%)	As Any Complaint (%)
Fatigue	20.0	59
Headache	9.0	44
Memory problems	6.0	40
Sleep disturbances	5.0	40
Rash	4.0	30
Joint pain	4.0	47
Shortness of breath	2.0	19
Abdominal pain	1.0	16
Muscle pain	1.0	22
Difficulty concentrating	1.0	31
Diarrhea	0.5	18
Depression	0.3	22
Cough	1.0	1

SOURCE: Joseph, 1997.

involvement but may explain only one or several of a set of symptoms in a veteran—who may have additional unexplained symptoms. Third, many conditions—perhaps most possible diagnoses—have known (and certainly unknown) environmental risk factors, so that having a "diagnosis" does not in itself preclude a contribution from Gulf War involvement. (For instance, increasing evidence suggests that past infection with chlamydia pneumonia (Grayston, Kuo, et al., 1993; Melnick, Shahar, et al., 1993; Puolakkainen, Kuo, et al., 1993; Saikku, 1997; Muhlestein, Hammond, et al., 1996; Wimmer, Sandmann-Strupp, et al., 1996) or some herpes viruses (Nieto, Adam, et al., 1996; Dummer, Lee, et al., 1994; Melnick, Adam, et al., 1993; Sorlie, Adam, et al., 1994) increases the risk of atherosclerosis, heart attacks, and strokes—as do exposures to environmental cigarette smoke and many other factors.) Further complicating the characterization of the number of those with symptoms "associated with" Gulf War involvement is the fact that many personnel who have symptoms have elected not to participate in Gulf War registries, for a host of reasons, including fear of job discrimination and the belief that enrollment confers few tangible benefits. These factors have complicated the ability to assess the degree to which symptom reports are greater in PGW veterans than in controls. They have also complicated the ability to do studies to investigate the relationship of factors (such as exposure to PB) to development of illnesses in PGW veterans because it is hard to define who constitutes a "case" and who constitutes a "control." (Some studies have used Registry participation per se to designate who is a case, and this strategy clearly produces misclassification. Others are beginning work on establishing a case definition for "Gulf War

Syndrome." Nonetheless, PGW veterans who do not meet the case definition should not automatically be considered suitable "controls," particularly if they report illness, because the validity of such case definitions remains to be ascertained.) This report will not cover the epidemiological evidence relating to illnesses in PGW veterans (which is the subject of a separate report). However, the available evidence does suggest that personnel deployed to the Gulf have an increase in self-reported symptoms compared to nondeployed controls, though they may have started out healthier. As a rough estimate, the number of PGW veterans—of the approximately 700,000 deployed—who may have "unexplained" symptoms, may range from 20,000 (those registered with no diagnosis to "explain" their symptoms) to 100,000 (those registered who are ill, assuming a small fraction of additional ill veterans who have not registered), or perhaps even higher.[1]

---

[1] For the purposes of study, subjects selected as representing ill PGW veterans should be those with more "characteristic" and more severe symptoms. It should be assumed that more than one illness or symptom complex may exist. (Separate study can ascertain whether the rates of these symptom complexes differ in ill PGW veterans and in controls. To define and distinguish among such illness complexes, statistical strategies to establish clustering should be performed. One group of investigators has performed a factor analysis of symptoms (Haley, Kurt, et al. 1997). Other viable strategies include cluster analysis, or use of unsupervised neural networks. After more-common symptoms in ill PGW veterans have been determined and "grouped," "healthy" controls should be selected who have none of these symptoms. (Common symptoms described in ill PGW veterans have included headache, fatigue, and difficulty with sleep, concentration, and memory; other symptoms have included diarrhea, rash, mood alteration, and chemical sensitivities.) The goal is to separate groups at extremes of symptomatology, just as studies of cardiovascular risk factors often compare those in the highest quintile on some factor to those in the lowest quintile to offer greater potential for separation along lines of associated exposures. Because the criteria employed for the purpose of study are intended to identify the more extreme cases, it should not be presumed that others with lesser symptoms are "free" of illness.

Is There a Syndrome? There is debate regarding whether a "syndrome" exists in PGW veterans. Some symptoms are more common than others in veterans, and veterans have different combinations of these more common and less common complaints. Many of the complaints are "nonspecific," such as fatigue, headache, rash, and diarrhea, which may occur in association with many known illnesses of infectious, collagen vascular, endocrine, toxic, or other causes. The picture of variable symptoms is not inconsistent with the presence of a single syndrome—many known medical conditions are characterized by a set of more common and less common symptoms, in which each individual with the syndrome has a different subset of symptoms and some have atypical presentations. (Conditions from widely varying categories of disease provide instances, such as tuberculosis, thyroid disease, B_{12} deficiency, or lupus. Adverse effects in response to drugs and medications are also variable, although some drugs—such as theophylline and digoxin—may have common sets of symptoms on overexposure. Individual presentations may differ, but a pool of common symptoms is recognized.) A "syndrome" is often defined either when unusual symptoms are present or when an objective "marker," such as a blood test, becomes available to which these varying symptoms can be tied. (It may also be defined by statistical grouping techniques such as those described above.) At present, there is no such marker in PGW veterans (see *A Review of the Scientific Literature As It Pertains to the Gulf War, Volume 3: Immunizations* (Golomb, forthcoming), section on mycoplasma, for one candidate). But the absence of an identified marker does not preclude the existence of a predominant syndrome; a marker or test for illness could, for instance, be identified in the future. Thus, at present the situation may be compatible with no predominant syndrome (but with a host of unrelated conditions having nonspecific symptoms, it remains necessary to explain why they are more common in PGW veterans); with one predominant syndrome and a smattering of less-common and unrelated complaints; or with several syndromes. Certainly, illness in PGW veterans includes incidental illness, which some

Although symptoms reported by ill veterans have not been accompanied by a demonstrable increase in hospitalizations (Gray, Coate, et al., 1996) or illness mortality (Kang and Bullman, 1996; Kang and Bullman, 1995), they are a source of continued concern to veterans, and efforts, including the present one, are under way to evaluate whether exposures of these veterans during the PGW might be linked to current reported symptoms.

This report presents PB's characteristics, the circumstances of its use, and an overview of theories relating PB to illnesses in PGW veterans; later chapters review these theories in detail. (A literature review was conducted first to identify theories that may relate PB use to illnesses in PGW veterans and then to identify evidence to allow assessment of these theories.) Current theories relating use of PB to illnesses in PGW veterans include, first, theories that suggest how the effect of PB may have been heightened in some individuals in the circumstances of the PGW. Mechanisms that have been theorized to promote heightened susceptibility in some individuals include individual differences in susceptibility to PB (and to other exposures), interactions between PB and other exposures present in the PGW, and increase in the permeability of the blood-brain barrier due to other exposures experienced by PGW veterans (such as stress), allowing access of PB (and other substances) to the brain. One or a combination of these factors may have acted to enhance the effect and the toxicity of PB and to enable access of PB to the brain, where additional toxic effects might have occurred. The next set of theories concerns what these hypothetical toxic effects, resulting from enhanced toxicity of PB, might have been. These include the possible relationship of PB to development of "multiple chemical sensitivity," effects of PB on the neuromuscular junction, and production of cholinergic dysregulation by administration of PB. One additional chapter reviews the evidence that such substances as PB could produce chronic neuropsychiatric effects. A final chapter briefly discusses other theories and considerations.

---

veterans would have been expected to develop irrespective of their involvement in the PGW. Certainly also some syndromes are associated with exposures experienced in the PGW: Posttraumatic stress syndrome has been diagnosed in a minority of ill veterans, as has viscerotropic leishmaniasis, providing examples of syndromes that account for symptoms in a few but not most ill veterans. Whether there are in addition one or a few dominant syndromes has not been settled. Despite the debate regarding existence of a syndrome, some groups have created working definitions of "Gulf War Syndrome" for research purposes.

The present review is concerned primarily with whether the existing scientific evidence is compatible with a contribution by PB to symptoms reported by PGW veterans. The term "syndrome" will be avoided; rather, we will refer simply to illness in PGW veterans, which intends no implication about the underlying causes.

METHODS

This effort can be divided conceptually into several parts. The first element concerns background information on characteristics of pyridostigmine bromide. This element comprises reviews of the nature, function, and past medical and military use of pyridostigmine.

The second element is a review of the circumstances surrounding the use of PB in the PGW. Information is presented regarding the production, storage and transport, and delivery of PB to troops, as well as decisions regarding who received PB. This information is important insofar as it demonstrates, or fails to demonstrate, irregularities in the circumstances of use that may have contributed to illnesses or differential effects among veterans. Data pertaining to circumstances of use have been gleaned primarily from government reports and interviews.

The third element consists of a review of theories and concerns associated with use of PB in the PGW. Existing theories were identified by searching the Internet, a popular venue for the airing of Gulf War hypotheses (see particularly the Gulflink and Chronic Illness sites) as well as through interviews with investigators of PGW illnesses, comments by veterans and veterans' advocate groups, and examination of the scientific literature.

The final conceptual element, comprising the bulk of the report, consists of chapters discussing evidence pertaining to specific theories regarding a relationship between PB and PGW illnesses. For this element, additional limited reviews of the literature were performed to identify data pertaining to theories that have been advanced concerning how PB and symptoms in PGW veterans are related.

The literature review process has been essential to every stage of this report and is particularly critical for the analysis of evidence pertaining to theories. A systematic literature review conducted by an experienced RAND librarian employed the following databases: Medline, Embase, Scisearch, Chemtox, CASearch, Pesticide fact file (for PB interaction with pesticides), Registry of Toxic Effects of Chemical Substances, Pharmaceutical News Index, Toxline, ADIS Newsletters, SEDBASE, BIOSIS Previews, PNI, RTECS, PASCAL, DTIC, the *New York Times* (via NEXIS), the *Wall Street Journal*, and the *Washington Post* (via DIALOG). The initial search was restricted to English language articles or those with English language abstracts, using the search word *pyridostigmine*. Articles and reports that appeared relevant, based on title, were identified and accessed. Initially, many additional articles were retrieved related to the Persian Gulf War and to diverse putative causes of illnesses in PGW veterans in order to gain an understanding of the topic's background and context. Subsequent, limited searches directed at specific theories were performed. These were supplemented by articles identified from a review of past reports on illnesses in PGW veterans (e.g., the Presidential Advisory Committee (PAC) and the Institute of Medicine (IOM)), articles identified by discussion with experts, and citations in evaluated articles. Cited government reports are restricted to those that are unclassified or declassified.

Chapter Two

FACT SHEET: PB PRETREATMENT FOR SOMAN EXPOSURE

The following synopsis serves as a brief review of PB, its function and mechanism.

WHAT IS PB?

- *Pyridostigmine bromide* is a chemical that blocks the nerve-signal-regulating enzyme *acetylcholinesterase* (AChE). It is given as a pill to military personnel during periods of high threat of chemical warfare attack to prevent death in the event of exposure to the nerve agent soman.

- It is used as an adjunct to postexposure administration of atropine and pralidoxime and confers no protection in the absence of these treatments.

HOW NERVE AGENTS WORK

- Soman, like other nerve agents, acts by inhibiting AChE, the enzyme that breaks down the body's acetylcholine (ACh), a neurotransmitter crucial to regulation of voluntary and involuntary muscles and to function of the brain.

- Once AChE is inhibited, ACh accumulates and may cause death from respiratory failure.

- In addition to spasms of the airways and reduced breathing drive, other effects of soman include slowed heart rate; increased secretions from the nose, eyes, intestines, salivary glands, sweat glands, and airways; increased movement of the intestines; twitching, weakness, and paralysis; loss of consciousness; and seizures.

HOW TRADITIONAL ANTI–NERVE AGENTS WORK

Atropine and Pralidoxime

- *Atropine* is the mainstay of postexposure antidote treatment for nerve agent exposure. Atropine opposes the effects of acetylcholine. (It opposes the "muscarinic effects"—see Chapter 3.) Rapid administration of atropine (by injection) is essential for severe nerve agent casualties.

- *Pralidoxime* (or other oximes), administered by injection, assists in postexposure treatment. Oximes have the ability to cause nerve agents to be removed from AChE. However, they are ineffective once a process called "aging" occurs.

What Is Aging?

- *Aging* is a chemical change that happens to the AChE-nerve agent complex. Aging results in permanent inactivation of the AChE. Aging happens quickly in the case of the soman-AChE complex—half of complexed agents will have aged within a couple of minutes—whereas it takes hours for comparable aging to occur for other nerve agents, such as sarin.

- Once aging has occurred, oxime therapy is ineffective.

How PB Works

- PB is a carbamate compound that is thought to protect AChE by reversibly binding to ("carbamylating") it, so that the nerve agent cannot bind to it. It may also assist in protection against nerve agent by "desensitizing" ACh receptors.

- PB is preferred over other carbamylators because it usually does not penetrate the central nervous system. Consequently, PB minimizes any harmful effects on brain function and does not significantly disable mental performance in those who take it.

PB Is Used When Soman Is a Danger

- *PB is needed for adequate protection against soman:* It takes only two minutes for 50 percent of the AChE-soman complexes to "age," permanently inactivating AChE. Since this reaction time is so short, personnel do not have enough time after they have been exposed to soman to realize they have been exposed to a nerve agent, to take oxime, and to allow oxime to pull nerve agent off AChE. Before all that can be done, most of the soman will have undergone aging, permanently inactivating the bound AChE. However, if personnel take PB in advance of exposure, soman will be prevented from binding to AChE in PB-bound AChE molecules, and aging cannot take place with permanent inactivation of these AChE molecules. The armed forces estimate that during a chemical attack, many personnel may be exposed to five times the lethal dose of nerve agent, so a "protective ratio" (the factor by which a treatment raises the lethal dose) of at least five is needed. Addition of PB allows the protective ratio to exceed five for soman, based on studies in monkeys.

- *PB is not needed against sarin:* It takes five hours for 50 percent of the AChE-sarin complexes to age. PB pretreatment does not confer an advantage against sarin, based on studies in animals; personnel have enough time to take oxime after exposure to this nerve agent before aging takes place, reactivating the AChE molecule. Indeed, soman is the only nerve agent for which PB is known to be necessary to produce an adequate protective ratio.

Chapter Three

CHARACTERISTICS OF PB

This chapter provides background on the drug PB (see Figure 3.1), which was used in the PGW as a pretreatment adjunct to protect against chemical warfare (CW) attack with the nerve agent soman. Topics include the chemical characteristics (and "pharmacokinetics") of PB, its prior Food and Drug Administration (FDA) approved and licensed use for the condition myasthenia gravis, its use in other medical conditions, and its use as a military CW defense agent.

Much of this chapter is technical. Information in this chapter is relevant to understanding some aspects of why PB was given and what was known about its safety and efficacy prior to the PGW. The rationale for treatment with PB is discussed briefly but does not constitute a focus of this report. Other documents focus more specifically on the rationale for use (Pyridostigmine, 1996; Pope, 1997) and the limitations in this rationale (Prendergast, 1997).

CHEMICAL CHARACTERISTICS

Action of PB: Inhibition of AChE

PB is a positively charged quaternary ammonium carbamate compound, which binds to ("carbamylates") two sites on acetylcholinesterase (AChE), a negatively charged site and an esteratic site, preventing acetylcholine (ACh) from binding to these same sites and being broken down by the enzyme (see Figure 3.1). This inhibition leads to buildup of ACh, which is not being hydrolyzed, resulting in increased action of ACh on its receptor.

Acetylcholine Receptors. Not all ACh receptors are alike. Receptors belong to one of two groups, "nicotinic" and "muscarinic," so termed because of specific chemicals—nicotine and muscarine—initially shown to bind to these receptors. Both types of receptors occur both in the CNS (central nervous system, including the brain and spinal cord) and peripherally (as part of the "PNS," or peripheral nervous system, which includes nerve cells and their connections located in the rest of the body).

11

RAND *MR1018/2-3.1*

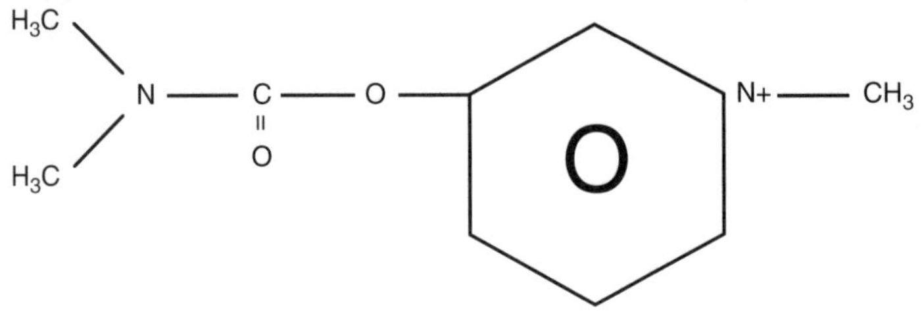

Figure 3.1—Structure of Pyridostigmine Bromide

Nicotinic Receptors. Nicotinic receptors exist in skeletal muscle (the "neuromuscular junction"), autonomic ganglia, the adrenal medulla, and the central nervous system. Nicotinic receptors consist of five protein subunits— classically, two alpha subunits, a beta, a gamma, and a delta. (At the nerve-muscle junction (neuromuscular junction), the alpha subunits are of type "$\alpha 1$" and an epsilon substitutes for the gamma subunit). Since at least 10 distinct subunit sequences for *neuronal* nicotinic ACh receptors have been identified in mammals ($\alpha 2$–$\alpha 7$, $\alpha 9$, $\beta 2$–$\beta 4$—again, this is as opposed to muscles, which use the fixed combination $[\alpha 1]_2 [\beta 1] [\delta] [\epsilon$ or $\gamma]$ in vertebrates), a great many subunit combinations are possible. These produce nicotinic receptors with different structures (though all share the property of having five subunits) and functional characteristics (Lena and Changeux, 1997). They also have different affinity for binding to different acetylcholine "agonists" (substances that bind to acetylcholine receptors and "activate" them) and show different predilections for desensitization (Corringer, Bertrand, et al., 1998). These characteristics are of importance in considering possible effects of PB on the acetylcholine system (see Chapter Thirteen, "Cholinergic Dysregulation").

Of note, receptors with the $\alpha 9$ subunit are actually stimulated by both nicotine and muscarine and have atypical "nicotinic/muscarinic" pharmacology (Changeux, Bessis, et al., 1996).

In each case the subunits are believed to form an "ion channel." Binding of ACh to the receptor produces signaling in the cell by leading to flux of ions through this channel. The different types of nicotinic receptors are not dis-tributed randomly but have characteristic localizations. The nicotinic receptors found at the neuromuscular junction (termed "N1" receptors) are different—in terms of structure and properties—from those at the autonomic ganglia (termed "N2" receptors, which mediate such functions as sweating); they in turn differ from the several varieties found in the CNS. The muscle receptors mediate "fast" effects (as electrical changes in the muscle fiber following ACh binding produce an "action potential," causing the muscle to contract), while central nicotinic effects may have a slower time-course, acting by influencing release of other neurotransmitters, such as dopamine, GABA (gamma amino butyric acid), and glutamate. Although "the nicotinic acetylcholine receptor is the best characterized neurotransmitter receptor" (it has been widely studied in the electric organ of eels and in the easily accessible neuromuscular junction in other animals) (Taylor and Brown, 1994) because of the differences in properties of different nicotinic receptors—and new nicotinic receptors have continued to be characterized—quite a lot remains unknown.

Muscarinic Receptors. Muscarinic receptors are found in the smooth muscle of viscera (internal organs), heart muscle, secretory glands, and in the "endothelial" cells lining blood vessels—as well as in the brain. Muscarinic receptors do not make up ion channels, as nicotinic receptors do. Rather, muscarinic effects are produced more indirectly, through chemicals termed "second messengers." There are at least five distinct muscarinic receptor types (at least five genes have been cloned and sequenced), which differ in their ability to couple to different second messenger "GTP binding proteins," or "G-proteins." These in turn exert other chemical effects, which lead ultimately to muscarinic actions. (The effects of G-proteins are fairly technical and include inhibition of cyclic AMP formation, stimulation of "phospholipase C," and regulation of ion channels—but in this case regulation is not direct, as with nicotinic receptors, but mediated by G-proteins.) (Taylor and Brown, 1994).

Functional Localization of ACh Receptors. As mentioned previously, nicotinic and muscarinic receptors predominate in different places in the body: for example, nicotinic receptors occur in skeletal muscle while muscarinic receptors are found in the smooth muscle of viscera. Moreover, different nicotinic receptors (and different muscarinic receptors) themselves are characteristically found in different parts of the rest of the body—such as "N1" nicotinic receptors at the neuromuscular junction, and "N2" receptors at the autonomic ganglia. Analogously, different receptors dominate in different functions and different parts of the brain. For instance, some areas of the brain (such as the "optic tectum") rely primarily on nicotinic receptors. Some areas—such as the hippocampus (which is critically involved in memory function) and the cerebral cortex—have predominantly muscarinic receptors of the type that bind with high affinity to the chemical "pirenzapine" (which antagonizes the action of ACh and serves as a major factor in distinguishing different types of muscarinic receptors), while the cerebellum and brainstem have predominantly muscarinic receptors that bind this chemical more sluggishly (Taylor and Brown, 1994). As scientists begin to understand more clearly what the effects are of AChE inhibition with such agents as PB on each different receptor type—

and begin to understand more clearly which brain effects rely on which receptors—a more satisfactory resolution to the possible contribution of PB to symptoms in PGW veterans may be obtained. This knowledge is still fairly rudimentary.

Terminology Issues. Actions on these receptors lead to characteristic effects, themselves sometimes termed muscarinic, nicotinic, or "central," depending on the type of receptor that produces these effects upon binding by ACh. When this admittedly loose terminology is used, "nicotinic" and "muscarinic" effects refer to effects from action on the *peripheral* nicotinic and muscarinic receptors. Although central effects themselves result from binding to central nicotinic or muscarinic receptors, it is often not well characterized which receptors are responsible for which effects, so that "central" effects are often referred to. (Nicotine addiction involves central effects that are clearly "nicotinic.") Similar effects—though not identical ones—occur whether increased action of ACh, resulting from inhibition of AChE, is produced by PB, by other carbamates (compounds which, like PB, reversibly "carbamylate" and inactivate the AChE), or by organophosphates (OPs), such as nerve agents or pesticides, which irreversibly "phosphorylate" and inactivate the AChE. A major difference is that since little PB normally crosses the blood-brain barrier into the brain, central effects from PB are normally minimal. In contrast, the related carbamate "physostigmine" does cross into the brain, as do many OPs.

Muscarinic, Nicotinic, and Central Effects of AChE Inhibitors. AChE inhibitors, including both PB and nerve agents, exert their effects by blocking AChE at ACh receptor sites, increasing ACh and ACh activity, causing first hyperactivity of smooth and of skeletal muscles (Medical Letter, 1990) and then paralysis (with high enough doses). If the agent penetrates the CNS, then CNS effects also occur. Nerve agents penetrate the CNS; however, PB does not, or at least not much, when taken under normal conditions. Limited evidence suggests that PB does penetrate the CNS when it is taken under stressful conditions. (See Chapter Seven, "Blood-Brain Barrier Passage.")

Skeletal muscle effects are among the so-called *nicotinic effects.* Early skeletal muscle symptoms include twitching and cramps and coincide with axonal "backfiring," in which a signal travels up the "axon," the nerve process that relays signals, in the reverse direction to that by which signaling ordinarily occurs. Twitching is first seen in eyelids, and it spreads to face and calves and then becomes generalized. This reaction occurs in the first 24 hours and may be followed by weakness or paralysis, depending on the severity of the intoxication. Paralysis involves all skeletal muscles, including the breathing muscles, and results in labored, shallow, and rapid breathing. Respiratory failure and cyanosis (turning blue) may ensue in some cases. Weakness of the tongue and pharyngeal muscles (muscles in the pharynx, or back of the throat) further enhances respiratory failure by promoting airway obstruction (Gutmann and Besser, 1990; Medical Letter, 1995; Whinnery, 1984).

Muscarinic receptors, as mentioned previously, are found in the smooth muscle of "viscera" (internal organs), heart muscle, secretory glands, and in the endothelial cells lining blood vessels—as well as in the brain. *Muscarinic effects* from action of ACh at smooth muscles, glands, and the heart include spasm of smooth muscles, increased glandular secretions, and slowing of the heart rate (Hardman, Limbird, et al., 1996). Specific examples of smooth muscle spasm and increased secretions include increased abdominal motility and intestinal secretions, with possible consequent abdominal cramping, nausea, vomiting, and diarrhea; excessive salivation (with drooling); lacrimation (increased secretions from tear ducts); rhinorrhea (runny nose); bronchorrhea (increased bronchial, or airway, secretions); bronchospasm (constriction of the airways); laryngospasm (constriction of the larynx area); diaphoresis (sweating); ureteral spasm with frequent urination or bladder incontinence; and sphincter relaxation, which may promote bowel incontinence. Miosis, or pupillary constriction, is almost always present. In addition, there may be reddening of the eyes and slowing of the heart (Gutmann, and Besser, 1990; Medical Letter, 1995; Whinnery, 1984; Taylor and Brown, 1994). Nicotinic and muscarinic effects on the heart rate are opposed, so theoretically either an increased or reduced heart rate may occur, but bradycardia (slowed heart rate) is more common.

ACh influences autonomic ganglia through both muscarinic and nicotinic mechanisms. Effects also include release of "catecholamines," such as adrenaline (nicotinic). Consequences of these effects may include pallor and transitory elevation of blood pressure followed by low blood pressure (Gunderson, Lehmann, et al., 1992).

So-called *central effects* result from accumulation of ACh at central synapses. As previously noted, central receptors are themselves characterized as muscarinic or nicotinic, but because it is often not well known which receptors are responsible for which effects, effects are commonly referred to simply as "central." Early signs include anxiety, restlessness, emotional lability, insomnia, and excessive dreaming. (Sleep EEG changes may also be seen—Janowsky, personal communication, 1997.) Larger doses may lead to headaches, tremor, drowsiness, memory impairment, apathy, fatigue, and depression. Severe intoxication results in confusion, ataxia, dysarthria and absent muscle-stretch ("myotatic") reflexes and progresses to coma, Cheyne-Stokes respirations (an abnormal breathing pattern), generalized grand mal–like seizures, and central respiratory depression (breathing problems produced by abnormal action of the breathing center in the brain) (Gutmann and Besser, 1990).

Delayed or chronic CNS effects (Gunderson, Lehmann, et al., 1992) may include giddiness, tension, anxiety, jitteriness, restlessness, emotional lability, excessive dreaming, insomnia, nightmares, headaches, tremor, withdrawal and depression, bursts of slow waves of elevated voltage in EEG (especially on hyperventilation), drowsiness, difficulty concentrating, slowness of recall, confusion, slurred speech, and ataxia (incoordination with walking) (Gunderson, Lehmann, et al., 1992).

Enzymes Regulate ACh Activity. ACh activity is regulated in large part by the enzyme acetylcholinesterase (also called "red blood cell cholinesterase" or "RBC cholinesterase" or "true cholinesterase" and abbreviated "AChE"), which binds to and breaks down ACh that has accumulated in the synapse, preventing inappropriate excessive signaling. *Butyrylcholinesterase* (also called "plasma cholinesterase" or "pseudocholinesterase," and abbreviated "BChE") plays a less critical role. It is made in the liver and circulates in the plasma. But it is thought that very little ACh will diffuse far from the synapse, so this enzyme plays a small direct role. A possible role for this enzyme in regulating chemicals like PB will be discussed in Chapter Eight ("Individual Differences in Response to PB").

Pharmacokinetics and Pharmacodynamics of PB

Pharmacokinetics refers to the study of the bodily absorption, distribution, metabolism, and excretion of drugs. *Pharmacodynamics* is a branch of pharmacology dealing with the reactions between drugs and living systems. This section will describe the pharmacokinetics, and to some degree the pharmacodynamics, of PB; these topics are important because they begin to illustrate individual differences in response to PB. Such individual differences could have relevance to symptoms in some PGW veterans.

PB is a positively charged compound that exerts its primary action by inhibiting the enzyme AChE. (It has other actions, including direct binding to, and stimulation of, the ACh receptor.) Because of its charge, PB has difficulty passing through biological membranes, which are relatively impermeant to charged molecules. Perhaps in part for this reason, PB is poorly and erratically absorbed from the gastrointestinal tract into the bloodstream. It has also been suggested that the "low oral bioavailability" of PB may result from "first pass" metabolism by the gut or liver (Leo and Grace, 1996). Recommended oral doses (per the manufacturer) are 30 times those of intravenous doses to achieve similar levels of activity in the body (Williams, 1984), and one author concluded that oral bioavailability amounted to only 7.6 percent—or one-thirteenth—of the administered dose (Aquilonius and Eckernas, 1980). However, other sources state, without citation, that about 40 percent of PB is absorbed following oral administration (Wannarka, 1984), indicating an oral dose would need to be 2.5 times the intravenous dose for the same amount to ultimately reach the blood.

PB makes its way to many sites throughout the body. After radioactive PB is given orally to animals, radioactivity (and, by presumption, PB) is detected in most tissues except the brain, intestinal wall, fat, and thymus (McEvoy, 1991). (PB has low oral bioavailability because of its ionic charge; although a fraction makes its way *through* the intestinal wall, it does not remain in residence in the intestinal wall.) PB has also been reported to cross the placenta and to decrease fetal plasma cholinesterase activity after large oral doses (McEvoy, 1991).

Most of the *orally administered* dose is eliminated in the feces (Whinnery, 1984). Most of the *absorbed* dose (the amount that enters the bloodstream from the GI tract) is eliminated through the kidneys unchanged or as the major metabolite, 3-hydroxy-N-methyl pyridium (3HMP) (Kornfeld, Samuels, et al., 1970; Somani, 1983); other metabolites, including 3-hydroxyphenyltrimethyl-ammonium (3HP) (Hennis, Cronnelly, et al., 1984), are present to a lesser degree (Kornfeld, Samuels, et al., 1970). Liver enzymes appear to play some role in metabolism at least in animals (McEvoy, 1991), particularly the microsomal glucuronidation of 3HMP (Somani, 1997), and there is a two- to threefold increase in concentration of PB in liver microsomes (Somani, 1977; Somani, 1997). According to one source, about 90 percent of the absorbed dose is metabolized by the liver on first pass (Wannarka, 1984) (data not referenced); however, other sources suggest that 75 to 90 percent is excreted unchanged in the urine (Cronnelly, Stanski, et al., 1980; Kornfeld, Samuels, et al., 1970; Keeler, 1990) or that as much as a third of the amount excreted may be the 3HMP metabolite. The 3HMP product is an acetylcholine antagonist (Yanaura, et al., 1993) and also inhibits AChE (Lee, Stelly, et al., 1992). Even after intravenous administration, in which there is no time burden getting the drug into the bloodstream, some PB activity can be detected in the urine 72 hours later (McEvoy, 1991). The half-time of elimination (estimates for the half-life with oral dosage are on the order of two to four hours; see Appendix A) is not stable but lengthens as PB is excreted; this could relate to the putative sequestering of PB in sites such as cartilage (see p. 19, "Accumulation of PB in the Body"). Because PB enhances the propulsive movement of the intestines, it may reduce its own absorption with continued use by encouraging its own elimination before the GI tract has had adequate time to absorb the PB.

Patients with severe myasthenia gravis seem to metabolize and excrete PB faster than patients with milder disease, which has been offered as an explanation for the resistance to anticholinesterase medication (that is, to the action of PB) that occurs with some severely ill patients (McEvoy, 1991).

Dosage requirements in myasthenia vary widely due to individual differences in absorption, metabolism, and excretion of PB (as well as differences in disease severity), so that dosage is usually determined individually for each patient. "Many of the same individual variations are probably present in normal subjects" (Whinnery, 1984); Chapter Eight explores whether these variations may be important for ill PGW veterans. PB reportedly has a variable duration of action in patients with myasthenia gravis, supposedly "depending on the physical and emotional stress suffered by the patient and the severity of the disease" (McEvoy, 1991), though other biological factors may be important. Moreover, individual muscle groups in the same patient may respond differently to the same dose of PB, producing weakness in one muscle group while increasing strength in another. The muscles of the neck and of chewing and swallowing are usually the first to be weakened by overdose, followed by the muscles of the shoulder and upper extremities, and finally the pelvic girdle, the muscles that control eye movement, and leg muscles (McEvoy, 1991).

The main "therapeutic" action of PB is AChE inhibition—that is, inhibition of the AChE enzyme, which breaks down ACh. The degree of AChE inhibition that occurs after PB administration is variable. In one small study, in which multiple doses of PB were given (30 mg every eight hours—the same dosing schedule given to PGW personnel deemed to be under threat of chemical warfare attack, but here given for six doses in eight healthy males), AChE inhibition was largely within the target range for nerve agent pretreatment, that is, 20–40 percent inhibition, following the first day of treatment (Sidell, 1990). However, other studies have shown substantial variability in response. In one study, peak inhibition varied from 20 percent to 39 percent of baseline activity, and the period of inhibition exceeding 20 percent varied from one-half hour to five hours—a difference of a factor of 10 (Sidell, 1990). In another study, AChE inhibition after a single dose ranged from 18 to 57 percent (Kolka, Burgoon, et al., 1991b). In a recent larger study of 90 healthy male and female volunteers ages 18 to 44, though ranges were not given, large individual differences were reflected by quite high standard errors in some groups of subjects, particularly for the time of maximum AChE inhibition after continued use (Lasseter and Garg, 1996). While significant differences in AChE inhibition did not occur as a function of sex or weight category in this study, this is likely a reflection of the large individual differences within each group obscuring any between-group differences. (More data regarding variability are discussed in Chapter Eight.)

Because of marked differences in the absorption of PB, the same administered dose may not lead to the same blood level of PB (Cohan, Drettchen, et al., 1977; Marino, Schuster, et al., 1996; Parker, Barber, et al., 1989). Indeed, one study found a more than sevenfold difference in steady-state plasma concentration between patients taking approximately the same daily dose of PB (Aquilonius,

Eckernas, et al., 1980). However, the relationship between blood levels of PB and RBC AChE activity is itself not as strong as one might suppose, leading to further variability in response. The correlation between PB and AChE inhibition was only –0.61 in one study (absence of correlation is 0, and a perfect correlation is 1 or –1), though in another the correlation was significant (r = –0.87, p < .05) (Kolka, Burgoon, 1991b). (A correlation of 0.61 implies that only about 36 percent of the variance in AChE inhibition can be explained by blood level of PB.) Moreover, percentage of RBC cholinesterase (acetylcholinesterase) inhibition was not highly correlated with weight, height, or body surface area (Kolka, Burgoon, et al., 1991b). Thus, in addition to marked variability in absorption of PB, the blood levels of PB following absorption do not necessarily predict the extent of AChE inhibition. Thus, variation in AChE inhibition following PB administration appears to be due to individual differences in amount of drug absorbed, in rate of elimination of the drug, and in sensitivity of AChE to inhibition by PB (Sidell, 1990). Later, evidence will be shown that AChE inhibition in turn does not strongly predict toxicity. Table 3.1 shows the several identified factors (in the pathway from administration of PB to response) which may lead to differences in individual response to PB for the same oral dose of PB.

Accumulation of PB in the Body. Some research has found that rats subcutaneously administered radioactive PB twice daily for 16 days do not excrete 100 percent of the daily dose of PB. On average, 76 percent was excreted as PB and its metabolites in urine and 7 percent in feces, leaving 17 percent unaccounted for, suggesting accumulation of the drug and its metabolites in the body with multiple dosing. Progressive increases in radioactivity per gram of tissue were also noted, and it was suggested that PB may bind specifically to chondroitin sulfate, since the radioactivity accumulated strongly in the ear and tail, which are cartilaginous tissues (Somani, 1977; Somani, 1983; Somani, 1997).

Pharmacokinetic and Pharmacodynamic Data: Extrapolation from Myasthenics to Normals. Some maintain that pharmacokinetic and pharmaco-

Table 3.1

Factors Leading to Individual Differences in Response to PB

Similar Exposure	Different Response
Same oral dose	Different amount entering blood (differences in absorption, peristalsis)
Same PB entering blood	Different levels of PB in blood over time (differences in clearance/metabolism)
Same PB in blood	Different levels of AChE inhibition
Same AChE inhibition	Different effect/toxicity

dynamic results, as well as toxicity information for healthy subjects and patients with myasthenia gravis, are similar, and the data from myasthenia gravis should be essentially applicable to all individuals (Whinnery, 1984). However, there are several reasons to be concerned that data from myasthenics and normals may differ (see Table 3.2).

First, high doses of PB are given to myasthenics in order to raise their neuro-muscular ACh activity toward normal. However, high doses of PB in non-myasthenics would raise neuromuscular ACh to supranormal—away from normal. Thus, it cannot be assumed that PB's safety for myasthenics would be the same for those without myasthenia—particularly with regard to nicotinic effects, the chief source of severe side effects. (Indeed, as long ago as 1984 it was observed that "the amount of pyridostigmine which can be administered without severe side effects appears to be related to the degree of impairment of neuromuscular transmission" (Williams, 1984).)   With regard to muscarinic side effects, these are often experienced by patients with myasthenia gravis (Hood, 1990); indeed, in one study, the reported side effect rate in myasthenics was 34 percent (Beekman, Kuks, et al., 1997). One analogy is the difference between how insulin affects diabetics and those not suffering from the condition. A severe diabetic may tolerate or require 60 units of insulin or more each day to bring his or her blood sugar *toward* normal. Yet far smaller doses may induce hypoglycemic coma or even death in a nondiabetic subject. Similarly, a high dose of PB may be harmless or indeed salutary in a patient with low acetylcholinergic activity (e.g., myasthenia gravis), but even a lower dose may be frankly harmful in an individual with normal ACh activity.

Second, patients with severe myasthenia appear to metabolize and excrete PB faster than those with milder disease (McEvoy, 1991). By extrapolation, myas-thenics may have a heightened metabolism of PB compared to normals (perhaps resulting from alterations in metabolism with regular use rather than because of the disease per se). For these reasons, and others presented at the start of Chapter Fourteen (explaining why cessation of PB may pose problems that will not be manifest in lifelong users like patients with myasthenia gravis), data from patients with myasthenia—or perhaps from those who use PB regularly—may not apply to those naive to PB.

Table 3.2

Reasons Extrapolation from Myasthenia to Normals May Not Be Valid

Myasthenia	Normal
PB restores nicotinic activity toward normal at the muscles	PB raises nicotinic activity away from normal
Accelerated metabolism?	Metabolism not accelerated
Use is continued indefinitely	Use is terminated

A third reason that data from myasthenia may not apply relates to the fact that patients with myasthenia use PB indefinitely, while Gulf War use was transient. Some evidence suggests that use of PB may lead to downregulation of the acetylcholinergic system (see sections on Downregulation and Motor Adapter Effects). Use of PB and other AChE inhibitors in animals has been shown to cause reduced ACh release, withdrawal of nerve fibers from junctional folds and reduced sensitivity of ACh receptors—effects that would be particularly offset by continued PB use (and indeed were generated by the body in an effort to restore regulation in the face of PB) but that might generate problems with PB discontinuation. The duration of these effects is not well characterized.

Additional differences in sensitivity to PB may result from the slow up-titration of PB in myasthenics. Those who have been brought to high doses may have heightened muscarinic activity (as a result of the higher dose of PB, since myasthenics do not have impairment in muscarinic cholinergic activity but only in nicotinic activity). This may result in faster peristalsis leading to reduced absorption of PB. For whatever combination of reasons related to absorption and elimination, it has been noted that myasthenics may develop a tolerance to, or loss of clinical response to PB (McEvoy, 1991). For these reasons, caution is warranted in extrapolating pharmacokinetic data, and evidence on side effects, from patients with myasthenia to nonmyasthenics. (This issue is discussed again in Chapter Fourteen, "Chronic Effects"; background from intervening chapters will allow additional material to be brought to bear.)

Other Actions on the Cholinergic System

Partial Agonist. PB is considered an AChE inhibitor. However, studies in diverse species (including amphibians, fish, and mammals) indicate that PB also reacts directly with the ACh receptor as a "partial agonist"; it produces some of the same effects that ACh itself would produce acting at the same receptor (Aracava, Deshpande, et al., 1987). Moreover, ion channel openings, which are normally stimulated by nerve signals that result in ACh binding to the receptor, show increased noise (Aracava, Deshpande, et al., 1987), which could theoretically adversely affect information-processing capabilities. (Opening and closing of ion channels is the means by which nerve signals are typically propagated.)

ACh Receptor Desensitization. Moreover, PB either alone or in combination with ACh induces an altered, "desensitized" species of the nicotinic receptor-ion channel complex (Aracava, Deshpande, et al., 1987). That is to say, PB use produces ACh receptors (binding sites) that are less sensitive to the action of ACh. (This has been proposed as one of the methods of conferring protection against nerve agent.) Normally, when ACh binds, certain ion channels open and produce an electrochemical signal. The frequency of these channel openings is decreased when PB is given, and ACh ion channel "currents" are modified (Sherby, Eldefrawi, et al., 1985; Akaike, Ikeda, et al., 1984). Other carbamates (chemicals in the same family as PB) produce similar but not identical effects (Sherby, Eldefrawi, et al., 1985; Shaw, Aracava, et al., 1985). This desensitization could have a role in cholinergic downregulation (see Chapter Thirteen).

Autoregulation. Most ACh receptors considered clinically are those that exist at the "postsynaptic" membrane—the membrane of a signal-receiving cell. ACh released from a signaling or "presynaptic" cell (a nerve cell or "neuron") binds to these receptors on the postsynaptic cell (typically either a nerve or muscle cell), allowing the presynaptic cell to communicate with the receiving cell. However, ACh receptors also exist at the presynaptic membrane—the membrane of the signaling cell—where they play an important role in "autoregulation" of ACh release from the terminal axon (the extension of the signaling cell that grows out and forms connections with the receiving cell). When ACh binds to and activates these presynaptic receptors, the effect is to inhibit further release of ACh from the presynaptic membrane (that is, from the signaling cell) (Gutmann and Besser, 1990). (However, nicotinic action presynaptically *increases* release in the brain of other neurotransmitters, including both glutamate and GABA.) The factors that regulate the degree to which this inhibition occurs are not understood. Thus, inhibition of ACh breakdown by PB will lead to increased binding by ACh on these presynaptic sites, potentially reducing continued release of ACh. No data were found to elucidate the strength or time-course of this autoregulatory effect.

ACh Receptor Heterogeneity. Neuronal ACh receptors exhibit "considerable heterogeneity with respect to their distribution, pharmacological sensitivity and functional role" (Albuquerque, Costa, et al., 1991). Many receptor types have been identified in the CNS (see the Chapter Thirteen discussion of neurotransmitter dysregulation); since these have different characteristics, they are presumably differently affected by such carbamates as PB, in the event that PB reaches the CNS.

Nonsynaptic Cholinergic Effects. It has been noted that "the presence of acetylcholine and its receptors at locations not related to synaptic activity raises the possibility that acetylcholine may have receptor-mediated cellular functions other than transmission of nerve signals, i.e., that acetylcholine may act as a local hormone modulating cellular functions" (Grando, Horton, et al., 1995). For example, both nicotinic and muscarinic ACh receptors, similar to those seen in the brain and autonomic ganglia, evidently regulate migration and cell stickiness of skin cells (epidermal keratinocytes). Immune and blood cells also have cholinergic mechanisms, as do sperm and ovaries (Schwarz, Glick et al., 1995).

Effects on Other Transmitter Systems

ACh (nicotinic) stimulation can cause release of neurotransmitters including GABA, dopamine, and glutamate (Kayadjanian, Retaux, et al., 1994; McGehee, Heath, et al., 1995; Role and Berg, 1996). Moreover, there appears to be a relation to serotonin action (Albuquerque, Pereira, et al., 1997a; Albuquerque, Pereira, et al., 1997b). It has been speculated that in addition to the actions of ACh in the usual signaling-cell/receiving-cell interactions (the "wiring" transmission mode), ACh may also be released in a "paracrine" or "volume transmission" fashion—acting more or less like a local hormone, drifting to modulate release of other neurotransmitters (not necessarily just at a site at which the ACh-releasing cell synapses) (Agnati, Zoli, et al., 1995; Changeux, Bessis, et al., 1996). Evidence in favor of this is that the "cell bodies" of the neurons that release ACh are restricted to a few nuclei located mainly in parts of the brain termed the basal telencephalon and dorsal pons, but the ends of the nerve cell processes from these cells are spread throughout the brain in a somewhat diffuse way, and no consistent match exists between the known distribution of the nicotinic ACh receptors in the brain and that of the acetylcholinergic "terminals" (release sites from the signaling cell) (Agnati, Zoli, et al., 1995; Changeux, Bessis, et al., 1996; Role and Berg, 1996). Further complicating matters, muscarinic receptors are known to regulate synaptic transmission in some instances with actions opposite to nicotinic receptors (Changeux, Bessis, et al., 1996), so that the effects depend on the relative distribution of these types of receptors. This distribution, however, has not yet been established (Changeux, Bessis et al., 1996). The information provided below should be considered with these provisos in mind.

As noted elsewhere (see Chapter Fifteen, Other Considerations, Hormone and Stress Effects), ACh may also stimulate release of catecholamines—epinephrine particularly, and also norepinephrine—and hormones, including cortisol, prolactin, growth hormone, beta-endorphin, and others.

Glutamate. The "glutamatergic" (i.e., glutamate-related) transmitter system shares elements with the acetylcholinergic system, including its ability to be influenced by carbamates (such as PB). In the mammalian central nervous systems, the NMDA (N-methyl-D-aspartate) type of glutamatergic receptor as well as the ACh receptor are involved in a number of processes. These range from control of transmitter release (described above), to postsynaptic membrane depolarization (changes occurring in the membrane of the signal-receiving cell) with mobilization of intracellular second messengers. Second messengers, such as calcium, in turn participate in mechanisms of protein synthesis, learning (through a process termed "long-term potentiation"), outgrowth of nerve processes to allow connections to other cells, cell death, and other functions (Albuquerque, Costa, et al., 1991). Glutamate receptor overactivation can induce delayed neuronal cell death (toxic effects by overactivation are termed "excitotoxicity"). Such effects may be mediated by breaking of DNA strands (Didier, Bursztajn, et al., 1996).

Indeed, it has been shown that low (nanomolar) concentrations of nicotine enhance both glutamatergic and acetylcholinergic synaptic transmission by activating presynaptic nicotinic ACh receptors that increase presynaptic calcium concentrations (McGehee, Heath, et al., 1995).

Studies have demonstrated that carbamates and OPs (including the OP agents diisopropylfluorophosphate (DFP) and the nerve agent VX) affect properties of the glutamate system, including such presynaptic properties (properties of the signal-sending side) as increasing transmitter release and such postsynaptic properties (properties of the signal-receiving side) as reducing the peak size of the current induced by binding of glutamate to its receptor. Moreover, carbamates may cause unstimulated endplate synaptic potentials, or voltage changes in the receiving cell side, large enough to provoke "action potentials" (full self-propagating signals down a nerve process that are normally produced in response to input from one or more signaling cells). This response could disrupt the specificity of signaling, since action potentials are more typically driven by specific inputs to the neuron. These data derive from work on insects' neuromuscular junctions, however, and insects employ glutamate rather than ACh at their neuromuscular junctions (Albuquerque, Deshpande, et al., 1985; Aracava, Deshpande, et al., 1987; Idriss, Aguayo, et al., 1986; Albuquerque, 1985). The degree to which PB per se affects glutamate neurons in the mammalian CNS remains to be evaluated but would likely depend in part on the degree to which PB has access to the brain. (It has been observed that ACh receptors and NMDA-sensitive receptors on central neurons share much functional homology with ACh receptors in muscle fibers (Albuquerque, 1988), suggesting that similar effects may apply if PB were to reach the CNS.)

GABA. Carbamates may also affect signaling through another neurotransmitter system, the GABA (gamma amino butyric acid) system. GABA is the chief inhibitory neurotransmitter in the mammalian nervous system (Hardman, Limber, et al., 1996). ACh acts presynaptically to modulate GABA release. Preterminal nicotinic receptors on GABAergic axons have been identified in rats (e.g., the interpeduncular nucleus (Lena, Changeux, et al., 1993)), and ACh has been shown to modulate the release of GABA (Albuquerque, Pereira, et al., 1995; Mukhopadhyay and Poddar, 1995; Kayadjanian, Retaux, et al., 1994).

Dopamine. By a similar mechanism, ACh acts via presynaptic nicotinic receptors to modulate the release of dopamine (Albuquerque, Pereira, et al., 1995; Kayadjanian, Retaux, et al., 1994). Indeed, in some parts of the brain (but not others), the release of GABA by nicotine is mediated by dopamine release (Kayadjanian, Retaux, et al., 1994). Nicotine evokes dopamine release (from the rat corpus striatum as well as frontal cortex) in vivo and in vitro. Chronic treatment with nicotine has been shown to increase the density of nicotine-binding sites (that is, nicotinic receptors) in the frontal cortex but to produce no increase in striatal preparations (Wonnacott, Marshal, et al., 1994). A reduction in dopamine release is evoked by the same amount of nicotine in the frontal cortex but not in the striatum (Wonnacott, Marshal, et al., 1994). There are also antidopamine muscarinic effects (Georguieff, Lefloch, et al., 1976)—and perhaps wholly or partly because of different distribution of muscarinic and nicotinic receptors, ACh stimulation regulation of dopamine activity may be opposite in different brain regions. (For instance, it is opposite in the "nigral" and "striatal" regions of the brain (Javoy, Agid, et al., 1974; Nose and Takemoto, 1974; Westernick and Korf, 1975; Davis, Faull, et al., 1979).) The clinical relevance of an effect of ACh on dopamine is suggested by reports of development and of exacerbation of parkinsonism (a condition of reduced motor movement combined with tremor that results from problems in the dopamine-rich nigrostriatal system in the brain (Wilson, Braunwald, et al., 1991)), following PB (Iwasaki, Wakata, et al., 1988) (Kao, Kwan, et al., 1993) and OPs (Davis, Yesavage et al., 1978) or unspecified pesticides (Butterfield, Valanis, et al., 1993; Hubble, Cao, et al., 1993)). Also, the ß2-containing neuronal nicotinic ACh receptor is believed to assist in mediating the reinforcing properties of nicotine (and other substances of abuse), by contributing to release of dopamine in the "mesolimbic" system of the brain (Picciotto, Zoli, et al., 1998).

Substance P. The cholinergic system, specifically AChE—and by extension PB—affects breakdown of "substance P" (Chubb, Hodgson, et al., 1980), a neurotransmitter involved in pain signaling.

Serotonin. Serotonin is known to be involved in important functions including regulation of mood, pain, impulsivity, and sleep. (See section on Sleep and Serotonin in Chapter Fifteen, "Other Considerations.") Of note: Several lines of evidence suggest important interactions between the ACh system and the serotonergic system. (A later section in Chapter Fifteen discusses considerations of illnesses in PGW veterans as they may relate to serotonergic dysfunction.)

Briefly, PB binds to the same site on the ACh receptor that serotonin is believed to bind to, a relatively new finding (Albuquerque, Pereira, et al., 1997a; Albuquerque, Pereira, et al., 1997b). (This site has also been called the "galanthamine binding site.") Although many identified classes of nicotinic receptors are in the brain that differ by which of a set of subunits make up their five parts, this binding site is highly "conserved" across different types of nicotinic receptors—that is, while other properties of the receptor change, this property remains constant. Carbamate and OP AChE inhibitors, including nerve agents and PB, have been shown to reduce platelet serotonin uptake, increase serotonin turnover, and reduce nighttime enhancement of serotonin in the pineal gland, and nighttime rise of melatonin measured in blood. Some serotonergic drugs have been found to augment the AChE-inhibiting effects of PB and slow the time-course of recovery. Others have been shown to have similar effects to PB in some circumstances, such as enhancing release of growth hormone from the pituitary gland in response to growth hormone releasing hormone from the hypothalamus. Finally, there has been an unsubstantiated (non–peer reviewed) report of benefit from combined serotonergic/dopaminergic treatment of ill PGW veterans (Hitzig, 1997). This treatment used the drug combination fenfluramine and phentermine. (Fenfluramine is no longer available, after reports of heart valve abnormalities with this drug or with the fenfluramine-phentermine drug combination.) Some issues related to serotonin are discussed in greater detail in Appendix B.

Opioids

The opioid codeine has, like serotonin, been shown to bind to the "galanthamine" binding site on nicotinic ACh receptors, acting as a modulation of central nicotinic function (Albuquerque, Pereira, et al., 1997b). (It is known that the opioid system, the serotonin system, and the acetylcholinergic system are all involved in regulation of pain. High levels of opioids and serotonin are related to increased tolerance to pain. More on the relationship between cholinergic function and pain will be discussed in Chapter Fifteen, in the section on "Sleep.")

Shelf Life

PB can be maintained for long periods without refrigeration (FDA, 1997). Because of the desire for long storage, the military policy is to maintain PB under refrigeration and dispose of PB that has remained unrefrigerated for a period exceeding six months. Refrigeration of PB is desired because prolonged storage without refrigeration may affect its potency. Discussion with FDA representatives indicates that PB does not break down into toxic products (FDA, 1997).

Breakdown Products

As noted above, the chief metabolite of PB is 3-hydroxy-N-methylpyridium. This product is discussed earlier in the section on pharmacokinetics and pharmacodynamics. Although it has traditionally not been thought to contribute to the action of PB, it may have some AChE inhibiting activity (Lee, Stelly, et al., 1992).

MEDICAL USE

Duration of Medical Use

PB was licensed by the FDA in 1955 for use in patients with myasthenia gravis and to reverse effects of nondepolarizing neuromuscular blockers (De Fraites, 1996).

Myasthenia Gravis

Myasthenia gravis is a disease characterized by increased weakness and fatigability of muscles caused by an autoimmune attack on ACh receptors at the junction of nerves and muscles. Antibodies are produced by the body to nicotinic ACh receptors at the neuromuscular junction (the junction at which the nerve joins the muscle and can signal the muscle to contract). These receptor antibodies attack the receptors and lead to the loss of functional receptors at which ACh can act. It is the action of ACh at the muscle's "motor endplate" that causes muscle fibers to contract; loss of the ability to contract produces muscular weakness (Drachman, 1994). Myasthenia gravis has a prevalence of 50 to 169 cases per million population, with approximately 25,000 affected persons in the United States (Antonini, Morino, et al., 1996; Drachman, 1994). The annual incidence is in the range of 2–10 per million population (Schon, Drayson, et al., 1996; Somnier 1996). It has a bimodal age distribution, with a primarily female early peak in the second and third decades and a late peak affecting predominantly males from 60 to 74 years old (Drachman, 1994; Antonini 1996, Morino, et al., 1996). Ten to 20 percent of patients do not have detectable antibodies, but it is believed that circulating antibodies are present even in these individuals, since passive transfer of immunoglobulins (antibodies) from these patients to mice leads to loss of ACh receptors at the mouse neuromuscular junction (Drachman, 1994). Experimental myasthenia has been developed in mice, in which there are antibodies to ACh receptors (Berman and Patrick, 1980).

PB is used as a treatment for myasthenia gravis. Myasthenics' loss of ACh receptors results in reduced ACh binding to receptors, which in turn results in reduced "cholinergic" activity. PB treatment increases the availability of ACh to bind remaining receptors (Drachman, 1994), partially restoring cholinergic activity. The maximal useful dosage rarely exceeds 120 mg each three hours; higher doses may increase weakness. Benefit is usually incomplete and often wanes after weeks or months of treatment (Drachman, 1994). Increasing doses are often needed, and patients may become unresponsive to PB after prolonged treatment (McEvoy, 1991). In some instances, responsiveness may be restored by reducing the dose or withdrawing the drug for several days under medical supervision (McEvoy, 1991).

Variant myasthenic syndromes with different mechanisms exist and patients with these syndromes respond poorly to PB (Engel, Lambert, et al., 1977, 1981). These syndromes are uncommon.

Reversal of Neuromuscular Blockade

PB is used to reverse a neuromuscular blockade (used in anesthesia) by "nondepolarizing neuromuscular blockers" (such as tubocurarine, metocurine, gallamine, pancuronium) following surgery, in intravenous doses ranging from 2 mg to 18 mg (Alisoglu, Nagelhout, et. al., 1995; McNall, Wolfson, et al., 1969). PB is not useful for reversing the action of "depolarizing" neuromuscular blockers (such as succinylcholine or decamethonium) and may actually prolong the action of these agents (McEvoy, 1991; Fleming, Macres, et al., 1996). This role for PB is relevant only in that it is another circumstance in which PB has been approved for use by the FDA and has been used with apparent safety. Its use in this circumstance, as in the instance of myasthenia (but in contrast to its use as a nerve agent pretreatment adjunct), also serves to bring muscle activity toward normal.

Treatment of Fatigue Due to Other Causes

It has been noted that carbamates (like PB) can temporarily increase clinical strength even for normal individuals (Rustam, Von Burg, et al., 1975). PB has been used with some reported success in the treatment of fatigue in non-myasthenic conditions.

PB has been used in treating the fatigue of patients with post-polio syndrome, in which presynaptic defects (defects in signal sending, rather than post-synaptic defects in signal receiving, as in myasthenia gravis) are thought to be present (Trojan and Cashman, 1995a; Trojan and Cashman, 1995b). The benefit may result from increased strength rather than reduced fatigability. Post-polio syndrome patients appear to have symptoms of both central and peripheral fatigue (Trojan and Cashman, 1995a).

PB has been found to benefit symptoms and quality of life in HIV-positive patients who test positive for ACh receptor antibodies (in open-label trials using 60 mg three times daily or four times daily), though the role of antibodies in these patients' symptoms is unknown (Cupler, Otero, et al.,1996).

PB has also been used for treatment of "drop attacks" in the elderly; elderly persons with drop attacks uniformly reported relief from falls with PB (Braham, 1994). It has been postulated that the postural righting reflex in these individuals requires a prompt neuromuscular response, which is aided by PB. Other individuals, including supposedly "neurotic" subjects with subjective weakness or fatigue in whom tests for ACh receptor autoantibodies are negative, have experienced relief with use of PB (Park, Kim, et al., 1993).

Neostigmine, a relative of PB, has been used with success in some Iraqi patients suffering from methylmercury poisoning. Use of this agent led to doubling of strength and large fluctuations in strength with administration and withdrawal of the drug, employing doses that might produce signs of toxicity in normal individuals (Rustam, Von Burg, et al., 1975). Again it seems that subjects with a clinical need for PB tolerate higher doses without apparent adverse effect than do "normal" individuals.

(Of note, other AChE inhibitors that penetrate the brain, such as tacrine, have been used to reduce symptoms of dementia in the elderly.)

Dose

In myasthenia gravis, dosing is usually initiated at 60 mg three times daily (twice the PGW dose), with dosage increased gradually until no further benefit to strength is seen (McEvoy, 1991). The average daily dose is 600 mg/d orally (60 mg 10 times per day, or about 7 times the PGW dose), with an acceptable dosage range of 360 to 1500 mg/d (up to ~17 times the PGW dose) (McEvoy, 1991). The literature reveals a de facto dose range from 30 to 2,000 mg/d, with up to 6,000 mg/d recorded in severe cases (~67 times the PGW dose) (Whinnery, 1984). In the reversal of a neuromuscular blockade, doses from 0.1 to 0.25 mg/kg, or 4 to 20 mg, have been quoted. These doses are quite different from those given to myasthenics in part because poor absorption of orally administered drug (in myasthenia) requires high doses compared to drug administered by injection (in reversal of neuromuscular blockade).

Possible Adverse Effects of PB Treatment in Myasthenia Gravis

Some concerns have been raised regarding possible deleterious effects of PB in the treatment of patients with myasthenia gravis, on the grounds that a decrease in the number of patients achieving complete remission after surgical thymectomy has occurred since 1961 (Scadding, Havard, et al., 1985). This effect was thought to be related to use of anticholinesterase therapy. It has been speculated that PB may cause damage to the neuromuscular junction and that this damage—unlike the immune effects of the myasthenia itself—cannot be corrected by surgical removal of the thymus. Symptoms of this damage may be difficult to distinguish from the effects of myasthenia per se (Rockefeller Report, 1997). (See Chapter Twelve, "Neuromuscular Junction Effects.")

MILITARY USE

Rationale for Use

PB is used as a "pretreatment" or, more precisely, as a "pretreatment adjunct" for poisoning by the nerve agent soman. It confers no protection on its own but enhances the protection conferred by postexposure treatment in the form of atropine and pralidoxime (2-PAM), when tested in animals.

Dose

Research in the United Kingdom has indicated that AChE inhibition of 20 to 40 percent should be maintained to provide "adequate" protection against death from soman poisoning; generally, 30 mg each eight hours orally has been found to provide that range of inhibition in people (Gall, 1981), although the inhibition may fall below 20 percent six hours after dosing. Dosing every eight hours has been estimated to leave five hours a day in which AChE inhibition falls below 20 percent (Whinnery, 1984). Nonetheless, the recommended dosing schedule for nerve agent pretreatment is 30 mg orally every eight hours.

Duration of Military Use

PB has been stockpiled by the U.S. military since 1986 (Dunn and Sidell, 1989), based on British data, for adjunctive nerve agent pretreatment protection. Though PB is approved by the FDA for use for myasthenia gravis, it remains an investigational new drug (IND) for nerve agent pretreatment by the military. (For more information on this issue, see Rettig, 1999). As noted previously, evidence from animal studies indicates that PB protects against lethality from the nerve agent soman (particularly in primates) and does not interfere in a meaningful way with protection against lethality from other nerve agents (studies done in rodents; no direct evidence in primates). Human studies demonstrating efficacy against nerve agent lethality would be clearly unethical, and this failure to demonstrate efficacy for use in humans—rather than safety concerns—had been the major stumbling block in the licensure of PB for nerve agent pretreatment. Thus, although PB has been stockpiled by the military and the decision was made to use PB pretreatment in the Persian Gulf, PB has not been licensed by the FDA for nerve agent pretreatment. The FDA granted a waiver for the requirement of informed consent for this drug prior to its use in the PGW. For more detail on the history of the U.S. use of PB in the military, and the respective positions of the FDA and DoD on this issue, see Rettig (1999).

What Are Nerve Agents?

Nerve agents include GA (tabun), GB (sarin), GD (soman), GF (cyclosarin), thiosarin, and VX (see Figure 3.2). These agents act by "irreversibly" (i.e., with a very long time-course) inhibiting the action of the enzyme AChE, which is involved in regulating (by breaking down) the neurotransmitter ACh. The resulting inhibition of AChE leads to a buildup of ACh at the synapse or at the motor endplate, the sites at which signaling between nerve cells, or between nerve and muscle, occur. This leads to increased action of ACh, discussed previously as nicotinic, muscarinic, and central effects. (For more information on CW agents, see Augerson, forthcoming.)

What Is the Effect of Postexposure Treatment for Nerve Agents?

Atropine, a muscarinic blocker, antagonizes the muscarinic effects of PB (see "Chemical Characteristics," above). 2-PAM (pralidoxime) enhances the protec-

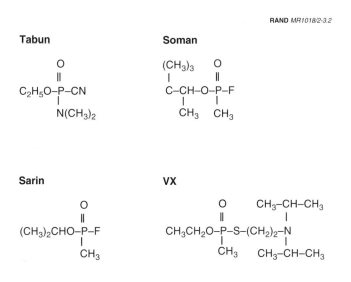

Figure 3.2—Structure of Nerve Agents

tion by pulling the nerve agent off AChE. Diazepam (Valium) may also be given by injection to prevent CNS effects, particularly seizures, and the long-term cognitive consequences that may ensue from prolonged seizure activity.

Atropine and pralidoxime were given to all troops in a "Mark I Nerve Agent Antidote" autoinjector kit (FORSCOM, 1990). Soldiers carried three 2 mg auto-injectors of atropine for use when symptoms first appeared and three 600 mg autoinjectors of 2-PAM for concurrent intramuscular use with atropine (Gunderson, Lehmann, et al., 1992). Military personnel at risk also carried a 10 mg intramuscular autoinjector of diazepam to administer to their companions if needed (Gunderson, Lehmann, et al., 1992).

Why Is PB Needed in Addition? Pralidoxime ceases to be effective once the effect called "aging" takes place (see Figure 3.3). Aging involves the release of a "leaving group" from the central phosphorus atom of the nerve agent in the nerve agent–AChE complex that permanently inactivates the AChE enzyme (Dunn and Sidell, 1989). (More specifically, there is "partial dealkylation" of the phosphorylated serine group at the active site in the enzyme (Mason, Waine, et al., 1993).)

RAND *MR1018/2-3.3*

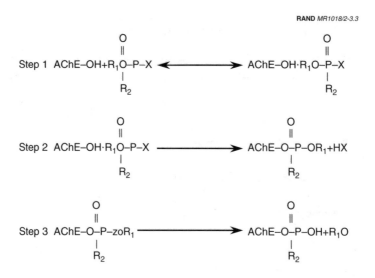

Figure 3.3—Reaction Between Nerve Agent Compounds (or Other OPs) and AChE

Step 1: Formation of AChE–nerve agent complex. Step 2: Phosphorylation and inactivation of the enzyme. Step 3: Aging reaction, in which a "leaving group" separates, providing a mono-phosphoric acid residue bound to the enzyme. Following the aging process, the nerve agent can no longer be pulled off the AChE molecule by pralidoxime (adapted from Sidell and Borak, 1992).

For those exposed to sarin, there is ample time following exposure to administer an oxime before aging of the nerve agent–AChE complex occurs. Sarin's half time to aging (time at which aging has occurred in half the sarin-AChE complexes) is several hours. The aging half-time is even longer for tabun, cyclosarin, and VX (Table 3.3). However, the half-time of aging for soman is approximately two minutes, inadequate for even highly trained personnel to administer atropine and oxime.

It has been estimated that, for adequate protection against nerve agents in combat conditions, a protective ratio of at least 5 is desired (Dunn, Hackley, et al., 1997; Dunn and Sidell, 1989). That is, the treatments we give must allow exposure to five times the usual lethal dose. The protective ratio (PR) is the LD_{50} with treatment (the dose that is lethal in 50 percent of subjects, if treatment is given) divided by the LD_{50} without treatment (the dose that is lethal in 50 percent if treatment is not given) (Sidell, 1990). In the absence of PB, the PR of atropine and oxime against the nerve agent soman does not reach this goal but is at best around 1.6 in primates (Dunn and Sidell, 1989). However, adding PB brings the ratio to in excess of 5 in primates (Dunn and Sidell, 1989), providing more adequate protection against death from soman (Table 3.4).

A PR of 5 was chosen as the target PR based on such findings as those in Table 3.4, taken from the New Drug Application for PB (Pyridostigmine, 1996). This shows results of computer models of possible battlefield scenarios based on U.S. weapons engineering that were used to estimate the level of exposure of troops to nerve agents in various combat situations. It indicates the percentage

Table 3.3

Aging Half-Time of Nerve Agents

Nerve Agent	Aging Half-Time	Source	Reference
Soman (GD)	2–6 min	Human, in vitro	Mager, 1984
	1 min	Marmoset, in vivo	Talbot, Anderson, et al., 1988
	8 min	Guinea pig, in vivo	Talbot, Anderson, et al., 1988
	9 min	Rat, in vivo	Talbot, Anderson, et al., 1988
Sarin (GB)	5 h	Human, in vivo	Sidell and Groff, 1974
	3 h	Human, in vitro	Mager, 1984
Cyclosarin (GF)	8 h	Human, in vitro	Hill and Thomas, 1969
	40 h	Human, in vitro	Mager, 1984
Tabun (GA)	13 h	Human, in vitro	Doctor, Blick, et al., 1993
	14 h	Human, in vitro	Mager, 1984
VX	48 h	Human, in vivo	Sidell and Groff, 1974

NOTE: Adapted from Dunn, et al., 1997, and New Drug Application to FDA for PB (Pyridostigmine, 1996; Dunn, Hackley, et al., 1997).

Table 3.4

Percentage of Population Within Target Area Exposed to Various Levels of Nerve Agent

	$10\,LD_{50}$	$5\,LD_{50}$	$1\,LD_{50}$
Soman (GD)			
Liquid artillery	≤43	≤22	≤3
Liquid bombs	≤65	≤62	≤56
Vapor artillery	≤90	≤86	≤77
Vapor bombs	≤78	≤70	≤63
Sarin (GB)			
Liquid artillery	≤40	≤15	≤1
Liquid bombs	≤24	≤15	≤7
Vapor artillery	≤100	≤100	≤90
Vapor bombs	≤99	≤92	≤72
Cyclosarin (GF)			
Liquid artillery	≤43	≤21	≤4
Liquid bombs	≤67	≤60	≤54
Vapor artillery	≤91	≤85	≤75
Vapor bombs	≤77	≤72	≤63
Tabun (GA)			
Liquid artillery	≤70	50	≤5
Liquid bombs	≤70	62	≤57
Vapor artillery	≤100	95	≤84
Vapor bombs	≤90	84	≤69
Vx			
Liquid artillery	≤70	≤47	≤14
Liquid bombs	≤40	≤25	≤14
Vapor artillery	≤2	≤2	≤1
Vapor bombs	≤4	≤4	≤3

SOURCE: Adapted from New Drug Application for PB (Pyridostigmine, 1996).

of the population within the "target area" that would be exposed to various levels of nerve agent. A "standard" target area for analysis for an artillery unit is 600 meters by 400 meters (Pyridostigmine, 1996). For soman (GD), with liquid exposure through either artillery or bombs, or with vapor exposure from bombs, a majority would be exposed to fewer than $5\,LD_{50}$s of nerve agent; and 7 percent or fewer would be exposed to more than $5\,LD_{50}$s but fewer than $10\,LD_{50}$s. That is, most of the people who would be protected if a PR of 10 could be obtained would also be protected by a PR of 5. For some personnel with higher nerve agent exposures, such as personnel near "ground zero" (the point of munition impact), CW exposure may not constitute the most serious injury.[1]

---

[1]For the present report, no attempt has been made to assess the validity of the models used, which reportedly predict the disposition and dosage footprints (ground laydown pattern) for a single munition and for multiple munition attacks. The NDA states that "Both models are accepted by the relevant military and scientific authorities for use in evaluating exposures and hazards, and in defining requirements for individual protection, detection, and doctrine for operations in a chemical warfare environment (Pyridostigmine, 1996).

How Does PB Confer Additional Protection? PB enhances the protection of oxime and atropine against a nerve agent, perhaps by reversibly binding to the AChE site at which the nerve agent or other cholinesterase inhibitors (like the OP DFP) would normally bind (Koelle, 1946; Sidell, 1990), preventing the nerve agent from binding. In particular, soman cannot bind to a PB-bound AChE molecule. This prevents aging of soman-AChE from taking place. (Without PB, this would lead to irreversible inhibition of the soman-bound AChE molecules, and recovery of AChE activity would require several weeks for full regeneration of AChE.) The stated goal of PB pretreatment is to bind (and thereby inhibit) approximately 30 percent of AChE; in animal studies, carbamylation of about 30 percent of circulating (RBC, or erythrocyte) AChE corresponds to a great increase in the effectiveness of the antidotes (Sidell, 1990). This 30 percent of AChE will be "protected" from binding and irreversible inhibition by soman and will be restored to normal function once spontaneous "decarbamylation" (dissociation of PB from the AChE molecule) occurs. (Meanwhile, there is enough time for oxime to be given, so that PB decarbamylates, and any residual nerve agent that binds the now-functional AChE can be pulled off.) In animal studies, however, a relationship between the rate of reactivation of AChE inhibited by a pretreatment compound (or the level of RBC AChE inhibition) and the protection against soman has not always been evident (Langenberg, De Jong, et al., 1996; Jones, Carter, et al., 1985), leading to some doubts regarding whether this mechanism adequately explains protection against soman (Prendergast, 1997).

Other mechanisms have been proposed that may contribute to protection by PB pretreatment, including desensitization of the neuromuscular endplate and ACh receptor; decreased quantal release of ACh; and decreased frequency of "miniature endplate potentials," small voltage changes in the cell receiving a signal (see also section on downregulation in Chapter Thirteen) (Gillies and Allen, 1977; Pascuzzo, Akaike, et al., 1984; Anderson, Chamberlain, et al., 1986).

Why Is PB Selected Instead of Other Carbamates? PB is preferred over other carbamates, particularly physostigmine, because it has fewer side effects, longer duration of action, and a greater margin of safety (Kolka, Burgoon, et al., 1991a). Physostigmine has been viewed as a candidate for pretreatment, but it has several disadvantages for field use: it has quite a short half-life in vivo, protecting dosing levels produce side effects, and it penetrates the CNS. CNS penetration leads to concerns that use of physostigmine could result in adverse effects on troops' performance.

PB does not cross the blood-brain barrier under ordinary circumstances, because of its positive charge (Kolka, Burgoon, et al., 1991b). Thus CNS side effects from PB are not thought to be an issue with normal use. While PB does not protect AChE in the CNS from nerve agents, it also presumably does not itself induce CNS symptoms and potentially deleterious performance changes (by inhibiting brain AChE. (Protection of the CNS is done postexposure, using atropine, oximes, and diazepam.) PB's ability to confer protection in doses without substantial side effects has made it the preferred pretreatment over physostigmine (Sidell, 1990).

Additive Effects of PB with Soman Have Not Been Clinically Reported. Because PB and nerve agents both inhibit AChE, it might be supposed that the toxicity would be additive—that a smaller amount of a nerve agent would be needed to produce toxicity if PB were given in advance. For reasons not well understood (which may relate to the ability of PB to desensitize the ACh receptor, as noted above), an additive effect on performance and on lethality evidently does not occur, at least for soman. (Studies in primates suggest that in the short term, prior to three hours after administration, AChE inhibition with soman is greater when PB pretreatment has been given—suggesting some additivity of effect; but in the longer term, beyond six hours, AChE inhibition with soman is substantially less if PB has been given (Blick, Murphy, et al., 1987). The dose of soman that proves lethal is not reduced in animals given PB before a soman challenge (instead, the lethal dose is markedly increased—that is, PB is protective). Moreover, pretreatment with PB in humans administered very small amounts of soman led to no change or fewer effects than without pretreatment (Sidell, 1990), consistent with primate studies in which sublethal doses of soman led to similar or slightly less effects if PB pretreatment had been given (Blick, Murphy, et al., 1987).

Similarly, prolonged miosis (constriction of the pupils) produced by the AChE-inhibiting OP DFP was prevented by pretreatment with physostigmine (a carbamate compound related to PB). The time-course of miosis was shortened to that of physostigmine alone, suggesting that DFP did not attach to the receptor site (Leopold and McDonald, 1948) and was protected from doing so by the carbamate (in this case physostigmine rather than pyridostigmine).

It should be noted, however, that if PB is given after nerve agent rather than before, additive effects might be expected (Pope, 1997).

Efficacy of PB Pretreatment for Soman

One primate study evaluated the effect of soman with and without PB pre-treatment: without PB, the AChE inhibition induced by soman was still complete (0 percent functional) at the termination of the study; for PB pretreated animals, though blockade was briefly complete at 10 minutes (0 percent functional), by 30 minutes AChE activity had been restored (Dirnhuber, French, et al., 1979). The time-course of blockade was consistent with that produced by PB alone. In another study, PB pretreatment markedly improved the protection conferred by atropine and oxime in primates: the protective ratio was increased with PB pretreatment from 1.6 to more than 40 in rhesus monkeys (Kluwe, Chinn et al., 1987). Lesser benefits against lethality from soman with PB pretreatment have been seen in other, nonprimate species (see Table 3.5).

No studies to assess protection by PB against death from soman, or any other nerve agent, have been done in humans, because experiments involving lethal doses of nerve agent obviously cannot be done in humans.

Efficacy of PB Pretreatment for Other Nerve Agents

As Table 3.5 shows, in rodents PB may slightly improve the protective ratio for tabun and maybe cyclosarin (based on studies in guinea pigs) and may slightly

Table 3.5

Effect of Therapy With and Without Pyridostigmine Pretreatment on Protective Ratios (PR) in Animals Exposed to Nerve Agents

Nerve Agent	PR:[a] No PB	PR:[a] With PB	Species	Reference
Soman (GD)	1.6	>40	Rhesus monkey	Kluwe, Chinn, et al., 1987
	1.5	6.4 (5.0[b])	Guinea pig	Jones, Carter, et al., 1985
	2.0	2.7 (7.1[b])	Guinea pig	Lennox, Harris, et al., 1985
	1.9	4.9	Guinea pig	Capacio, Byers, et al., 1993; Capacio, Koplovitz, et al., 1995
	1.7	6.8	Guinea pig	Inns and Leadbeater, 1983
	1.4	2.7	Rabbit	Joiner, Dill, et al., 1989
	2.2	3.1	Rabbit	Sultan and Lennox, 1983
	1.9	2.8	Rabbit	Koplovitz and Stewart, 1994
	1.1	2.5	Mouse	Sultan and Lennox, 1983
	1.2	1.4	Rat	Anderson, Harris, et al., 1992
Sarin (GB)	36.4	35 (24[b])	Guinea pig	Koplovitz, Harris, et al., 1992
	2.1	2.2 (2.0[b])	Mouse	Koplovitz, Harris, et al., 1992
Cyclosarin (GF)	NA	>5	Rhesus monkey	Koplovitz, Gresham, et al., 1992
	2.7	3.4	Guinea pig	Stewart and Koplovitz, 1993
	1.4	1.4	Mouse	Stewart and Koplovitz, 1993
Tabun (GA)	4.4	7.8 (12[b])	Guinea pig	Koplovitz, Harris, et al., 1992
	2.4	3.9	Rabbit	Joiner, Dill, et al., 1989
	4.2	>8.5	Rabbit	Koplovitz and Stewart, 1994
	1.3	1.7 (2.1[b])	Mouse	Koplovitz, Harris, et al., 1992
VX	58.8	47 (45[b])	Guinea pig	Koplovitz, Harris, et al., 1992
	7.8	6.0 (3.9[b])	Mouse	Koplovitz, Harris, et al., 1992
	2.5	2.1	Rat	Anderson, Harris, et al., 1992

SOURCE: Adapted from Dunn, et al., 1997; and Pyridostigmine, 1996.

[a]With atropine plus oxime treatment.

[b]PR with two doses of PB given.

reduce the protective ratio for sarin and VX. Nonetheless, the protective ratios remain well over 5 for these agents, in rodents, so that PB has been perceived as not exerting a particularly concerning detriment on the very good protection provided by atropine and 2-PAM for these agents.

The presumption is that reduction in benefit occurs because both PB and nerve agent are binding to, and inhibiting, AChE. (1) PB confers added immediate detriment for peripheral AChE sites, by binding and inhibiting *additional* molecules of AChE, over and above those inhibited by nerve agents, with little or no offsetting benefit. Because there is time for oxime to be given after nerve agent exposure and before significant aging can take place (e.g., for sarin-AChE complexes), irreversible AChE inhibition is not expected; the oxime will have pulled off the sarin before the complex has aged. (PB is not needed to block and protect some fraction of the AChE from permanent inactivation, since the inactivation would presumably not be permanent.) (2) Additional peripheral AChE blockade will occur because PB in addition to nerve agent will bind and inhibit AChE, and increased binding of the peripheral sites by PB may "drive" increased central binding by nerve agent. (More nerve agent may be available to cross into the brain, because it has not been tied up by binding to peripheral sites that are already occupied by PB.) Tabun also has a long half-time of aging but may be somewhat less oxime-sensitive, at least in guinea pigs. Whether other mechanisms of protection are in play remains a matter of debate.

The actual evidence regarding the effect of PB on protection against nerve agent lethality is limited, in major part because it is based on studies in animals. Indeed, for most nerve agents, the evidence is based on studies in rodents and lagomorphs, which are not closely related to humans. One study in primates compares protective ratios with and without PB, in the context of postexposure treatment with atropine and pralidoxime (analogous to the regimen available to military personnel); this represents a relatively limited body of data. No studies were identified in which the protective ratio against sarin of standard nerve agent pretreatments were examined with and without PB treatment in primates.

There are differences in results from one study to another within an animal species and marked differences across animal species (differences that are not always in the same direction from one nerve agent to another). PB pretreatment, as previously stated, is presumed to markedly enhance protection against lethality in the event of soman exposure, based on (limited) evidence in monkeys.

PB pretreatment hampers protection against nerve agent lethality for other, nonsoman nerve agents (in the context of atropine and pralidoxime treatment). It is presumed to do so only to a minor and unimportant extent, but this supposition appears to be based solely on evidence from nonprimate animals (Anderson, Harris, et al., 1992; Koplovitz, Harris, et al., 1992). The effects of PB pretreatment on treatment efficacy—enhancement or reduction of treatment benefit—have not been studied for most nonsoman nerve agents in primates, and the PRs that result with PB pretreatment in primates for these other agents are not known. That is, no studies have been identified that assess protection with and without PB pretreatment in primates, in the context of atropine and pralidoxime postexposure treatment, for the nerve agents sarin or tabun; for cyclosarin, the apparent benefit of PB in rodents was reversed to detriment in primates. This offers the problematic possibility, which evidence should be obtained to preclude, that just as there is an exaggerated response to PB for soman pretreatment in primates versus rodents in the direction of increased protection, so there may be an exaggerated response to PB for sarin pretreatment in primates versus rodents in the direction of reduced protection. However, no evidence supports severely reduced protection in primates. Nonetheless, in a war situation, in which *both* soman and other nerve agents, such as sarin, may represent threats, the possible reduction in sarin protection (of a severity that remains to be quantitated in primates), considered together with the likelihood of sarin (or other nerve agent attack), should be pitted against the possible increase in soman protection multiplied by the likelihood of a soman attack.

The issue of whether a PR of 5 should continue to be considered the consistent goal of nerve agent pretreatment and treatment, across all nerve agents, is not addressed here, but should be reevaluated.

Guinea pigs are presumed to be a good model for primates with regard to nerve agent treatment studies (Wetherell, 1992). For instance, PB provides higher PR for primates and guinea pigs than for other rodents (order: primates, guinea pigs, rabbits, rats (Sidell, 1990; Dirnhuber, French, et al., 1979)), which may relate to the fact that pralidoxime does not confer significant protection against soman in these two species (Inns and Leadbeater, 1983); efforts to standardize testing of nerve agent countermeasures advise using guinea pigs for initial studies followed by nonhuman primates (Koplovitz, Gresham, et al., 1992). Although widely used as models for nerve agent defense studies, guinea pigs represent a problematic model; oxime efficacy is dramatically different in guinea pigs compared to primates for instance, pralidoxime confers benefit against GF in primates but not in guinea pigs, so that the slight benefit PB confers vis-à-vis tabun in guinea pigs might not be present in primates, which appear to be more oxime-sensitive.

Another limitation in current evidence is that the effect of PB in rhesus monkeys is not known to reflect the effect of PB on other primates, and particularly on humans; more confidence would be achieved if studies were performed—

and showed similar findings—in other primate species and in species more closely related to humans. There is some theoretical cause for optimism, since aging rates in several species of primates—in marmosets, squirrel monkeys, and cynomolgus monkeys—differ from those in rodents—rats and guinea pigs—in a consistent direction (Talbot, Anderson, et al., 1988), providing some rationale to think that similar effects may occur across primate species. However, there are also several reasons for concern in extrapolation of results from primates. First, doses of protective agents in primate studies have been higher than those in humans; doses of PB three times (Koplovitz, Gresham, et al., 1992), 10 times (Dirnhuber, French, et al., 1977), or even 20 to 50 times higher (Dirnhuber, Green, et al., 1977) than those used in humans have been employed (perhaps most commonly 10 times higher), with the argument that since these higher doses produce AChE inhibition comparable to that with the 30 mg thrice a day regimen in humans, these doses are therefore "physiologically similar" (Dirn-huber, Green, et al., 1978). Atropine doses are also four times higher, due to the "reduced sensitivity" of the monkeys to atropine, which is presumed to also hold for central effects (Dirnhuber, Green, et al., 1978). Results from these different dose studies, which also typically combine the three possible post-exposure doses, are used in representing the expected PRs. However, for many reasons these doses cannot be presumed to be physiologically similar.

First, the very fact that higher doses of PB and atropine are needed in nonhuman primates to gain comparability on one physiological measure suggests the monkeys may not represent a good model. Second, it is known that when multiple measures are used to rank treatments, not all measures show effects in the same direction (D'Mello, Cross, et al., 1994); in particular, a higher PB dose may be needed in primates to generate comparable AChE inhibition but may produce highly noncomparable effects in some other measure. This is important because AChE inhibition might not represent the sole mechanism of benefit. Third, in vitro studies in primate and human muscle tissue suggest that 10 times lower, not 10 times higher doses of PB in primates are needed to generate protection against soman in vitro (although this now refers to pipetted doses, rather than oral doses—10^{-6}M is needed in human intercostal muscle tissue to produce somewhat comparable benefit to that of 10^{-7}M PB in primates, although it is possible that this is a function of different sensitivity to, and perhaps incomplete ability to wash off, soman (Smith, 1981). No data were identified that assessed whether comparable oral doses of PB in humans and primates lead to comparable muscle concentrations. If they do, it would imply that the primate studies on which we base estimates of PRs for humans use 100 times the "physiologically equivalent dose" of PB given to humans, if physiological equivalence is defined by the metric of soman protection, presumably the metric of interest. This makes the simplifying assumption of linearity of response. Undoubtedly several of these assumptions, e.g., of comparable muscle concentration after the same weight-adjusted oral dose, will be found to be incorrect. Unfortunately they cannot be assumed to be incorrect in any given direction. This adds substantial uncertainty to estimates of protective benefit of PB even against soman, the nerve agent it is presumed to have protective efficacy against.

In short, the use of PB as a pretreatment adjunct improves survival in tested species of primates with soman exposure, but these tests employ substantially higher mg/kg doses of PB than employed in humans, as well as higher mg/kg doses of atropine; data from other mammals suggest PB does not materially hamper survival with exposure to other nerve agents in these mammals, though there is no direct evidence of this in primates for some nerve agents, including sarin and tabun.

It should be noted that "protection" by PB against lethality from soman attack does not appear to be accompanied by protection against incapacitation from soman, so that mission completion will not necessarily be abetted by PB pretreatment. The aim of maintaining 20 to 40 percent RBC ChE inhibition is "only recommended for counteracting the lethal effects of nerve agent poisoning and are not necessarily appropriate in maintaining combat effectiveness (a desirable characteristic)" (Moylan-Jones, Parks, et al., 1979). Animal studies have reliably shown that even "low" doses of nerve agent, on the order of one to two LD_{50}s, are associated with profound incapacitation despite PB and posttreatment regimens that markedly reduce lethality (Dirnhuber Green, et al., 1978; Moylan-Jones, Parks, et al., 1979; Hayward, Wall, et al., 1990; Wetherell, 1992).

There remain issues regarding whether AChE inhibition by PB (and "protection" of bound sites from nerve agent attachment) actually represents the mechanism of protection by PB. A new drug application for PB as military pretreatment, filed in May 1996, suggests that the degree of AChE inhibition relates to the degree of protection (Pyridostigmine, 1996). Higher doses may produce more average cholinesterase inhibition and more protection, up to a point, and in guinea pigs and rats, a positive correlation exists between the degree of cholinesterase inhibition and protection (Lennox, Harris, et al., 1985). But this need not actually imply a causal connection: at the individual level, the animals with a greater degree of enzyme inhibition do not necessarily experience more protection. In guinea pigs, though PB dose correlated strongly with AChE inhibition, there was no clear relation of the PR to either the PB dose and/or to the level of AChE inhibition (Jones, Carter, et al., 1985). In primates, the level of AChE inhibition was reported not to be critical to effectiveness (Koplovitz, Gresham, et al., 1992). The FDA, in failing to approve the 1996 submission of the New Drug Application, has expressed concern that the evidence from studies in monkeys and guinea pigs does not permit the conclusion that RBC acetylcholinesterase inhibition is either proportional to the degree of protection or necessary for protection:

> "the data . . . did not allow us to reach the conclusion that the extent of protection is proportional to the extent of red blood cell acetylcholinesterase inhibition, or even that red blood cell acetylcholinesterase inhibition is a necessary concomitant of protection. To the contrary, there is a dissociation between the two. In the monkey studies, the enzyme inhibition is unrelated to the extent of protection. Furthermore, in guinea pigs, for example in one published study (in *Fundamental and Applied Toxicology*, 5, S242–S251 (1985)), red blood cell acetylcholinesterase inhibition rates from 5 percent to 80 percent were associated with PRs of 5.0 to 6.4 with little or no suggestion of a dose relationship." (Prendergast, 1997.)

Time-Course of Effectiveness. Studies in guinea pigs show a maximum protective benefit of PB pretreatment when soman exposure occurs 60 minutes after pretreatment. PRs (the ratio of LD_{50} with treatment divided by LD_{50} without treatment) for different time intervals following exposure are listed in Table 3.6 (Sidell, 1990; Gordon, Leadbeater, et al., 1978). Because of metabolic and other differences, the time-course in humans may be somewhat different.

Chemical Warfare Threat. The decision to employ PB as a nerve agent pretreatment was based on the information available regarding the perceived threat of chemical warfare. At least 23 nations are reported to have stockpiles of nerve agents, though these are prohibited for use in war by the 1925 Geneva Convention and the 1989 Paris Convention on Chemical Weapons (which not all nations have signed) (Gunderson, Lehmann, et al., 1992). The nations reported to have chemical weapons include not only Iraq and Iran, but Egypt, Syria, Libya, Israel, Ethiopia, Burma, Thailand, North Korea, South Korea, Cuba, Vietnam, Taiwan, China, and South Africa (Barnaby, 1985; Gunderson, Lehmann, et al., 1992). In addition, the Iraqis not only have CW capability, but have militarized nerve agents and used them against Iranians and against the

Table 3.6

PB PRs for Soman Exposure (Guinea Pigs)

Interval from PB to Soman	Protective Ratio (PR)
10 minutes	3.4
30 minutes	8.0
60 minutes	12.5
2 hours	6.0
3 hours	4.7
4 hours	3.2

Kurds (Barnaby, 1985; Gunderson, Lehmann, et al., 1992). Use of nerve agent was confirmed by chemical examination of casualties (Barnaby, 1985). Typically, Iranian casualties were exposed after the explosion of artillery shells or bombs between 4 and 200 meters away (Barnaby, 1985). After 1984, chemical warfare intensified and became more frequent, despite numerous UN missions to investigate use of CW in the Iran-Iraq conflict, and repeated appeals by the UN). Iraq used chemical weapons more extensively and more frequently than Iran. Therefore, CW was justifiably understood to represent a valid Iraqi threat in the PGW. This threat was subsequently confirmed by the discovery of nerve agent munitions, including those containing sarin and cyclosarin, in the Khamisiyah ammunitions storage facility in Iraq (Gulflink, 1997).

Although no direct intelligence indicated that soman stockpiles were present in Iraq, it was known that the former Soviet Union had stockpiled soman. With the dissolution of the Soviet Union and the consequent political and economic destabilization and fragmentation, the military was concerned that arms of many sorts were for sale to the highest bidder, possibly including Iraq.

How Nerve Agents Work. Nerve agents include the G agents (GA or tabun; GB or sarin; GD or soman); and VX. The G agents are viewed as "nonpersistent" since they evaporate and disperse over several hours in temperate conditions. The oilier VX is construed as "persistent" since it may linger for weeks or longer, continuing to pose a hazard (Dunn, 1989). Other nerve agents such as cyclosarin (GF), or thiosarin, are derivatives of these G nerve agents. Nerve agents work by "irreversibly" inhibiting AChE (that is, with very long half-life), as described above, leading to excess cholinergic activity in the brain and the "periphery" (skeletal muscles, smooth muscles and glands), producing respiratory failure and death.

How Long Have Carbamates Been Used for AChE Inhibitor Pretreatment? The first use of a carbamate for pretreatment for lethal effects of an organophosphorus compound was in 1946; physostigmine was reported to protect cats against an otherwise lethal dose of the organophosphate DFP (Koster, 1946). The first use of a carbamate as pretreatment for a *nerve agent* occurred later, in sarin-challenged rats. Atropine alone was unsuccessful as a therapy (one of five rabbits lived), but pretreatment with physostigmine led to enhanced survival (five of five rabbits lived) (Wills, 1963; Sidell, 1990). PB was considered a candidate pretreatment drug as early as the mid-1950s (Wannarka, 1984), and a major effort to develop a useful formulation was under way at the Biomedical Laboratory at Edgewood, Maryland, in the early 1970s (Wannarka, 1984), though enthusiasm for chemical warfare defense waned in the mid 1970s, stalling progress. An IND (investigational new drug) application for PB for pretreatment use was filed with the FDA in February of 1984 (Wannarka, 1984).

Subsequent interactions between the FDA and DoD on this issue are detailed in a separate RAND report (Rettig, 1999).

Side Effects

In two decades of PB testing in the military, the incidence of side effects with PB administration was reputedly under 1 percent. Most side effects were mild, principally involving the GI tract (increased flatus, loose stool).

In pre-PGW military tests of PB, there is some suggestion that incidence of side effects may not have been as low as supposed; use of small samples may have obscured even relatively pervasive effects. For example, in one study containing a list of 38 symptom questions, each at four times, in a small set of subjects, it was stated that no symptoms were significantly more common in those assigned to PB compared to a placebo (Gleadle, Kemp, and Wetherell, 1983b). In fact, however, symptom reporting was typically more common in PB patients compared to placebo patients. Symptoms were reported more often in PB than placebo cases 97 times, compared to 18 times with placebo patients reporting a symptom at a higher rate than PB patients. The ratio becomes 100:18 if one includes the query to patients that they attributed the symptoms to their pill; the results, using the sign test, are $z/2 = 7.37$, $p < .0001$. If each time period is not considered separately, the resulting value is $z/2 = 4.96$, $p < .001$. This suggests that across a wide range of symptoms, in patients blinded to PB versus placebo status, symptom reporting was indeed significantly more common in those receiving PB (Gleadle, Kemp, and Wetherell, 1983b).

The PGW experience entailed a substantially higher incidence of reported side effects than those anticipated from pre-PGW studies. As part of the legal requirement for use of PB as an investigational new drug, DoD was required to collect data on the safety and efficacy of PB (Federal Register, 1997). Three surveys have been conducted to determine the incidence and severity of side effects associated with the use of PB as a nerve agent pretreatment. The first was a questionnaire sent to 42 selected medical personnel involved in Operation Desert Shield and Operation Desert Storm; 23 of the questionnaires were completed and returned. Among the 23, 10 responded that the drug was tolerated either very well or well. The most common side effects reported were gastrointestinal (abdominal cramps, nausea, and diarrhea), with other effects including weakness, light-headedness, exacerbation of asthmatic symptoms, fatigue, sleep disturbances, and reduced mental concentration. Of the many thousands of military personnel reported on,[2] eight were hospitalized for side effects

---

[2]The source cited states that 5,825 personnel were reported on. Dr. Ronald Clawson, in reviewing this report, states, "There is a misconception that the number of personnel reported on in this study

attributed to PB, with reasons for hospitalization including cholelithiasis (gallstones), asthma, and allergic skin reaction (Federal Register, 1997).

The second survey was a questionnaire given to an unspecified number of soldiers deployed in the PGW; 149 responded. Of those who took the drug, 37.5 percent reported side effects, most frequently gastrointestinal. Nausea was reported most frequently (11 percent of subjects), followed by headache (7.5 percent) (Federal Register, 1997).

The third survey was designed to document the effect of PB on aviators' ability to carry out combat missions. Of the 118 aviators who participated, 48 were taking other medications, most commonly the antibiotic ciprofloxacin, and 26 of the 108 who reported taking the drug experienced side effects they attributed to PB, most commonly headaches and diarrhea (Federal Register, 1997).

In one published retrospective study, 30 medical officers from the Army's XVIII Airborne Corps were questioned regarding symptoms in personnel they oversaw during the PGW. These officers oversaw 41,650 soldiers and 234,000 person-days of PB use and were reportedly in daily close contact with these units (Keeler, Hurst, et al., 1991). Based on their recall, 50 percent of troops had GI changes (including flatus, loose stools, abdominal cramps, and nausea). Urinary urgency or frequency was also common. Less than 5 percent complained of headaches, runny nose, sweating, and tingling of the extremities. However, these symptoms did not noticeably interfere with performance of "the full range of demanding physical and mental tasks required" (Keeler, Hurst, et al., 1991).

Few (one percent) perceived a need for medical attention and about 0.1 percent discontinued PB based on medical advice. A total of 483 aid station or clinical visits related to PB occurred, usually within hours of taking the first tablet. In some patients, these effects continued as long as PB was taken. In others, it abated after one to two days of use. Reported problems leading to medical attention are listed in Table 3.7.

Later information from hospital personnel indicated that two women of low weight (45–50 kg) reported increased salivation, severe abdominal cramping, nausea, sweating, and muscle twitching. The presence of symptoms in these individuals was taken to suggest a possible effect of body weight, since lower-weight individuals receiving the same fixed dose in fact are subject to a higher

---

was 5,825. Due to unclear wording in the survey, the responders identified the number of people who worked for them (i.e., medical personnel) rather than the number of people in the units that they supported. The survey forms were mailed to the commanders of every major medical unit in the theater, covering hundreds of thousands of personnel."

Table 3.7

Problems Leading to Medical Attention After PB Use in the PGW

Complaint	Number
GI disturbances severe enough to prompt medical visits	313
Urinary frequency	150
Bad dreams	5
Worsening of acute bronchitis	3
Headache	3
Slurred speech but normal neurological exam	3
Rashes, one of these with urticaria (hives) of hands and feet	2
Vertigo	1

SOURCE: Keeler, Hurst, et al., 1991.

dose-per-body-weight. During the PGW, administration of PB with meals was reported by some to reduce GI complaints and was instituted by some units (Keeler, Hurst, et al., 1991).

A second published report included both a cross sectional study of 213 Israeli soldiers from one unit, regarding symptoms and severity 24 hours after starting PB; and a case-control comparison of AChE inhibition, with the same survey questionnaire, for nine soldiers with and 12 without complaints from a different unit (Sharabi, Danon, et al., 1991; see Table 3.8). The most frequent symptoms were nonspecific and included dry mouth, malaise, fatigue, and weakness. The more predictable symptoms were infrequent, including nausea, abdominal pain, frequent urination and runny nose. Symptoms were mild, and there was no correlation of subjective symptoms with BChE inhibition (Sharabi, 1991).

Another study (unpublished), by the British Medical Services of 208 British PGW personnel, found that 25 percent of the study group suffered side effects serious enough to consider discontinuation of PB (Martin, 1994). More than half missed at least one tablet in first 48 hours of treatment—"a time when one would have expected compliance to be close to 100%." It is noted that "Anecdotal evidence suggests that symptoms attributable to NAPS [nerve agent pretreatment system] therapy may continue for some time after cessation of treatment." These studies of individuals who took PB during the PGW are observational and uncontrolled but may reflect the PGW experience.

Studies outside the PGW venue are more likely to be controlled but may lack the potential interactions between PB and other exposures, including stress. (In addition, individual reports of adverse responses that could reflect individual differences have been discounted in some studies. In one study, it was stated that "A man [in the PB group] who complained of persistent fatigue, headache, poor concentration and irritability had domestic problems" (Kemp and Wetherell, 1982), as though causality can be imputed. Finally, the nature of the

Table 3.8

**Symptom Frequency: Cross-Sectional
Survey of 213 Israeli Soldiers**

Symptom	Percentage of Frequency
Malaise	53.4
Fatigue, numbness	37.0
Weakness	37.0
Headache	29.0
Dizziness/imbalance	19.0
Moodiness	18.0
Restlessness	18.0
Heavy extremities	10.0
Excessive sweating	9.0
Altered mood	8.0
Sense of fear	6.0
Dry mouth	71.0
Nausea	22.1
Abdominal pain	20.0
Lack of appetite	14.0
Diarrhea	6.0
Rhinorrhea	10.0
Hot flushes	20.0
Rapid heartbeat	8.0
Frequent urination	11.0

SOURCE: Sharabi, Danon, et al., 1991.

"placebo" chosen was stated in only one study identified; the placebo was lactose (Moylan-Jones, Parkes, et al., 1981). Lactose is known to cause gastrointestinal problems among members of the population who are "lactose intolerant" (and this has led to problems in placebo-controlled trials in the past in which lactose was employed as a placebo) (Golomb, 1995); a true increase in GI and perhaps other symptoms could be obscured by employment of lactose as a placebo.

One double-blind crossover study of seven soldier volunteers who received one week each of a placebo and of PB, with daily exposure to four hours of heat, two hours of rest, and two hours of moderate exercise (40 percent maximum aerobic power), failed to detect differences in symptoms (based on a questionnaire) between PB and placebo, though the PB group demonstrated reduced hand grip strength ($p < .05$), higher rectal temperature ($p < .01$) and smaller pupil diameter ($p < .01$) (Cook, Kolka, et al., 1992).

Another study followed 45 male and 45 female subjects in various weight categories who received 30 mg of PB or a placebo every eight hours, for 22 days (Lasseter and Garg, 1996). Controls reported more headaches than the active treatment group (10 of 30, $p < .05$). While diarrhea and abdominal pain were reported by four of 15 subjects in each active treatment group, the difference between PB and placebo in this small sample was not significant (p = .068).

Less directly germane is information on nine PGW veterans who attempted to overdose on PB, consuming 13 to 30 tablets of 30 mg of PB (390–900 mg) (Almog, Wingler, et al., 1991). Findings included the following:

- No correlation was seen between serum cholinesterase inhibition and severity or incidence of cholinergic symptoms in this self-selected group.

- Plasma cholinesterase (pseudocholinesterase, or BChE) levels were decreased 30 to 50 percent before other signs or symptoms were evident. Pseudocholinesterase inhibition was therefore construed as "a reliable and sensitive diagnostic tool" in PB poisoning.

- Major clinical symptoms went away within several hours, while cholinesterase levels returned to normal within one to two days. Thus clinical recovery was faster than enzyme recovery. This was felt to match findings in organophosphorus poisoning: "neuroadaptation" leads to tolerance to continuing low AChE activity (Almog, Winkler, et al., 1991).

Physiologic Effects. A number of small studies report effects on physiological parameters, including pupil size, heart rate, temperature, sweating, skin blood flow, and motor strength. Some also examine the impact of exercise or decompression on the effect of PB. Others have investigated performance effects.

Findings relating to physiological parameters at rest or with exercise include no change (Sidell, 1990) or a reduction (Kolka and Stephenson, 1990; Stephenson and Kolka, 1990; Gall, 1981; Sidell, 1990; Lasseter and Garg, 1996) in heart rate (of about five beats per minute); no change (Gall, 1981; Sidell, 1990) or reduction (Cook, Kolka, et al., 1992) in pupil size; no change (Roberts, Sawka, et al., 1994) or increase (Kolka and Stephenson, 1990; Stephenson and Kolka, 1990; Cook, Kolka, et al., 1992) in temperature; no change (Glikson, Achiron, et al., 1991) or reduction (Cook, Kolka, et al., 1992) in motor strength; no change (Sidell, 1990) or increase (Kolka and Stephenson, 1990; Stephenson and Kolka, 1990) in sweating; and no change or reduction (Kolka and Stephenson, 1990; Stephenson and Kolka, 1990) in skin blood flow. Effects may vary by ambient temperature, work load, duration of exercise, and other factors.

Acute effects are indirectly relevant to the issue of possible delayed and chronic effects, but are not directly the focus of this report. Nonetheless, Appendix B shows results of several studies of the effects of PB in humans on physiological parameters, performance, and side effects.

Chapter Four

PB USE IN THE PERSIAN GULF WAR

This chapter briefly reviews circumstances of use of PB in the PGW, including production and storage of PB, training of personnel with regard to PB use, decisions regarding use, and actual use of PB. (This does not include such circumstances of use as concurrent exposures, which are reviewed elsewhere—see Chapter Nine, "Interactions.") A review of the circumstances of use was undertaken to ascertain whether any irregularities in these circumstances might pertain to illnesses in PGW veterans and to evaluate ways in which circumstances may be improved in future deployments. This chapter relies heavily on non–peer reviewed sources (government reports and personal communication), because much information regarding circumstances of use is rare in the peer-reviewed literature.

PRODUCTION

PB for use in the PGW was produced overseas. No 30 mg PB tablets are manufactured in the United States. Duphar BV in Holland and Roche Products, Ltd., in England produced PB tablets used in Operation Desert Shield and Operation Desert Storm in the PGW (Brake, 1997). Discussion with FDA officials indicates that drugs manufactured overseas for use in the United States are required to meet the same criteria and are subject to the same oversight as drugs manufactured in the United States. PB was distributed in blister packs of 21 30 mg tablets (a one-week supply), each termed a Nerve Agent Pretreatment Pack (NAPP).

PACKAGING

The NAPP states the agent and dose (21 tablets PB USP 30 mg). Dutch packaging from 1990 contained the following directions:

1. Commence taking only when ordered by your commander.

2. Take one every eight hours.

3.   It is dangerous to exceed the stated dose.

The PB packaged at Duphar in Amsterdam, the Netherlands, included the manufacture date and lot number.

Current packaging (not that used in the Gulf War) on PB packaged at Roche Products Ltd., U.K., states "For Military Combat Use and Evaluation" and contains the following additional warning:

Warning

If you have asthma, are pregnant or are taking medications for high blood pressure or glaucoma, see your unit doctor before taking pyridostigmine.

Pyridostigmine may cause stomach cramps, diarrhea, nausea, frequent urination or headaches.

Seek medical attention if these or other symptoms persist or worsen.

STORAGE

Under Forces Command (FORSCOM) guidelines, following FDA/DSCP directives, PB in NAPP must be stored refrigerated in temperatures ranging from 2° to 8° C (35° to 46° F) to retain potency for the full shelf life. Those that have exceeded their expiration date or have remained unrefrigerated for more than six months are not to be used (FORSCOM, 1990; Field Manual, 1990). According to discussion with some in-theater personnel, PB, once overseas, was not refrigerated, although others report that PB that remained in the hands of the medical/logistics community was reputedly refrigerated (Clawson, 1999); nor was there any indication that PB required refrigeration during what proved to be a short conflict. Discussion with FDA officials indicates that no concerns regarding toxic products were related to a lapse in the refrigeration of PB (FDA, 1997). PB is refrigerated only to ensure efficacy with extended storage. PB given in the PGW was primarily made for the PGW and manufactured shortly prior to it. Other PB was manufactured approximately five years earlier (Clawson, 1999). PB is on a "shelf life extension program" through the FDA. PB from 1985 has continued to undergo testing, and has continued to pass all tests, receiving successive one- to two-year shelf life extensions (Clawson, 1999).

TRAINING AND EDUCATION

As part of granting a waiver of informed consent to DoD for use of PB as a nerve agent pretreatment during the PGW, the FDA required DoD to disseminate information to all military personnel concerning the risks and benefits of PB (Federal Register, 1997; Friedman, 1997).

Efforts were made to train medical personnel in the use of PB and in the recognition and treatment of side effects related to use of PB. According to FORSCOM regulations, unit medical personnel must be trained to recognize the signs and symptoms of PB overdose, allergic reactions, and side effects and to give emergency treatment if necessary (FORSCOM, 1990). A "Field Manual" was produced (and has since been updated) that describes the purpose of nerve agent pretreatment; the NAPP Tablet Set; effects of PB; principles of use; administration in an uncontaminated environment; signs and symptoms of overdose, adverse reactions, and contraindications; emergency medical treatment for PB's adverse side effects, allergic reactions, and overdose; and responsibilities of corps/division/wing commanders, the units, and the unit medical personnel (Field Manual, 1995; Field Manual, 1990).

Evidence suggests there was wide variation in the education of personnel in the combat setting. A survey by DoD, of an unspecified number of military personnel, queried their views on the adequacy of the training and information they received regarding PB (Federal Register, 1997). Of 149 respondents, 43.7 percent responded to the question "Was training about pyridostigmine adequate?" in the negative. Most expressed the desire for more information on side effects, long-term effects, and the drug's mechanism of action. The following list is a sample of comments from those who felt the training was inadequate, and from those who felt it was adequate but could have been better (Federal Register, 1997):

- "No standard side effects were given."

- "No training on side effects."

- "People were worried about the drug's side effects. Many people avoided taking it. Some people would double dose after missing one."

- "Combat lifesavers brief it and said it was FDA-approved."

- "Many soldiers didn't take the tablets due to the fact that they weren't FDA approved or thought not."

- "Didn't know what it did, what it was for. Disregarded instructions to take it."

- "Training was not enough in layman's terms. You would need to know more about nerve agents."

Veterans made similar remarks regarding the adequacy of the information they received, at hearings before the Senate Committee on Veterans' Affairs and the Presidential Advisory Committee on Gulf War Veterans' Illnesses (Federal Register, 1997).

As part of a DoD survey of medical personnel (described in Chapter Three, sub-section on "Side Effects"), 15 of 23 medical officers who returned the survey indicated that the information sheet on PB was not distributed to personnel instructed to take the drug. Two respondents said the information was dis-tributed, and one, whose unit was not instructed to commence treatment with PB, indicated that he had the sheet available for distribution (Federal Register, 1997). The FDA has expressed concern about several features of PB training. These include the high rate of dissatisfaction regarding education, the responses indicating that the Army's educational activities were uneven and possibly not targeted to the education level of all personnel; and the indication that the information sheet on PB was not provided and disseminated to military personnel in the Gulf as conditioned in the commissioner's letter granting the waiver of informed consent under the interim rule (Federal Register, 1997). (See also Rettig, 1999.)

DECISION REGARDING USE

Under FORSCOM guidelines, the corps or division commander determines whether to begin, continue, or discontinue the NAPP medication with advice from the intelligence officer or chemical officer and the surgeon (FORSCOM, 1990). Unit commanders had discretion on whether and when to order use of PB and could delegate this authority to the lowest level of field command (Federal Register, 1997). Documentation does not exist on how far down the command chain the authority was delegated in each unit (Federal Register, 1997). The decision to use PB was to be reevaluated each three days, and administration beyond 21 days was not recommended without a thorough evaluation of the situation (FORSCOM, 1990). There is no documentation regarding adherence to these directives.

USE

Some unit commanders reportedly advised troops to take more than the stated amount of PB. Veterans' self-reports of pills taken, based on telephone inter-views conducted by the Office of the Special Assistant to the Deputy Secretary of Defense for Gulf War Illnesses (OSAGWI), range from one tablet daily to five tablets every four to six hours (Brake, 1997). The troops did not necessarily take PB as advised (Federal Register, 1997); monitoring was variable, ranging from strict enforcement, with pills taken while in formation, to use of the honor sys-tem (Brake, 1997). Some individuals report having taken more than 60 tablets in total (Zeller, 1997), or in one "Open Letter" on the Internet, 500 tablets over six months (Hamden, 1997).

Although several reports states that "most" or "nearly all" or "a great majority" of U.S. troops received PB (Defense Science Board, 1994; National Institutes of Health, 1994) or that most allied coalition troops and Israeli civilians received PB pretreatment (De Fraites, 1996), the actual usage appears to be substantially less comprehensive. One estimate, in use by the Office of the Special Assistant for Gulf War Illnesses is that 250,000 to 300,000 U.S. personnel received some PB, an estimate based on number of tablets delivered but not returned in the system (Brake, 1997). (This estimate is subject to uncertainty based, among other factors, on uncertainty in average duration of use.) Tablets were taken primarily in January 1991 in preparation for the air war, and again in February 1991 in preparation for the ground war (Brake, 1997). Based on the author's discussions with Israeli military personnel and leaders, conducted in concert with the OSAGWI, Israeli military but not civilians received PB during the PGW.

There is no documentation on whether or when each unit issued orders to begin taking PB or on who took it (Federal Register, 1997).

OTHER NATIONS

PB nerve agent pretreatment was used by the United Kingdom and Canada as well as the United States; perhaps 45,000 U.K. troops received PB (Defense Science Board, 1994). The French evidently dispensed PB to their troops but did not issue the order to use it. However, not all PB was returned, and some French troops took PB. Saudi Arabian and Egyptian troops did not take it.

PB TIMETABLE IN THE PGW

The following timetable is adapted primarily from De Fraites (1996) with additional input. (The accuracy of the statements has not in each case been independently verified.)

Aug. 2, 1990: Iraq invades Kuwait. At the onset of Operation Desert Shield, the threat of chemical weapons, including exposure to nerve agents is recognized.

Aug. 7, 1990: FORSCOM message provides guidance for issue and use of PB, IAW FM 8-285 during Operation Desert Shield. PB tablet to be used when risk of imminent nerve agent exposure is evident, and only on direct order of division or corps commander.

Oct. 11, 1990: U.S. Army Medical Research and Development Command identifies the need for FDA waiver for use of PB in Operation Desert Shield. Though PB has been licensed by FDA, it had not been specifically approved for use as NAPP.

Dec. 21, 1990: FDA publishes interim regulation in Federal Register allowing waiver of informed consent for investigational new drugs (IND) for DoD use during Operation Desert Shield. This statement explains FDA position on specific waivers to DoD under circumstances when informed consent is considered unfeasible.

Dec. 28, 1990: Assistant Secretary of Defense (Health Affairs) submits to FDA a specific request for waiver of informed consent for PB pretreatment for Operation Desert Shield.

Jan. 8, 1991: FDA approves the waiver of informed consent for PB for Operation Desert Shield. The FDA's Informed Consent Waiver Review Group supports the DoD use of PB as the only potentially useful nerve agent pretreatment available. The group "had no specific safety concerns" with the dose of 30 mg each eight hours (only 15 percent of the dose often used to treat myasthenia gravis). The only substantial FDA concern expressed in this memo is that DoD instructional materials (Field Manual 8-285 and Training Manual 90-4) implies that PB pretreatment had been proven effective in human trials. FDA agreed with the text of a supplemental information sheet produced by DoD that stated that PB had been shown effective in animal studies.

Jan. 16–17, 1991: Operation Desert Storm (air war) begins. PB use was ordered on at least two separate occasions in the subsequent 30 days. The soldier information sheet gets very limited distribution.

Feb. 23, 1991: Ground war begins and concludes after 100 hours. Results of a survey involving 40,000 XVIII Corps (Airborne) soldiers conducted shortly after cessation of hostilities indicated that though minor symptoms such as abdominal cramps and frequent urination were quite common, only about 1 percent of people taking PB sought medical care, and fewer than one in 1,000 had to discontinue PB pretreatment.

May 24, 1996: New Drug Application for PB use in NAPP filed with FDA.

SUMMARY

Circumstances of PB use were appropriate in several respects. A waiver of informed consent was obtained from the FDA prior to administration of PB to personnel without informed consent. Conservative strategies for use of PB with the threat of nerve agent exposure were devised, requiring repeated reevaluation of PB use every several days, with decisionmaking regarding use of PB by high-level commanders with medical, chemical, and intelligence consultation. A training manual was devised and training programs were implemented in an effort to ensure that medical and chemical personnel had knowledge regarding the use and side effects of PB. Agreement in principle was made to educate troops regarding the function and side effects of PB. No irregularities were identified in storage or delivery that would have altered the characteristics of PB to render it unexpectedly deleterious.

The circumstances of PB use were suboptimal in several respects. Training in the use and side effects of PB was not in all cases reflected in practice in the field. The FDA's requirement of information distribution regarding PB to all military personnel as a condition of the waiver of informed consent was not upheld. Personnel perceived the education they received to be inadequate. Because of these problems, wide variations in de facto use occurred across and within units, with irregularities in orders given regarding dosage in some units and with some personnel electing to alter the dosing schedule or refrain from use of PB. Record-keeping to allow a determination of which units received PB, for how long, and when is not available; neither are records regarding which level of command made the decision regarding the use of PB.

Overall, many circumstances of PB use—including its manufacture, transport, and storage—do not appear to have contributed materially to illnesses in PGW veterans. For instance, there is no evidence that manufacture was flawed and resulted in an inferior or toxic product; or that adverse storage conditions were present and led to toxic substances or byproducts of PB. Whether other types of "circumstances" of PB use—such as coexposure with other PGW exposures—could have been contributory is the subject of subsequent sections (e.g., Chapter Nine, "Interactions Between PB and Other Exposures").

SCIENTIFIC RECOMMENDATIONS

Scientific recommendations for the circumstances of PB use constitute policy recommendations, which are not the primary focus of the present report. However, certain recommendations can readily be made:

- Advance planning and training should be improved regarding education and the consent process.

- Medical personnel should instruct soldiers regarding PB side effects.

- Consistent strategies should be adopted for handling those who "decline" to take PB when ordered.[1]

---

[1]The military has held that refusal by personnel to take PB under orders, when the threat of chemical warfare is perceived, potentially compromises the welfare of the whole unit in the event of nerve agent attack and is therefore untenable. This position is made less persuasive by the limited corpus of evidence regarding benefits of PB in the event of nerve agent attack. Evidence of benefit vis-á-vis soman derives from only a few studies in primates: in one study, the effects of atropine and

- Careful planning should be undertaken to ensure accurate generation and coordinated maintenance of records regarding who received which agents, from what lots, in what doses, and when.

- Testing of PB pretreatment for nerve agents other than soman should be performed in primates. The effects of pralidoxime and atropine postexposure treatment should be compared with and without PB pretreatment to ensure that PB pretreatment does not in fact enhance lethality to an important degree.

---

oxime postexposure treatment were tested with and without PB pretreatment to calculate protective ratios. Of more concern, there is *no* primate evidence regarding the effect of PB pretreatment in the event of nerve agent attack with other nerve agents. (That is, no studies have evaluated lethality with atropine and pralidoxime, with and without PB pretreatment.) The beneficial effect of PB pretreatment against soman occurs in other mammals but is magnified in primates. It is conceivable that the *detrimental* effect of PB on death from *sarin and VX* that is seen in other mammals is also magnified in primates, and there is no primate evidence to preclude this possibility. (Neither is there evidence from close primate relatives to humans that benefit against soman is preserved, though evidence from some other primate species suggests that primates may share similar characteristics related to aging of AChE–nerve agent complexes.) It is also possible, however, that PB provides benefit in primates against all nerve agent threats. Because neither the mechanism of benefit of PB for soman nor the mechanism of "harm" for sarin and VX are fully understood, this determination cannot be made without empirical testing. Thus, the existing state of knowledge is consistent with the possibility that refusal to take PB either compromises *or enhances* the viability of the unit in the event of nerve agent attack, particularly when the threat includes nonsoman nerve agents. It might be appropriate to consider this element of uncertainty in making judgments about the right of personnel to refuse the pretreatment drug.

Chapter Five

HEALTH PROBLEMS IN PGW VETERANS

The epidemiology of illness in PGW veterans is not the focus of this report, and indeed was the subject of a distinct RAND effort. A summary of some factors related to epidemiology is provided here. This is in no way intended to be a complete review of the epidemiological data.

GULF WAR VETERANS REPORT HEALTH PROBLEMS

Many PGW veterans (on the order of 100,000) have participated in health registries through the VA or DoD, and most of these veterans report having health problems. A variety of studies have characterized the symptoms and diagnoses in PGW veterans. Table 5.1 shows, as an example, the most frequent principal diagnoses in PGW registry personnel as of February 1997 (n = 74,653). Findings, while generally consistent, vary somewhat with the wording and category boundaries employed to define the symptoms and diagnoses.

SYMPTOMS IN PGW VETERANS

Findings will be similarly reported from a single study examining symptoms in PGW veterans. Findings from other studies evaluating symptoms are qualitatively similar. "SSID," or "signs, symptoms and ill-defined conditions," constituted the primary diagnosis for 17.2 percent of the veterans, and the primary or secondary diagnosis for 41.8 percent.

Although the authors state that "more definitive, often psychological, diagnoses can be made by increasing the intensity of the evaluation and by multidisciplinary input," no evidence was provided that psychological diagnoses would be made on intensive scrutiny at a higher rate than in non-PGW personnel, or in personnel without symptoms (or perhaps those for whom symptoms were falsely "assigned," to deal with the possibility that diagnoses may be given precisely because of illness reporting).

Table 5.1

Most Frequent Principal Diagnoses in PGW Registry Personnel
February 1997 (N = 74,653)

Symptom	Frequency (%)
No diagnosis	22.8
Missing diagnosis	5.1
Pain in joints	4.0
Person with feared complaint in whom no diagnosis was made	2.7
Psychalgia	2.0
Other specified adjustment reaction	1.9
Depressive disorder, not elsewhere classified	1.8
Contact dermatitis and other eczema, unspecified cause	1.6
Asthma, unspecified	1.6
Lumbago	1.6
Essential hypertension	1.5
Migraine	1.5
Malaise and fatigue	1.4
Allergic rhinitis, cause unspecified	1.3
Unspecified sinusitis (chronic)	1.3
Other and unspecified noninfectious gastroenteritis and colitis	1.3
Osteoarthritis, unspecified	1.1
Sleep disturbance	1.0
Irritable colon	0.9
Alopecia	0.9
Anxiety states	0.8
Headache	0.7

COMMENT ON HEADACHE

Of the approximately 10 percent of all subjects who had a primary diagnosis of headache, 35 percent were regarded as migraine (classified as neurological), 38 percent as tension (classified as psychological), and 27 percent as ill-defined SSID (Roy, Koslowe, et al., 1998). To further convey the element of arbitrariness in these designations, there was wide variation in diagnosis by region with migraine representing from 23 percent to 50 percent of all veterans; tension, 19 percent to 48 percent; and ill defined, 4 percent to 41 percent (Roy, Koslowe, et al., 1998). Table 5.2 lists the symptoms in order of prevalence.

In those with a primary diagnosis of good health, prevalences were as shown in Table 5.3.

Table 5.2
Symptom Prevalence as Primary and Any Diagnosis

Symptom	Primary Diagnosis (%)	Any Diagnosis (%)
Fatigue	26.8	30.3
Headache	14.5	21.3
Sleep disorders	11.7	19.0
Memory loss	9.9	16.9
Sleep apnea	7.4	5.5
Rash	3.8	5.7
Dyspnea	4.7	8.0
Chest pain	2.4	3.9
Digestive	1.8	2.6

SOURCE: Roy, Koslowe, et al., 1998.

Table 5.3

**Symptom Prevalence in Those with a
Primary Diagnosis of Good Health**

Symptom	Percentage
Fatigue	20.7
Joint pain	20.1
Headache	12.5
Sleep disturbance	11.2
Memory loss	14.7
Problems concentrating	9.2
Rash	10.9
Depressed mood	7.1
Muscle pain	6.7
Diarrhea	6.7
Hair loss	5.9
Dyspnea	4.9
Abdominal pain	5.3
Bleeding gums	3.6

SOURCE: Roy, Koslowe, et al., 1998.

Symptoms for those given a diagnosis other than SSID (Table 5.4) and those diagnosed with SSID (Table 5.5) are qualitatively similar, and roughly similar in ordering, to those of other reports on symptoms in ill PGW veterans. Results from other studies will not be reviewed here.

Table 5.4

Symptom Prevalence in Those Given a Diagnosis Other Than SSID

Symptom	Percentage
Fatigue	47.1
Joint pain	55.7
Headache	41.7
Sleep disturbance	34.6
Memory loss	35.6
Problems concentrating	27.9
Rash	32.2
Depressed mood	24.0
Muscle pain	23.7
Dyspnea	20.7
Diarrhea	19.2
Abdominal pain	17.9
Hair loss	13.2
Bleeding Gums	9.1
Weight loss	7.2

SOURCE: Roy, Koslowe, et al., 1998.

Table 5.5

Symptom Prevalence in Those Diagnosed with SSID

Symptom	Percentage
Fatigue	59.5
Joint pain	47.4
Headache	44.3
Sleep disturbance	41.0
Memory loss	40.6
Problems concentrating	31.1
Rash	29.8
Depressed mood	21.5
Muscle pain	21.5
Dyspnea	20.2
Diarrhea	18.0
Abdominal Pain	15.6
Hair loss	13.0
Bleeding gums	8.5

SOURCE: Roy, Koslowe, et al., 1998.

INCREASED SYMPTOM REPORTING IN PGW VETERANS

Many of the problems reported by ill PGW veterans occur also in the general population. It is desirable to know whether and to what degree PGW veterans experience higher rates of illness than those who did not serve in the PGW. Several studies have shown that those deployed to the Gulf have higher rates of self-reported physical symptoms compared to those who were not deployed (Centers for Disease Control and Prevention, 1995; Stretch, 1995; Iowa Persian Gulf Study Group, 1997; Canadian Department of National Defence, 1998; Fukuda, Nisenbaum, et al., 1998; Lange, Tiersky, et al., 1998a; Lange, Tiersky, et al., 1998b; Tiersky, Natelson, et al., 1998; Wolfe, Proctor, et al., 1998c). Symptoms commonly reported by deployed veterans include those that might be expected from the diagnoses above: fatigue, joint pain and stiffness, diarrhea, unrefreshing sleep or sleep difficulties, diarrhea and abdominal discomfort, weakness, cognitive symptoms including difficulty remembering, problems with word finding, or impaired concentration, headaches, and weakness. Some recent efforts have been made at devising case definitions. One researcher has articulated case definitions for each of three syndromes identified by factor analysis (Haley, 1997). Another, from the CDC, requires symptoms in two of three major categories of fatigue, musculoskeletal symptoms, and mood-cognition (Fukuda, Nisenbaum, et al., 1998). Others have used criteria involving chronic fatigue, fibromyalgia, or chemical sensitivity (Lange, Tiersky, et al., 1998a; Lange, Tiersky, et al., 1998b; Tiersky, Natelson, et al., 1998).

Regarding findings of increased symptom reporting, one study conducted by the CDC evaluated symptoms in an Air National Guard unit from Pennsylvania ("Unit A") and three comparison units from Pennsylvania and Florida chosen for similarity in mission responsibility (Centers for Disease Control and Prevention, 1995). A total of 3,927 personnel from four units participated in a survey with response rates from 36 percent to 78 percent. In all units, the prevalence of each of 13 chronic symptoms (lasting six months or more) was significantly greater among subjects deployed to the Gulf than among those not deployed. (The symptoms most frequently reported and considered "moderate" or "severe" included fatigue (61 percent), joint pain (51 percent), nasal or sinus congestion (51 percent), diarrhea (44 percent), joint stiffness (44 percent), unrefreshing sleep (42 percent), excessive gas (41 percent), difficulty remembering (41 percent), muscle pain (41 percent), headaches (39 percent), abdominal pain (36 percent), general weakness (34 percent), and impaired concentration (34 percent). The prevalence of five symptom categories—diarrhea, other GI complaints, difficulty remembering or concentrating, "trouble finding words," and fatigue—was significantly greater among those deployed from Unit

A than the other units. Both self-report and selective participation could have biased these results, however.

A second, more complete evaluation of the cohorts examined by the CDC entailed a cross-sectional survey of 3,273 currently active volunteers from four Air Force units (including 1,155 Gulf War veterans and 2,520 nondeployed personnel), together with a cross-sectional clinical evaluation of 158 PGW veterans from one unit, irrespective of health status (Fukuda, Nisenbaum, et al., 1998). A clinical case definition was determined, in which criteria were satisfied for a "case" if one or more chronic symptoms were present from at least two of three categories: fatigue, mood-cognition, and musculoskeletal symptoms. Severe cases were those in which there were "severe" symptoms from each category. A factor-derived case was defined as one in which the combined factor score was in the top 25 percent of questionnaires, including non-PGW veterans. Forty-five percent of PGW veterans and 15 percent of nondeployed personnel were symptom-category cases. Forty-seven percent of PGW veterans and 15 percent of nondeployed were factor score cases. This suggests that the authors selected the 25 percent cutoff to match the symptom-derived cases. The authors stated that the syndrome should be such that it embraces at least 25 percent of PGW veterans, but this is at once arbitrary and inappropriate; 25 percent of legionnaires or Four-Corners residents would obviously not need to be ill for Legionella pneumonia or hantavirus to have produced an illness syndrome in those groups. For symptom-derived cases, 39 percent of PGW veterans and 14 percent of nondeployed personnel met criteria for mild to moderate illness; while 6 percent versus 0.7 percent met criteria for severe illness. Illness was reportedly not associated with time or place of deployment or with duties during the war. There were no differences in lifetime report of medical illness of 35 medical and psychiatric conditions, including heart disease, hypertension, diabetes, alcohol and substance abuse, anorexia/bulimia, migraine or severe headache, anxiety, diarrhea, irritable bowel syndrome, or impotence. History of prior depression was significantly more common in severe cases (15 percent) than in noncases (0 percent; $p < .05$). Severe illness was associated with Gulf War service, female sex, enlisted rank, and smoking, on multivariate analysis. There was no association between illness and number of deployments, month/season of deployment, duration of deployment, military occupational specialty, direct participation in combat, or self-reported locality in the Gulf region (most were in Riyadh).

The Iowa Persian Gulf Study Group (1997) assessed the prevalence of self-reported symptoms in Iowa Gulf-deployed veterans and nondeployed personnel. From 238,968 persons, 4,886 were randomly selected from one of four groups: Gulf-deployed active-duty military, Gulf-deployed National Guard/Reserve, non-Gulf-deployed active-duty military, or non-Gulf-deployed

National Guard/Reserve. A total of 3,695 completed a telephone interview. Symptom reporting was higher for Gulf-deployed veterans for fibromyalgia (19.2 percent versus 9.6 percent), cognitive dysfunction (18.7 percent versus 7.6 percent), alcohol abuse (17.4 percent versus 12.6 percent), depression (17 percent versus 10.9 percent), asthma (7.2 percent versus 4.1 percent), anxiety (4.0 percent versus 1.8 percent), bronchitis (3.7 percent versus 0.8 percent), Post-traumatic Stress Disorder (PTSD) (1.9 percent versus 0.8 percent), sexual discomfort (1.5 percent versus 1.1 percent), and chronic fatigue (1.3 percent versus 0.3 percent).

Another group distributed 16,167 survey questionnaires of which 31 percent were returned; they reported that deployed veterans had significantly more of any of 23 physical health symptoms than nondeployed veterans, an effect not significantly altered by controlling for smoking and drinking, age, rank, education, marital status, and branch of military service (Stretch, Bliese, et al., 1996a; Stretch, Bliese, et al., 1995; Stretch, Bliese, et al., 1996b).

A study examining exposures and symptoms in Gulf War veterans from a Fort Devens ODS Reunion Survey did not include a nondeployed control group, but found that the five most commonly endorsed symptoms among the 2,119 who returned the survey (of 2,313 subjects surveyed), were aches/pains, lack of energy, headaches, insomnia, and feeling nervous/tense (Wolfe, Proctor, et al., 1998c). PTSD was associated with health symptoms, but those with combat exposure were not more likely to report increased health symptoms.

A health survey returned by 3,113 PGW-deployed (73 percent) and 3,439 non-deployed (60.3 percent of those solicited) Canadian Forces veterans, from 9,947 personnel to whom the survey was sent (all Canadian Gulf-deployed and a sample of those serving elsewhere during the Gulf War) found that Gulf-deployed veterans reported higher prevalences of symptoms of chronic fatigue, cognitive dysfunction, multiple chemical sensitivity, major depression, PTSD, anxiety, fibromyalgia, and respiratory diseases (bronchitis and asthma together) (Canadian Department of National Defence, 1998). They also reported higher numbers of children with birth defects (before, during, and after the PGW).

Because these studies are based on self-reported illness, it is possible that reporting bias and self-selection could have influenced results. Although the degree to which these factors may influence self-reported symptomatology is unknown, it can by no means be assumed that bias serves as the sole explanation for the higher rates of symptom reporting in those deployed to the Persian Gulf.

FACTORS ASSOCIATED WITH REGISTRY PARTICIPATION

Symptoms, then, appear more common in those deployed to the Gulf, although similar symptoms and illness may occur at lower rates in other military and civilian persons. Determination of what constitutes the cause or causes of illness may be helped by analysis of factors associated with illness development. Registry participation is not equivalent to illness. Many PGW veterans who have not participated in registries report health problems, and some who have participated in registries report no health problems. However, a rough relation between illness and registry participation is present. Table 5.6 shows predictors of registry participation and their associated odds ratios, from one study.

The degree to which predictors of registry participation predict illness as opposed to inclination to participate can only be determined by evaluating these predictors against more definitive criteria for illness. Indeed, others cite increased participation of reservists, who in one account represented nearly half of those reporting the problem, while making up only 17 percent of the troops serving there (Thompson, 1996). However, "the Pentagon attributes this discrepancy to the reluctance of active-duty soldiers to complain for fear of losing their jobs in a shrinking military, on the reservists' greater age and on the fact that the war disrupted their lives more severely than those of active-duty troops" (Thompson, 1996).

LIMITED EVIDENCE IS CONSISTENT WITH THE POSSIBILITY THAT PB, OR ADVERSE RESPONSE TO PB, MAY BE ASSOCIATED WITH ILLNESS

A definitive link between PB and illness in PGW veterans is not present. Two factors have complicated determination of such a link. First, outcome data have been poor; until recently, no case definitions for illness in PGW veterans

Table 5.6

Registry Participation Predictors

Factor	Odds Ratio
Stationed in PGW theater	2.2
Age: younger than 31/older than 22	2.1
Enlisted	2.0
Construction worker	1.3
Female	1.3
Hospitalized during 12 months prior to PGW	1.2
Army	4.7 (4.6–4.9)
National Guard	2.6 (2.5–2.6)

SOURCE: Gray, 1998.

had been devised. Second, data on exposure have been poor; no records were made and preserved of who received PB, to permit a more definitive association between PB and illness to be identified or excluded. Two lines of information are available that are consistent with the possibility of a link between PB and illness, although they are not definitive for a causal connection.

One study found that two of three syndromes, derived by factor analysis in a group of ill PGW veterans, were significantly associated with self-report of adverse response to PB during the PGW (Haley, 1997). This study is described in somewhat more detail in Chapter Seven, "Individual Differences in Reactions to PB." This finding might suggest that individuals with a combination of exposure and special susceptibility may have had increased risk of illness, although recall bias could contribute to the finding.

One recent report found that, among British servicemen (findings for men only were reported), service in the PGW was associated with increased risk of illness (using the CDC case definition for Gulf War Illness (Fukuda, Nisenbaum, et al., 1998)) more than could be accounted for by deployment to an unfamiliar hostile environment (based on comparison to Bosnia and nondeployed PGW-era cohorts): an odds ratio of 2.5 (2–2.8) (Unwin, 1999). Among PGW, Bosnia, and Era cohorts, 61.9 percent, 36.8 percent, and 36.4 percent met CDC PGW illness criteria, respectively, with 25.3 percent, 11.8 percent, and 12.2 percent meeting criteria for severe symptoms (Unwin, 1999). As seen in Table 5.7, various self-reported exposures were associated with illness in PGW veterans. In particular, self-report of PB exposure in British veterans was associated with increased odds ratios for CDC-defined PGW illness (Unwin, 1999). For Gulf War and Bosnia troops, the odds ratios associated with PB were comparatively high, constituting the highest odds ratios for the Bosnia-deployed; and for PGW troops, coming in an approximate tie to use of nuclear, biological, and chemical warfare protective suits (which could represent a proxy for PB use or heavy PB use, signifying perceived threat of imminent CW attack). Recall and reporting bias remain possibilities; and many other exposures were also apparently associated with likelihood of illness. The degree to which recall bias is likely to be responsible for the findings is, however, small: confirmation in official records of vaccination status was present for some veterans, and for these personnel the odds ratios of illness as a function of vaccination status were similar to those in the population overall, suggesting that illness status did not strongly influence recall of exposures.

In summary, many PGW veterans report health problems, and reporting of health problems occurs at a higher rate in PGW veterans compared to other deployed and nondeployed veterans. Moreover, self-reported exposures in the

Table 5.7
Odds Ratios for CDC-Defined Persian Gulf War Illness, in Veterans from the PGW,
Bosnia, or Gulf-Era Veterans Not Deployed to the Gulf

Factor	PGW	Bosnia	PGW Era (not deployed)
PB	2.6 (2.2–3.1)	3.4 (1.7–6.8)	1.9 (1.4–2.8)
Pesticides on clothes or bedding	1.9 (1.6–2.2)	1.7 (1.4–2.2)	1.9 (1.5–2.3)
Personal pesticides	2.2 (1.9–2.6)	1.8 (1.5–2.2)	1.8 (1.5–2.2)
Exhaust from heaters or generators	1.9 (1.6–2.2)	2.8 (2.1–3.7)	2.4 (1.9–2.8)
NBC suits (indicator of higher PB usage?)	2.7 (2.3–3.3)	2.7 (1.6–4.8)	2.3 (1.5–3.7)
Anthrax vax	1.5 (1.3–1.7)	1.5 (0.7–2.9)	NA
With records	1.4 (1.0–1.8)	2.6 (0.9–7.4)	NA
Any biological	1.5 (1.3–1.7)	1.5 (0.8–2.8)	NA
With records	1.4 (1.1–1.9)	2.5 (0.9–6.6)	NA
Yellow fever	1.3 (1.1–1.7)	1.0	NA
With records	1.4 (0.9–2.0)	0.8	NA
Tetanus	1.3 (1.1–1.5)	1.0	NA
With records	1.1 (0.8–1.4)	1.0	NA
Any routine	1.2 (1.1–1.4)	1.1 (0.9–1.3)	NA
With records	1.0 (0.7–1.3)	1.0 (0.7–1.3)	NA

PGW are associated with increased likelihood of illness, with PB showing a particularly strong odds ratio. The likelihood that this is the result of recall bias in ill veterans is reduced by information showing that for risk factors for which records are available for some (British) veterans, comparable odds ratios are seen.

Chapter Six

THEORIES LINKING PB TO ILLNESS IN PGW VETERANS

Several theories relate PB to illnesses in PGW veterans. Following a general discussion of these theories in this chapter, a chapter devoted to each theory will discuss the evidence in greater detail. The first three theories relate to how some individuals, or individuals in some conditions of the PGW, may have had increased susceptibility to effects of PB. The next four theories relate to how PB—perhaps enabled by heightened susceptibility in some individuals—could have produced chronic symptoms. One chapter discusses evidence relating to whether agents like PB could plausibly produce chronic effects, and a final chapter discusses other considerations or theories that have been examined in lesser detail. The descriptions of the theories and their presumed rationales in this chapter are not intended to reflect conclusions or balanced assessment of those theories after examination of the evidence. (See chapters corresponding to the respective theories for such assessment.)

BLOOD-BRAIN BARRIER PASSAGE: DOES PB CROSS THE BLOOD-BRAIN BARRIER DURING CONDITIONS OF STRESS?

PB is normally viewed as having minimum potential for CNS toxicity, due to its failure to cross the blood-brain barrier. However, recent evidence suggests this failure to cross the blood-brain barrier is vitiated under conditions of stress (Friedman, Kaufer, et al., 1996; Hanin, 1996) and possibly with administration of multiple chemicals. Therefore, central effects of PB may contribute to symptoms.

INDIVIDUAL DIFFERENCES IN RESPONSE TO PB: DO PHYSIOLOGIC DIFFERENCES INFLUENCE SUSCEPTIBILITY TO PB?

Genetic polymorphism or phenotypic differences in enzymes that may help to break down PB, as well as other individual differences in action of PB, influence its effect and toxicity. Examples of enzymes for which individual variations occur include butyrylcholinesterase (Gentry, Bitsko, et al., 1996; Loewenstein-

Lichtenstein, Schwarz et al., 1995; Lotti, 1995) and paraoxonase (Davies, Richter, et al., 1996). Symptoms occurring in some PGW veterans but not in others who experienced similar exposures may have resulted in part from these and other individual differences.

INTERACTIONS WITH OTHER EXPOSURES: DO INTERACTIONS BETWEEN PB AND OTHER EXPOSURES ENHANCE THE TOXICITY OF EFFECTS?

PB in interaction with pesticides and insect repellents (permethrin and DEET) may lead to synergistic nervous system toxicity (McCain, 1997; McCain, 1995a; Abou-Donia, 1996a, 1996b, 1996c), which may contribute to symptoms seen in PGW veterans. Interactions with other drug and chemical exposures may be germane, and a "toxic cocktail" of many exposures may possibly have contributed to illnesses in PGW veterans. A possible PB interaction with nicotine use in tobacco merits evaluation.

BROMISM: DOES ACCUMULATION OF THE BROMIDE FROM PB PRODUCE BROMISM?

Excessive use of PB may lead to symptoms of bromism from accumulation of bromide in the body. Bromide intoxication may cause various combinations of a host of neurological and psychiatric symptoms, including confusion, irritability, tremor, memory loss, concentration difficulties, incoordination, vision changes, and psychotic behavior. An acne-like eruption of the face and hands ("bromoderma"), or other rash may also occur. Some of these symptoms were seen in PGW veterans who received PB.

MULTIPLE CHEMICAL SENSITIVITY (MCS): DOES PB LEAD TO MCS?

PB, together with other chemical exposures, may contribute to the condition termed "multiple chemical sensitivity syndrome," or "toxicant-induced loss of tolerance" (Miller and Hitzel, 1995; Miller, 1996a, 1997; Miller, Ashford, et al., 1997). Some evidence suggests that symptoms in some PGW veterans are compatible with this "syndrome."

NEUROMUSCULAR JUNCTION EFFECTS: DOES PB PRODUCE NEUROMUSCULAR JUNCTIONCHANGES?

PB, as with other AChE inhibitors, may lead to motor endplate degradation (Gebbers, Lotscher, et al., 1986; Glickson, Achiron, et al., 1991). Changes can be detected in the signaling cell side ("presynaptic"), as well as at the side of the receiving muscle cell ("postsynaptic"). Gross changes in the muscle are seen under a microscope and with testing of synaptic function, and these changes may contribute to symptoms in PGW veterans.

NEUROTRANSMITTER DYSREGULATION: DOES PB ALTER REGULATION OF NEUROTRANSMITTERS, PARTICULARLY ACETYLCHOLINE?

Heightened ACh activity from PB use may lead to changes in regulation of the cholinergic system, such as "desensitization" of cholinergic receptors, reduced release of ACh, and other strategies of "adaptation" to high levels of ACh. Regulatory effects may persist after cessation of PB, producing subsequent symptoms of low ACh. Such symptoms might be expected to include fatigue, memory loss, and sleep difficulties—symptoms prominent in PGW veterans.

CHRONIC EFFECTS

It has been questioned whether PB, in conjunction with other AChE inhibitor exposures (Gordon, Inns, et al., 1983), could lead to delayed and/or chronic neuropsychiatric effects, perhaps through mechanisms described in other chapters. This chapter reviews the plausibility and evidence regarding long-term neuropsychiatric effects following PB and other AChE administration.

OTHER CONSIDERATIONS

An assortment of other topics possibly relating PB to symptoms and complaints in PGW veterans are briefly reviewed. These include

- Fertility

- Hormone effects (PB has been shown to lead to effects on growth hormone, thyroid-related hormone, and ACTH that vary by sex, age, circadian timing, presence of dementia, or cognitive, affective, or anxiety disorder (Giustina, Bresciani, et al., 1994; O'Keane, Abel, et al., 1994; Murialdo, Fonzi, et al., 1993; Llorente, Lizcano, et al., 1996; Lucey, Butcher, et al., 1993)

- Sleep (regulated by ACh and serotonin)

- Violent death (especially from unintentional injury)

- Teratogenicity (effects on fetal development) .

COMMENT ON PB DOSES

In subsequent chapters, when doses of PB are given in mg/kg, they will be translated to the corresponding number of PGW doses, calculated assuming a 30 mg dose was given to a 70 kg (154 lb) man, for 0.43 mg/kg. (This assumes that the equivalent mg/kg dose is the physiologically equivalent dose, which unfortunately need not be the case, as discussed below.) It is important to note that the mg per kilogram dose given to a 45 kg (100 pound) serviceperson (of which there were some)—is a full 54 percent higher (0.66 mg/kg). The same per kilogram dose will be a smaller multiple of the small-person-PGW dose: the stated number of PGW doses will overstate the small-person multiple by 54 percent (multiply by 0.43/0.66, or 0.65 to get the number of small-person PGW doses). (Although the stated number of PGW doses will understate the large-person PGW multiple, this is less relevant to concerns about amplified risk in some individuals.)

This correction may deviate from the "true" dose equivalent particularly when a mode of administration other than oral is used, resulting in a higher dose to the blood with than when PB is given orally. Because of widely different estimates of the multiplier, an adjustment for route of administration will not be calculated into the PGW dose. For a more accurate presentation, the stated PGW multiple may need to be further multiplied by a factor in the range of two to 30, and the reader is invited to bear this in mind. For instance, as stated earlier, PB manufacturer Roche Products, Ltd., has recommended that one-thirtieth of the oral dose should be used when giving PB intramuscularly or intravenously; whereas one study based on eight humans reported that an average of 16 percent of the oral dose was absorbed (16 percent ±4 percent, range 10–22 percent in that sample) (Moylan Jones, Parkes, et al., 1979), suggesting a multiplier of five or six.

Although some animal studies that find PB to be toxic use many times the PGW mg/kg dose, some animal studies on which efficacy of PB is based also do so. The dose of PB in animals that is "equivalent" to that in people cannot simply be determined by administering the same number of mg of PB per weight. Just as the same mg/kg dose leads to different levels of AChE inhibition from one person to another, so there are differences from one species to another in the amount of AChE inhibition conferred, on average, by a given mg/kg dose of PB. Since the "benefit" of PB is presumed to result from the AChE inhibition produced by PB, the percentage of AChE inhibition rather than the PB dose may be used to determine a "pharmacologically equivalent dose." In short, producing the same average percentage of AChE inhibition in a different species may require a different PB dose. (Unfortunately, what is pharmacologically equivalent for therapy may not be identical to what is pharmacologically equivalent for adverse effects, unless these effects are also predicted exclusively by AChE inhibition.)

As an example, in studies showing PB to be effective for soman pretreatment in primates, the "equivalent" dose has often been chosen to be the dose of PB that produces a degree of inhibition of AChE comparable to that sought in humans (e.g., approximately 30 percent), rather than the same mg/kg dose given to humans (1.2 mg/kg/day, for a "typical" person). The consequence is that higher doses of PB are administered per weight in monkeys compared to man— three times as high (Hayward, Wall, et al., 1990), 10 times as high (4.13 mg/kg PB intragastric single dose "to produce" blood ChE carbamylation of 30 percent, comparable to that expected with 30 mg/man) (Dirnhuber and French, 1978; Dirnhuber, French, et al., 1977), or even an individualized 21–50 times as high a mg/kg dose in monkeys (25–60 mg/kg/d (Dirnhuber, French, et al., 1977) versus 1.2 mg/kg/d in people) to achieve an AChE inhibition range of 20 percent to 50 percent, similar to the AChE inhibition range seen in humans on the designated pretreatment dose of 30 mg three times a day (Moylan-Jones, Parkes, et al., 1979, 1984).

Analogously, while the dose of atropine given to the "typical" human is 2 mg, a dose four times higher (on a per weight basis) of atropine is administered to primates to produce the "equivalent" dose in testing the protective effect of post-nerve-agent atropine, on the grounds that they are less "sensitive" to the effects of atropine. Much higher doses of atropine—e.g., 17 mg/kg—have been used in other animal models, such as guinea pigs (Gordon, Maidment, and Leadbeater, 1974).

Therefore, if higher doses per kg of PB are used in animals and considered pharmacologically equivalent when showing the benefits of PB (an assumption that is optimistic in extrapolating benefit to humans with lower doses), they should surely also be considered clinically equivalent in evaluating toxicity (the conservative and therefore prudent assumption which supposes that comparable AChE inhibition in primates—as reflected in a higher dose—is required to fairly show possible toxicity).

Chapter Seven

BLOOD-BRAIN BARRIER PASSAGE

DOES PB CROSS THE BLOOD-BRAIN BARRIER DURING CONDITIONS OF STRESS?

Pyridostigmine bromide is a carbamate AChE inhibitor with a positively charged "quaternary ammonium" group, which is believed to prevent its penetration through the "blood-brain barrier," a layer of cells that controls which substances may penetrate from the general circulation into the brain. Therefore, side effects of PB are typically those of heightened peripheral cholinergic activity (nicotinic and muscarinic). PB has been perceived as having an enhanced safety profile relative to such other carbamates as physostigmine, because of its relative disinclination to penetrate the blood-brain barrier. However, recent evidence suggests that PB can cross the blood-brain barrier under some circumstances, specifically in the context of stress or chemical combinations.

The ability of PB to cross the blood-brain barrier under circumstances of stress may render data on side effects of PB obtained during peacetime inadequate to predict effects that occur during war. Moreover, PB itself has been shown to enhance permeability of the blood-brain barrier, allowing penetration of normally excluded agents.

EVIDENCE

Published Research

In military reports dating at least to 1981, it was noted that the assumption of blood-brain barrier impermeability was not absolute (Kemp and Wetherell, 1981), that the blood-brain barrier was known not to be uniform even within individuals of the same species (Rapoport, 1976); and that evidence from animal studies suggests that PB can enter the midbrain, medulla, cerebellum, and cerebral cortex (Clement, 1977). Studies relating to PB penetration occurring in *specific conditions* of blood-brain barrier disruption (such as stress), and blood-brain barrier disruption resulting from PB administration are few and, to our knowledge, recent. Results of the several published studies abstracted will be reviewed in turn. The first shows evidence that PB crosses the blood-brain barrier in a stress protocol in mice. The second suggests that there may be increased central and reduced peripheral side effects of PB in humans under war stress as compared to peacetime, suggesting similar stress-induced crossing of the blood-brain barrier. The third shows that PB itself enhances penetration of the blood-brain barrier by a virus. A fourth shows that heat-stress markedly increases blood-brain barrier permeability, though permeability to PB was not tested per se. The fifth abstract shows that concomitant exposure to chemicals amplifies the effect of stress on enhancing permeability of the blood brain barrier.

Forced Swim Study in Mice

The first study found that "stress" in the form of a forced swim increased PB penetration of the blood-brain barrier in mice. Researchers found that PB did not penetrate the blood-brain barrier in mice under normal conditions. However, in a four-minute forced swim (shown previously to simulate stress), an increase in permeability of the blood-brain barrier to PB was seen (Friedman, Kaufer, et al., 1996). This was demonstrated by a reduction in the dose of PB needed to achieve 50 percent inhibition of brain acetylcholinesterase (AChE). The dose needed for 50 percent inhibition was reduced from 1.5 mg/kg (~3.5 times the PB dose a 70 kg PGW vet would have received) in the absence of "stress" to 0.01 mg/kg (two-hundredths of the 70 kg PGW veteran dose) in the presence of stress—more than a hundredfold difference. A tenfold increase in penetration through the blood-brain barrier of compounds ordinarily relatively excluded by the blood-brain barrier was seen with these low levels of PB in stressed animals.[1] More than a hundredfold increase in an indirect marker of brain neuronal activity[2] was seen in stressed animals. A comparable effect occurred with 0.01 mg/kg PB (two-hundredths of the PGW dose) in *stressed* animals as occurred with 2 mg/kg PB (five times the PGW dose) in *unstressed* animals (in both instances leading to 95 percent inhibition of AChE in the cortex of the brain) (Friedman, Kaufer, et al., 1996).

It appears likely that these effects were the result of PB obtaining access to the brain, since PB was found to influence brain function similarly when applied directly to slices of brain tissue: application of PB (1 mM) to hippocampal slices

---

[1]These compounds consisted of dye bound to albumin or of AChE plasmid DNA, including the cytomegalovirus promoter.

[2]This indirect marker of brain neuronal activity is brain c-fos mRNA determined by reverse transcription followed by polymerase chain reaction amplification.

reduced AChE activity within 30 minutes with similar efficacy to that observed in vivo at a dose of 2 mg/kg and induced a parallel hundredfold increase in brain levels of "c-fos oncogene" (the indirect marker of neuronal activity in the footnote 2). Moreover electrophysiological recording in slices of mouse brain showed increased stimulated neuronal activity in part of the mouse hippocampus (an area called "CA1") following PB application (Friedman, Kaufer, et al., 1996).

Central effects of PB (that is, brain effects) were relatively more prominent than peripheral effects in conditions of stress, as compared to the unstressed condition. Control mice injected with 0.1 mg/kg PB (0.23 times the PGW dose) showed inhibition of serum butyrylcholinesterase (BChE) activity similar to that measured in humans in peacetime (18.8±3.5 percent human; 20.4±5.5 percent in mice), with no inhibition of brain AChE. The same dose in stressed mice (restraint stress) appeared to produce a lesser inhibition of BChE—with relatively suppressed peripheral nervous system (PNS) effects and relatively enhanced central nervous system (CNS) effects.

The studies were performed in mice, and on small samples (three to 11 mice per group; n = 8 with PB and forced swim). Also, "p values" and confidence intervals were not provided (a common "omission," or difference in convention, in basic science literature). Nonetheless, the size of the effect precludes doubt regarding its importance in the animal model used. It remains to be determined what forms of "stress" produce such effects, to confirm that such an effect occurs in primates (and humans), and to determine what classes of agents normally excluded by the blood-brain barrier may gain access under conditions of stress.

Comparison of Human and Mouse Data

The second study compares human data during war and peace to data on stressed and unstressed mice. It found that human data in war (stress) and peace (nonstress) appear analogous to rodent data in forced swim (stress) versus none (nonstress); in both instances peripheral effects of PB appear to predominate in the unstressed case, while central effects become more pronounced in the presence of stress.

Friedman, Kaufer, et al. (1996) compared results from human studies on symptoms produced by PB in 35 healthy young volunteers during peace and on symptoms occurring during use of PB in 213 soldiers treated during the PGW. In peacetime volunteers, peripheral nervous system symptoms predominated. Symptoms included abdominal pain, diarrhea, frequent urination, increased salivation, rhinorrhea, and increased sweating, with an average of 18.8 percent complaining (range 5.5–38.9 percent). Only 8.3 percent (range 1–16.6 percent) of participants reported symptoms related to CNS function (headache, insomnia, drowsiness, nervousness, difficulties in focusing attention, impaired calculation ability). In treated Gulf War personnel, CNS symptoms predominated: 23.6 percent (range 6.2–53.4 percent) reported CNS symptoms, while only 11.4 percent (range 6.1–20.4 percent) reported PNS symptoms. Results were felt to be consistent with the differential effects of stressed and unstressed conditions on mouse BChE and AChE, noted above.

However, the humans compared in peace and in war derive from different databases and are not necessarily comparable. Moreover, treated Gulf War veterans' reactions, if they indeed result from PB (there was no placebo control group), might not reflect the effects of PB in war stress on others who did not present for treatment.

This study's findings could have implications for possible long-term consequences of PB or of stress. The enhanced capacity of systematically administered *plasmid DNA* to reach the brain under stress may explain the vulnerability of stressed animals to viral infections (see Study 3, below). The time-course for this vulnerability remains to be determined. *Transcriptional responses* observed in this study were postulated to predict induction of secondary and tertiary processes with uncertain consequences and time-courses—effects that could conceivably have a role in long-term effects of PB on symptoms (Friedman, Kaufer, et al., 1996). At present, however, all long-term effects remain speculative. (See Chapter Fourteen, "Chronic Effects.")

Effect of Cholinesterase Inhibition on the Blood-Brain Barrier

A third study on the effect of cholinesterase inhibition on the blood-brain barrier found that PB given to mice in subtoxic doses led to changes in the blood-brain barrier, allowing an infectious agent to gain entry to the brain and produce lethal CNS infection in a subset of animals not identifiably different from those not so affected.

A study conducted in Israel demonstrated that PB at doses of 0.4 mg/kg, about equal to one PGW PB dose (actually, 0.93 of a dose) and approximately a tenth of the LD_{50} (the LD_{50} is the dose lethal in 50 percent of animals), led to increased blood-brain barrier permeability in mice, as gauged by ability of a peripherally introduced nonneuroinvasive neurovirulent Sindbis virus strain (SVN) to cause CNS infection (Grauer, Ben Nathan, et al., 1996). (A strain that is "nonneuroinvasive is one that does not ordinarily invade the CNS. A "neurovirulent" strain may cause disease in the CNS once there.) Though a single oral dose in PGW veterans was 0.4 mg/kg, perhaps 7 percent of the oral dose is available as blood PB, so that the injected dose given to mice is in fact substantially larger than that given to humans, on a per-weight basis (see

Chapter Three). $0.1 \, LD_{50}$ of soman and physostigmine led to similar effects. CNS infection occurred six to eight days following inoculation in about 40 percent of mice in which $0.1 \, LD_{50}$ of PB had been introduced at the time of peak viremia (the peak of virus detectable in the blood, which occurred at about one day following inoculation) and in about approximately 20–40 percent of mice exposed to soman and physostigmine. High viral titers (levels of virus) were recorded in brain tissue of sick mice, with up to $5.2 \cdot 10^6$ PFU (plaque-forming units, a measure of the amount of virus) in sick mice as compared to no virus in mice that appeared healthy. Survival was 100 percent in mice exposed to PB or SVN alone but only about approximately 60 percent in those exposed to both. The differences were not due to changes in viral traits, e.g., neuroinvasiveness or neurovirulence, since no virus was observed when the virus isolated from brains of soman-treated mice was injected intraperitoneally to nontreated mice. Since there are cholinesterases located in the blood-brain barrier, the effect described was speculated to result from direct inhibition of the enzymes located in the capillary wall.

One could speculate whether a similar effect could underlie part of the observed increase in toxicity reported when PB is mixed with other agents, such as insecticides (see Chapter Nine, "Interactions Between PB and Other Exposures"). No virus was detected in the 60–70 percent of mice that appeared healthy following the same soman treatment. (See Chapter Eight, "Individual Differences in Reactions to PB.)

Effect of Heat on the Blood-Brain Barrier

Heat stress in rodents (exposure to 38° C for four hours, not out of range of possible experience in the PGW) has been shown to markedly increase blood-brain barrier permeability to tracers, including Evans Blue albumin and labeled sodium (Sharma, Nyberg, et al., 1992); PB was not a focus of that study. Another study, published as an abstract, found no increase in PB penetration with heat alone in guinea pigs (25° C, 39° C, or 43° C for two hours). This was interpreted as demonstrating that penetration of PB into the brain under stress depends on the experimental conditions used. Differences in animal species, duration of stress, and nature of stressor may be pertinent factors. Both heat stress and restraint stress had been shown to markedly increase blood-brain barrier permeability in rats and mice, respectively, although heat stress was maintained for four hours for the rats.

Effect of Chemicals and Heat on the Blood-Brain Barrier

Dr. Abou-Donia (Duke University) is currently conducting animal studies on effects of physical/emotional stress (restraint stress, involving placement of an animal in a Plexiglas restraint tube each morning after chemical treatment, if any), heat stress, and chemicals on the blood-brain barrier in animals. Combinations of PB (5 mg/kg/d orally, or 3.8 times the PGW dose) with high doses of other chemicals agents (DEET 500 mg/kg/d subcutaneous; permethrin, 500 mg/kg/d in oil, daily for 30 days) influence the blood-brain barrier such that PB can cross and produce central cholinesterase inhibition (inhibition that is region-specific), and charged (radioactively labeled) chemicals that ordinarily do not cross the blood-brain barrier may do so. Findings suggest that addition of restraint-stress increased the effect of chemicals alone on the blood-brain barrier (Abou-Donia, Abdel-Rahman, et al., 1997). The smallest effect occurs with stress followed by chemicals, the largest when stress and chemical exposures occur concomitantly (Abou-Donia, 1998). One investigator found in preliminary work that heat stress (exposure to 38°C for four hours prior to sacrifice) may produce effects on the blood-brain barrier similar to those produced by restraint stress in mice (Abou Donia, 1998).

An abstract by another group found that shorter heat exposures (two hours) in guinea pigs, even at higher temperatures, did not lead to detectable entry of intravenously injected radiolabeled PB into the CNS, as evaluated autoradiographically. However, exposure to 43° C did itself result in partial inhibition of brain AChE activity (Lallement, Foquin, et al., 1998). At present, no direct evidence supports or refutes the possibility that heat might increase blood-brain barrier penetrability in humans.

Blood-Brain Barrier Breaches

Blood-brain barrier permeability is increased in other settings that continue to be defined. For example, headache may actually produce neurogenic inflammation (through antidromic stimulation to the trigeminal-vascular junction leading to release of pro-inflammatory peptides); indeed, it is thought to be for this reason that the antimigraine drug sumatriptan is ineffective for mild headache, in which the drug cannot penetrate the CNS, but is effective for moderate or severe headache, in which neurogenic inflammation permits CNS access for sumatriptan (Rothrock, 1999).

OTHER RESEARCH

In one peer-reviewed study, intracranial placement of heat-killed BCG (bacillus Calmette-Guerin), which normally would not cross into the brain, followed by subsequent peripheral exposure to BCG (in the presence, however, of a powerful adjuvant), precipitated a demyelinating response in rats (Matyszak and Perry, 1995). This is a case in which proximal events allowing substances entry to the CNS led to temporally distant responses.

Another peer-reviewed study demonstrated that aluminum levels in mouse brain increase following administration of aluminum adjuvanted vaccines (Redhead, Quinlan, et al., 1992). Moreover, the paper cites increasing evidence that aluminum ions can contribute to increased permeability of the blood-brain barrier, acting synergistically with iron ions.[3] Therefore, it is conceivable that aluminum-adjuvanted vaccines, such as the anthrax and botulinum toxoid vaccines administered to some military personnel during the PGW, could have increased blood-brain barrier permeability independently from—and perhaps in addition to—effects produced by PB, chemicals, heat, or stress. However, such effects remain to be demonstrated in humans, and it is unknown whether effects from these sources would be additive, synergistic, or neither.

DISCUSSION

Our understanding of the possible immediate and delayed consequences of the introduction to the brain of foreign substances normally excluded from the CNS is limited at best. Data are consistent with the possibility that some neuroactive substances, including PB, may gain access to the CNS through impaired blood-brain barrier function in conditions of heat (around 100° F), chemical combinations, and/or physical/emotional stress. The scope of definitions of "stress" that may produce leakiness in the blood-brain barrier continues to be characterized. It is not clear how many well and ill PGW veterans may have been exposed to comparable or "relevant" forms of stress. The doses of chemicals used in these experiments are extreme, and it is difficult to compare their stress protocols to experiences of PGW veterans.

It is also possible that breaches in the blood-brain barrier could lead to enhanced susceptibility to neurovirulent infectious agents or neurotoxic effects from concurrent chemical exposures. Therefore data on side effects from PB obtained without "stress," or sustained heat, or perhaps chemical combinations, may not adequately reflect effects that may occur in the presence of these factors. Consequently, it is possible that data on acute (and chronic) effects of PB obtained using PB alone, in peacetime conditions, may not adequately reflect effects that occur in an environment in which such factors as stress, heat, or chemical exposures are also present.

---

[3]Refer to *A Review of the Scientific Liturature As It Pertains to Gulf War Illnesses*, Vol. 3: *Immunizations* (Golomb, forthcoming), in the chapter relating to effects of aluminum in vaccines.

CONCLUSIONS

At present, evidence from animal studies suggests that disruption of the blood-brain barrier in situations of heat, chemical exposure, and physical/emotional stress, some of which may have been present in the PGW, may lead to central effects from drugs, chemicals, and infectious agents normally denied access to the CNS. The practical effect of this disruption in such conditions as those seen in the Gulf War is uncertain. Moreover, whether chronic or delayed consequences of these exposures may occur is a matter for further study.

SCIENTIFIC RECOMMENDATIONS

Further research should help provide the following information:

- The nature of the "stresses" and chemical combinations that disrupt the blood-brain barrier.

- The nature and duration of blood-brain barrier disruption following stress.

- The classes of normally excluded agents that gain access to the CNS with such blood-brain barrier disruption.

- The effects of stress using drugs and chemicals in doses and through administration routes more similar to those used by military personnel.

- A determination of whether such effects occur or continue with subacute or subchronic exposures similar to those expected in combat.

- What becomes of agents that cross the blood-brain barrier due to a leaky barrier after the barrier function has been restored; are such agents "trapped" in the CNS, and if so, what are the implications, if any?

SUMMARY ANALYSIS

Exposure: It is unknown whether PGW veterans would have been "exposed" to breaches in the blood brain barrier. Animal data indicate that some forms of stress, high-dose chemical combinations, heat, AChE inhibitors, and aluminum all may contribute to enhanced blood-brain barrier permeability. Different veterans would have experienced different combinations and different "doses" of these factors. Whether these would be adequate to significantly enhance blood-brain barrier permeability in some instances is not known.

Compatible symptoms: Increased symptoms compatible with central AChE inhibition were reported following PB administration during the PGW compared to peacetime. This is consistent with the existence of breaches in the blood-brain barrier.

Link between exposure and symptoms: There is no information to determine whether factors thought to promote breaches in the blood brain barrier were more likely to be present in individuals reporting central symptoms following exposure to PB.

Chapter Eight

INDIVIDUAL DIFFERENCES IN REACTIONS TO PB

DO PHYSIOLOGIC DIFFERENCES INFLUENCE SUSCEPTIBILITY TO PB?

This chapter addresses evidence about the existence of individual differences and the possible relation of individual differences to illnesses in PGW veterans. Differences have been demonstrated in side effects with PB administration, in chemical response to PB, and in the relation of chemical response to side effects. Some evidence suggests a connection between differences in response to PB and subsequent development of illnesses in PGW veterans. Possible sources of individual differences are discussed.

Individual differences in properties that may influence PB metabolism and effects have been identified (such as quantitative differences in BChE levels), and others are likely. The existence of individual differences in response to PB in the short term is illustrated by the wide variation in symptoms (symptom character and severity) reported in response to PB in the PGW. One study suggests a correlation between these short-term differences (gauged by self-report of adverse response to PB administered during the PGW) and symptom reporting in PGW veterans (Haley and Kurt, 1997), although this result remains to be confirmed and, if confirmed, to be understood. Differences in levels of such enzymes as BChE that are thought to scavenge PB have also been found and have been reported to correlate with symptoms (not confined to acute symptoms) following exposure to carbamates.

The potential for individual differences in response to an exposure to such carbamates as PB is great. Empirically, differences in response to PB are known to occur; and biological differences that may contribute to this individual variability are beginning to be understood (though current understanding remains limited). A great variety of classes of factors have been identified that have potential for contributing to individual differences. Whether individual differences in sensitivity to PB contribute meaningfully to differences in long-term clinical outcomes in PGW veterans remains to be determined. However, evidence can be cited that suggests a possible role for such differences, supporting the need for further scientific inquiry. Because of these factors, the same oral dose of PB may lead to different blood levels of PB and to different "therapeutic" and toxic effects.

CHEMICAL FINDINGS

Differences in the inhibition of AChE in response to PB are marked. First, absorption of PB may be affected by clinical differences in response to PB itself (see below). For instance, PB itself may increase gastrointestinal peristalsis, speeding transit of PB from the gut to the feces and limiting absorption of PB into the blood stream. This process may occur at different rates in different individuals because of the variability in effect of PB (discussed below)—a variability which this effect will amplify. Second, once PB is absorbed, there may be differences in rates of clearance from the bloodstream due in part to differences in enzymes (different types and different amounts) that assist in clearance of PB. This may help account for the approximately threefold differences in plasma PB levels measured at comparable times after a single 30 mg dose of PB—values of about 10 ng/ml to about 30 ng/ml at two hours after the dose (Parker, Barber, et al., 1986)—and even larger differences reported in other studies (see Chapter Three for more data).

Moreover, the same plasma level of PB may be associated with substantially different degrees of RBC AChE inhibition; the correlation in several studies has been rather low, with 2 percent inhibition associated with 14 ng/ml PB in one subject, compared to 24 percent AChE inhibition in another, despite a lower plasma level of 11 ng/ml (Parker, Barber, et al., 1986). Because of these various factors, the same oral dose of PB has been associated with quite different degrees of AChE inhibition—with AChE inhibition in one study ranging from 18 percent to 57 percent (Kolka, Burgoon, et al., 1991); and in another study of 19 subjects, ranging from 0 percent to 49 percent at two to three hours after a single 30 mg dose (Parker, Barber, et al., 1986). (For the three subjects measured at exactly two hours after dosing, the figures ranged from 2 percent to 49 percent inhibition. Plasma PB levels were not even monotonically related to RBC AChE inhibition among these three cases.) Presumably even larger ranges would be uncovered if larger populations were tested. (In the study cited, subjects with greater than 40 percent inhibition were excluded from further evaluation—including further use of the drug. In the PGW, personnel who may have had excessive AChE inhibition would not have had access to this information, because testing was not performed, and they would therefore not have been told to terminate or modify PB use.)

Moreover, in another study, the duration of effect in which AChE inhibition exceeded 20 percent ranged from 0.33 to 5.0 hours, a fifteenfold difference (Sidell, 1990). The range of individual differences might be seen to be even greater if larger samples were tested. (Quite large standard deviations were seen in some subgroups in a larger study of 90 volunteers who took PB (Lasseter and Garg, 1996).) These differences may be in part the consequence of differences in absorption leading to different blood levels of PB and may in part relate to differences in sensitivity of AChE to PB, because the correlation between PB and AChE inhibition has been as low as –0.61 (signifying that only about 37 percent of the variance in AChE inhibition is accounted for by the blood level of PB) and because marked individual differences were not highly correlated with weight, height, or body surface area (Kolka, Burgoon, et al., 1991; Lasseter and Garg, 1996). Moreover, differences may arise from different AChE levels on RBCs or even different RBC counts. Differences in the rate of elimination of absorbed PB may also play a role (Sidell, 1990). (These differences are also described in Chapter Three, "Characteristics of PB.") Another potential issue is that of accurate measurement of AChE inhibition, potentially producing erroneous results—perhaps accentuating apparent variability.

CLINICAL FINDINGS

Differences in *acute* response to PB are reflected in differences in side effect profiles noted at the same dose of PB. Different subjects develop different side effects with the same dose of PB, and many develop no side effects. The side effects of PB are reviewed in Chapter Three, "Characteristics of PB." Baseline differences in personality predicted side effects in response to the related chemical physostigmine (Janowsky, 1997). Since "personality" is substantially influenced by neurochemistry, this is consistent with the possibility that baseline neurochemical profile may in part determine acute effects.

RELATIONAL FINDINGS

There are differences in clinical symptoms in response to PB and differences in AChE inhibition in response to PB. Differences in AChE inhibition might be presumed to directly produce the differences in clinical symptoms. However, differences in AChE inhibition do not explain the differences in clinical effect, although they may participate in the production of these differences. Cholinergic side effects from PB do not correlate well with AChE inhibition. For instance, in one clinical report of nine PGW veterans who attempted to overdose on PB, consuming 390 to 900 mg of PB (13 to 30 tablets), no relation was found between AChE inhibition and cholinergic symptoms (Almog,

Winkler, et al., 1991). This clinical report suggests that variation in factors other than AChE inhibition play a role in the effects of PB. These variable factors remain to be fully elucidated (although potentially contributory factors, such as individual susceptibility to psychological stress and disruption of the blood-brain barrier, are discussed elsewhere). It should be remembered that PB participates in numerous effects distinct from AChE inhibition: For example, PB acts as an ACh "partial agonist," binding to the site on AChE to which serotonin normally binds; PB influences other neurotransmitter systems, such as the GABA and glutamate systems; PB participates in "autoregulation" of ACh release from the nerve terminals; and PB enhances the desensitization of ACh receptors. (See Chapter Three, "Characteristics of PB.") Individual differences in these additional effects have not been explored, but they could further explain the differences in symptoms in persons with comparable levels of AChE inhibition.

INDIVIDUAL DIFFERENCES IN BASELINE CHOLINERGIC STATUS

Substantial evidence supports the existence of baseline differences in acetyl-cholinergic "status" and responsiveness, which could influence response to PB. The imaged brains of some individuals demonstrate increases in choline, the rate-limiting factor in ACh synthesis (Janowsky and Overstreet, 1995). More-over, some individuals show heightened behavioral effects (for instance, depression, which commonly occurs acutely after being given AChE inhibitors, or other ACh-promoting agents (Tammings, Smith, et al., 1976)) in response to ACh "agonists" (agents that promote the action of the ACh system) (Janowsky and Overstreet, 1995). Perhaps not surprisingly, ACh stimulated depressive effects occur more readily and more commonly in persons with depression (75 percent)—who have been shown to have cholinergic (muscarinic) "supersensitivity" in many studies (Risch, Janowski, et al., 1981; Sitaram, Nurnberger, et al., 1982; Risch, Kalin, et al., 1983; Janowsky and Risch, 1984; Sitaram, Jones, et al., 1985; Sitaram, Jones, et al., 1987; O'Keane, O'Flynn, et al., 1992; Steinberg, Weston, et al., 1993). However, they also occur in many normal individuals (25 percent) (Risch, Cohen, et al., 1981; Janowsky and Overstreet, 1995). Exemplifying the increased effect of cholinergic agents in groups with baseline cholinergic supersensitivity, administration of the PB-like agent physostigmine led to increased changes in rater-evaluated "behavioral inhibition" and in self-rated anxiety, depression, hostility, and confusion in patients with mood disorders—the class of patients shown to more commonly have the cholinergic supersensitivity—compared to other psychiatric groups or normals (Janowsky, Risch, et al., 1980; Janowsky, Risch, et al., 1981).

"Altered" responsiveness of the ACh system is common not only with depression but in association with many other conditions. For instance, the surge in growth hormone that occurs following delivery of PB or physostigmine is more marked than in normals not only in those with mood disturbances but in people with high cortisol levels, either naturally or through drugs; Alzheimer's patients, those with obsessive-compulsive disorder or panic disorder, and schizophrenics; and age may also influence the responsiveness (Raskind, Peskind, et al., 1989; Corsello, Tofani, et al., 1991; Rapaport, Risch, et al. 1991; O'Keane and Dinan, 1992; O'Keane, O'Flynn, et al., 1992; Borges, Castro, et al., 1993; Ghigo, Nicolosi, et al., 1993; Lucey, Butcher, et al., 1993; O'Keane, Abel, et al., 1994; Thakore and Dinan, 1995).   Thus, many lines of evidence confirm strongly that the effects of AChE-inhibiting agents (or ACh-stimulating agents) may relate in part to the underlying state of the ACh system, which has been shown to be highly variable.   Although this may in part reflect genetic differences (Janowsky, Overstreet, et al., 1994), it is also possible that past exposures to chemicals that affect the ACh system may play a role (see Chapter Thirteen, "Neurotransmitter Dysregulation").   Chronic effects of PB, if PB gains central access, may be more likely in those whose ACh sensitivity is high to begin with. This would be compatible with the report that those with self-reported acute response to PB are more likely to have developed chronic symptoms.   (It may be only in these individuals that the heightened ACh action was sufficiently "out of range" of normal to induce alterations in regulation or that those individuals reflect a susceptible subset in some other way.)

INDIVIDUAL DIFFERENCES AND ILLNESSES IN PGW VETERANS

Haley, Kurt, and Hom (1997) examined a set of ill PGW veterans and conducted a factor analysis in which six clinical "syndromes" (three they view as predominant) were identified in ill persons who served in the PGW. Two of the three main syndromes, termed by the authors "confusion ataxia" and "arthro-myo-neuropathy," were significantly associated with self-report of adverse response to PB at the time of PB administration during the PGW. (These syndromes were derived by Haley et al. using factor analysis, and the symptoms included—as the labels suggest—confusion and gait disturbance in the former case, and joint/muscle/nerve pain in the latter.) The "exposure" here is not use of PB but adverse experience associated with use of PB. These findings suggest that individual differences in tolerance may be linked to long-term adverse consequences. These could, for instance, reflect individual differences: in PB absorption, metabolism, or action; in cholinergic regulation; or in concomitant exposures that influence the effect of PB.

Limitations

There are several limitations to the analysis by Haley, Kurt, and Hom (1997). First, factor analysis has the potential to create "syndromes" or factors that may not be reproduced when a new sample is examined. Second, Haley's sample was small, exacerbating the potential to produce irreproducible factors. Third, determination of adverse response to PB was made by self-report and thus may be subject to recall bias (Lees-Haley and Brown, 1992). Recall bias has the potential to produce the spurious appearance of a relationship between an exposure and an adverse outcome due to the selective recollection of the exposure in an affected group.

Regarding the first limitation, there is a strong need to determine factors using one sample and to validate them with another (cross validation). (This process is rendered more difficult by the small sample size.) Moreover, other methods for identifying natural groupings of data (in this case "syndromes" or symptom complexes) can also be employed, such as unsupervised neural networks (Bishop, 1995), and it would be instructive to see whether these alternative methods would replicate the findings of Haley's factor analysis on the same and on new databases of ill PGW veterans. If individuals identified as having one factor-analyzed "syndrome" are found to share common objective neurological findings, particularly findings that distinguish them from those with other factor analysis–derived syndromes, it may enhance confidence in the legitimacy of the syndromes. Such work is currently being done using sensitive neurological tests (Haley, 1998).

Because records of who received PB in the theater were not made and maintained, self-report is the best method available for determining exposure to PB (and to many other putative exposures) in PGW veterans. Moreover, while recall bias might influence recall of exposure in persons with and without illness (Lees-Haley and Brown, 1992), there is no compelling reason to suppose that recall bias would result in differential recall of exposures for persons with one symptom complex compared to another (though such differential recall cannot be excluded). Therefore, if the differential association between these syndromes and exposures were replicated in another sample, it might favor a true association. Moreover, a study in PGW veterans (discussed in Chapter Fourteen, "Chronic Effects") does not support a connection between symptom reporting and an overall exposure index (in which PB is not included) in PGW veterans (Sillanpaa, Agar, et al., 1997), suggesting that biased recall of exposures may not be prominent.

SOURCES OF INDIVIDUAL DIFFERENCES IN RESPONSE TO PB

If experiencing an adverse, acute response to PB is indeed associated with subjects' likelihood of developing subsequent illnesses, it remains to be determined which factors contribute to individual susceptibility. Differences in susceptibility to longer-term consequences of PB (if longer-term consequences exist) could occur in the absence of differences in acute symptoms, if different mechanisms are at play. Similarly, as will be shown in the case of bromism (Chapter Ten), persons who apparently develop chronic sequelae of bromide intoxication could not be predicted on the basis of initial blood levels of bromide or on the basis of acute symptoms.

Several sources for differences in response to PB have been, or could be considered. Butyrylcholinesterase (BChE) *polymorphism* (differences in structure of the chemical BChE) has been particularly emphasized as a source of possible individual differences, though the numbers of persons who are either homozygous (< 1 percent) or heterozygous (< 5 percent) for the "atypical" variety of BChE—the variety that has been looked at in this context—are probably too small to account for the numbers of ill veterans. These may constitute 5 to 20 percent of PGW veterans, employing very crude estimates derived from numbers of registry participants with unexplained illness (lower number) and all registry participants assuming additionally some unregistered ill persons (higher number); both figures potentially omit some ill PGW veterans and may include veterans with illness unrelated to PGW service. Other sources of individual differences include other polymorphisms, such as the far more common K-variant (~20 percent of the population); quantitative (rather than qualitative) differences in BChE (that is, differences in amount rather than type of BChE); differences in other "esterases" (enzymes that participate in breakdown of ACh and AChE inhibitors); native differences in cholinergic responsiveness; differential hormonal effects; and differences induced by concurrent, antecedent, or subsequent exposures. Other chapters (such as "Characteristics of PB," "Chronic Effects," and "Interactions Between PB and Other Exposures") make reference to additional sources of individual differences.

The possible contribution of several of these sources of individual differences are discussed here—particularly the contribution of enzyme polymorphism and of differences in enzyme levels. Because there is a moderate amount of literature regarding BChE polymorphism and the effect of PB, a moderate amount of text will be devoted to BChE polymorphism, though it will be concluded that the most commonly discussed polymorphism—relating to the "atypical" BChE—is unlikely to play a major role in explaining selective susceptibility to illnesses in PGW veterans. Quantitative differences in levels of enzymes, and perhaps other polymorphisms of BChE, or polymorphisms related to other enzymes, may play a more important role.

BChE Polymorphism

Terminology. BChE "polymorphism" refers to the presence of different forms of the chemical BChE in different individuals, resulting from genetic differences in coding for BChE. To understand polymorphism more fully, it is helpful to distinguish between "genotype" and "phenotype" and to understand the difference between "homozygotes" and "heterozygotes. The "genotype" is determined by which genes are present in an individual to code for the enzyme. There is a most-common form of the gene, termed "U" or "usual" and less-common forms of the gene, one of which is termed "A" or "atypical." Because people have two copies of each gene, that is two "alleles" (one from each parent), the genes may both be the same, or they may be different. A "homozygote" is a person for whom the genes encoding the enzyme, one gene obtained from mother and one from the father, are the same. Thus, a homozygous "usual" person would be designated as "UU." Persons who are homozygous for the atypical allele ("AA") are quite rare. A "heterozygote" is a person for whom the genes coding the enzyme, obtained from the mother and father, differ; thus, a person carrying a U allele from one parent and an A (or other) allele from the other parent would be a "heterozygote." The "genotype" for BChE refers to which genes a person has to encode the enzyme. In some instances, different "genotypes" may nonetheless result in the same "phenotype," or appearance and amount of the chemical—because some DNA mutations do not affect which amino acids make up the enzyme. In other instances, individuals with the same "genotype" may nonetheless have differences in expression or "phenotype"—most commonly in the amount of the enzyme (presumably due to environmental or other genetic factors), though generally the form of the enzyme will be the same.

BChE. BChE is also called pseudocholinesterase or plasma cholinesterase, as opposed to acetylcholinesterase (AChE), also called red blood cell cholinesterase, or true cholinesterase. BChE is a plasma enzyme thought by some to be involved in the scavenging of—and removal of—PB (among other chemicals) from the circulation (Schwarz, Glick, et al., 1995; Soreq, 1995), and more generally in protecting AChE at brain synapses and neuromuscular junctions from anticholinesterases (Schwarz, Glick, et al., 1995).

It has been suggested that pralidoxime (2-PAM), used in the treatment of nerve agent poisoning after exposure, may act by regenerating BChE and allowing it to react with more of the organophosphate (OP) nerve agent before the OP has a chance to inactivate neuromuscular AChE; this reaction effectively turns BChE into an organophosphatease (or agent that metabolizes OPs) (Schwarz, Glick, et al., 1995). Because of BChE's ability to scavenge PB and assist in its elimination, BChE polymorphism has been postulated to be involved in the large differences in PB dose required by patients with myasthenia gravis

(Schwarz, Glick, et al., 1995)—although Chapter Three shows evidence that differences in absorption of PB play a major role. In a report of one PB-exposed soldier, although BChE has less affinity for PB than does true AChE, differences in BChE appeared to lead to differences in the clinical effect of PB (that is, to cholinergic toxicity) (Loewenstein-Lichtenstein, Schwarz, et al., 1995).

BChE Polymorphism: Qualitative Differences in BChE. "Atypical BChE," produced by several alternative genetic mutations, has been the focus of some interest following the PGW. BChE (an enzyme) is a protein and as such consists of a chain of amino acids. Atypical BChE has a substitution of the amino acid "aspartate" (D) at position 70 in the chain of amino acids that comprises the BChE protein, by the amino acid "glycine" (G). The result is termed D70G. This enzyme is much less sensitive than the normal enzyme to several inhibitors, particularly to positively charged compounds such as PB (Gentry, Bitsko, et al., 1996). "Atypical" BChE has received more attention than have other genetic polymorphisms of BChE (Loewenstein-Lichtenstein, Schwarz, et al., 1995; Leon-S, Pradilla, and Vezga, 1996).

Altogether, since the gene was cloned, 22 different mutations have been identified in the coding region of the human BChE gene (Soreq, Ehrlich, et al., 1994). Some produce mutations that do not influence the amino acid sequence or the BChE effect. "Nonexpressing" BChE mutations—in which no BChE is produced—occur rarely (Taylor and Brown, 1994). Still other mutations alter amino acids and produce phenotypic changes in the resultant enzyme, in some cases producing BChE that is incapable of metabolizing ("hydrolyzing") the muscle relaxant succinylcholine, so that patients may develop failure to breath ("apnea") when given succinylcholine during anesthesia (e.g., Loewenstein-Lichtenstein, Schwarz, et al., 1995).

Estimates of BChE Variants in the Population. It has been estimated that approximately 96 percent of the population has the normal genotype (UU, or homozygous "usual") and that four to five percent are heterozygous for the atypical form (UA) (Gentry, Bitsko, et al., 1996). This information suggests that approximately 0.2–0.25 percent are homozygous atypical (AA). Other reports cite a rate of 0.04 percent homozygous carriers in Europe overall, but cite rates of up to 0.6 percent in certain subpopulations (Loewenstein-Lichtenstein, Schwarz, et al., 1995). In fact, however, recent research suggests that a much more common variant, the "K" variant, occurs in about 20 percent of the population and is, like atypical BChE, associated with decreased BChE activity (Jenson, Nielsen, et al., 1996; Lehmann, Johnston, et al., 1997; Russ, Powell, et al., 1998). No efforts have been made to examine the frequency of the K-variant in ill Gulf War veterans.

Effect of Atypical BChE. Differences in BChE associated with different genotypes not only are structural, but also affect persons' response to certain chemicals. The clinical effects of homozygous atypical BChE include postanesthesia
apnea (for instance, induced by succinylcholine), hypersensitivity to the anticholinesterase insecticide parathion, and reportedly severe effects with administration of PB in one soldier (Loewenstein-Lichtenstein, Schwarz, et al., 1995).
Here, differences in hydrolysis of certain chemicals with the atypical as
compared to the typical form are shown. These chemicals include the test
chemical butyrylthiocholine, PB and carbamates, and the drug tacrine.[1]

Biochemical effects of atypical BChE (whether native or "recombinant") include
low rates of hydrolysis of the test chemical butyrylthiocholine.[2]

Atypical BChE, in those homozygous for the atypical form, has been found to
react much more slowly with PB and other carbamates (based on differences in
the rate of inactivation of PB); heterozygotes demonstrated intermediate rates
of reaction (Loewenstein-Lichtenstein, Schwarz, et al., 1995), between those of
homozygous usual and homozygous atypical individuals. It has been suggested
that cholinergic symptoms in patients receiving treatment with tacrine may
occur in up to 15 percent due to BChE heterozygotes and to patients with liver
abnormalities who consequently have low BChE levels (Loewenstein-
Lichtenstein, Schwarz, et al., 1995). While a recommended dose of PB (for
myasthenia gravis, for example) may be 90 percent hydrolyzed by "wild-type"
(UU) BChE in the blood, the same dose may not be appreciably hydrolyzed by
homozygous atypical BChE. This difference could result in higher levels of PB
in the circulation and hence to increased likelihood of symptoms from PB, or
increased likelihood of PB "overdose" (Gentry, Bitsko, et al., 1996). Thus, BChE
may have an important role in elimination of PB from the circulation, and differences in BChE genotype and phenotype could lead to substantial differences

---

[1]Atypical BChE had one two hundredth the affinity for tacrine. (Tacrine is a reversible
cholinesterase inhibitor used to improve cognitive function in Alzheimer's disease.) Heterozygotes
showed intermediate inhibition curves with tacrine (Loewenstein-Lichtenstein, Schwarz, et al.,
1995). A two orders of magnitude increase was found in the 50 percent inhibitory concentration
(IC50) for tacrine with atypical BChE—that is, in the amount of tacrine required to inhibit 50 percent of BChE. The concentration of cholinesterase in the blood is approximately 50 nM; 75 percent
is due to soluble BChE and 25 percent to RBC AChE ("true" cholinesterase); plasma tacrine levels
are 21 nM in patients under treatment. Dissociation constants of 40 nM for normal BChE and 8000
nM for atypical BChE, calculated from this study (Loewenstein-Lichtenstein, Schwarz, et al., 1995),
suggest that while 40 percent of tacrine is bound to BChE in persons with the normal allele, only 1
percent is bound in atypical homozygotes (Loewenstein-Lichtenstein, Schwarz, et al., 1995).

[2]The rate of hydrolysis of butyrylthiocholine in those with the homozygous atypical BChE was
approximately one-third the "normal" rate found by averaging the results for 20 normal individuals.
(This rate was 81 ± 23 nmol/hour/microliter serum, assayed at 2 mM substrate.) Heterozygotes
(average of three cases) had activity approximately 60 to 70 percent of normal (intermediate
between homozygous atypical and homozygous normal) (Loewenstein-Lichtenstein, Schwarz, et
al., 1995).

in PB concentrations in the blood. See Table 8.1 for different effects of usual and atypical BChE on PB. As this table shows, the inactivation rate for PB is substantially lower with atypical BChE than with normal BChE—about a seventh; although both rates are considerably slower than inactivation rates with either RBC or brain-type AChE, clinical evidence suggests that BChE still plays an important role in PB inactivation.

Persian Gulf Veteran with Atypical BChE.[3]   A case report has described an Israeli soldier homozygous for "atypical" BChE who suffered severe symptoms following PB prophylaxis during the PGW (Loewenstein-Lichtenstein, Schwarz, et al., 1995) His symptoms included nausea, insomnia, weight loss, and fatigue, which worsened consistently with continued PB administration and were accompanied by a deep depression. These symptoms improved gradually over the weeks following discontinuation of PB (Loewenstein-Lichtenstein, Schwarz, et al., 1995). Serum BChE from the patient, as well as recombinant "atypical" BChE were far less sensitive than normal BChE to PB and several other carbamate cholinesterases. Heterozygotes for BChE were determined to have intermediate activity, as noted above.

Comparison of Atypical BChE in PGW Veterans Versus Controls. A comparison of rates of "atypical" versus usual BChE in (only) 20 PGW veterans enrolled in the Comprehensive Clinical Evaluation Program (CCEP) who had received PB, compared to 20 volunteer controls (of unstated origin) matched for sex and age (within five years) did not reveal differences in BChE phenotype between

Table 8.1

Effects of Different Esterases on PB Inactivation

	Normal BChE	Atypical BChE	Brain type AChE	RBC AChE
PB second-order inactivation rate constant (per M per minute times 1/1,000) PB: 10^{-5} M	1.4±0.5	0.2±0.3	22±9	25±7
Time-dependent reactivation (percentage original activity after 30 minutes), PB	9	8	32	24

SOURCE: Loewenstein-Lichtenstein, Schwarz, et al., 1995).

---

[3]The chemical "dibucaine" is used as a diagnostic tool to evaluate the presence of atypical BChE. Dibucaine inhibits BChE by 70–85 percent in homozygous normal individuals (approximately 96 percent of the population); by 50–65 percent in heterozygotes, (approximately 4 percent of the population); and by only 16–25 percent in those who are homozygous for atypical BChE (approximately 0.03 percent of the population). The atypical enzyme is also resistant to inhibition by carbamates at doses which inhibit the typical enzyme by about 35 percent in normal homozygotes (Sidell, 1990). Other strategies for evaluation of BChE phenotype are also used.

the two groups or in blood cholinesterase levels or spontaneous reactivation times for AChE after PB administration. Fourteen veterans recalled symptoms while taking PB; seven felt ill; six sought medical attention. Seventeen complained of chronic symptoms during the CCEP, including fatigue, rash, joint pain, memory problems, sleep disturbance, depressed mood, diarrhea, shortness of breath, headache, hair loss, difficulty concentrating, muscle pain and others (Gentry, Powell, et al., 1992; Gentry, Bitsko, et al., 1996).

Prior to this study, it was possible to surmise that the interaction of PB with atypical BChE would be unlikely to be responsible for illnesses in most ill PGW veterans because of the low frequency of the atypical BChE allele (~5 percent) and the high rate of reported illnesses in PGW veterans (perhaps 4–20 percent of all PGW veterans, or if all illnesses were in those who had received PB, then perhaps 14–70 percent of those). This study corroborates that prior knowledge, albeit in a small sample. To extend this knowledge, to determine whether a small (but still increased) fraction of ill veterans might have one or more atypical BChE allele, would require a larger study, perhaps confined to confirmed *ill* PGW veterans with self-reported exposure to PB versus healthy controls who also report PB use. (Only 17 of these 20 CCEP cases complained of chronic symptoms.) Additional subjects have been recruited for the study noted above.

It remains possible that *selected* instances of illness in PGW veterans are associated with atypical BChE genotype (heterozygous or homozygous). Moreover, it remains possible that substantial phenotypic variability in BChE activity within a genotype, specifically in regard to the amount of BChE, could influence susceptibility to effects of PB.

Other BChE Mutations. As mentioned previously, another relatively inefficient variant of BChE termed the K variant—with 30 percent reduced scavenging activity relative to the UU variant (Soreq, 1994; Bartels, Jensen, et al., 1992)—has been identified and shown to be common—e.g., 20 percent frequency—in some populations (Russ, Powell, et al., 1998). There is conflicting information regarding whether the presence of this variant contributes to risk of Alzheimer's disease. This variant has a higher prior probability of contributing to susceptibility to PB effects in PGW veterans, because of its higher prevalence in the population. But to date there is no information regarding the relative frequency of this gene in ill versus well veterans exposed to PB in the PGW; testing for this variant in Gulf War veterans has not been performed.

Other Putative Links Between BChE Variability and Illness. A syndrome termed "Intermediate Syndrome" has been described (Senanayake and Karielledde, 1987), which generally occurs 24–96 hours after exposure to OPs, and which may also be seen with carbamate intoxication (Leon-S, Pradilla, et al., 1996). It is characterized by cranial nerve palsies, neck and proximal limb weakness, and respiratory paralysis, and its frequency, mechanism, and long-term deleterious effects remain unknown (Leon-S, Pradilla, et al., 1996). It has been suggested, based on published reports from 1965 to 1995, that intermediate syndrome "and the like" occurred in "between 20 percent and 68 percent" of patients with insecticide intoxication (Leon-S, Pradilla, et al., 1996); and, moreover, that BChE activity was usually more depressed than AChE and that "the lower the BChE concentration (usually less than 10 percent of normal values), the stronger the possibility of developing the intermediate neurotoxic syndrome" (Leon-S, Pradilla, et al., 1996). Although the data have certain limitations (see below), differences in ability to metabolize carbamates and OPs (through variability in BChE, toxin interactions, and variability in other detoxifying enzymes) serve as a plausible factors that could influence why only some persons with apparently similar AChE-inhibitor exposure develop intermediate syndrome and others do not. (Of note: OPs are themselves believed to reduce BChE activity, so that cause and effect are difficult to sort out after the fact.)

Although PB is a carbamate, intermediate syndrome has not been reported with use of PB. In addition, it is not possible to distinguish whether low BChE was a cause or effect in this finding, presuming that the finding of depressed BChE in those with intermediate syndrome is valid (data were not given; the source was a non-peer-reviewed letter). Moreover, illnesses in PGW veterans do not strongly correspond in either time-course or symptomatology to intermediate syndrome, a finding that suggests against a role of BChE variability acting through intermediate syndrome as a cause of illnesses in PGW veterans. However, this does not preclude a role for BChE variability influencing the toxicity of PB, nerve agent, and pesticide exposures, individually or in combination, in PGW veterans.

Quantitative Differences in BChE. Although functionally important BChE polymorphisms (differences in form of BChE) have been presumed to be uncommon, based on data regarding "atypical BChE" without more-recent knowledge of the "K variant," differences in the quantity of BChE (BChE levels) are common (Loewenstein-Lichtenstein, Schwarz, et al., 1995). Because BChE may serve in a scavenger role, quantitative differences in BChE might result in differential susceptibility to cholinesterase inhibitors, including PB. BChE levels in serum of people homozygous for the "usual" BChE allele have been shown to vary with a standard deviation of 25 percent in the normal non-exposed population (Soreq, Ehrlich, et al., 1994; Altland, Goedde, et al., 1971). Decreased BChE levels have been attributed to burn injuries, and kidney or liver dysfunction, while increases have been seen in obesity, asthma, and alcoholism, suggesting variable sensitivity of individuals affected with these and other conditions to PB (or to OP poisoning) (Soreq, Ehrlich, et al., 1994).

Such variability may contribute to differences in results, and consequently to dispute regarding long-term neurological and psychiatric effects of OP poisoning in humans (Soreq, Ehrlich, et al., 1994). Some studies report abnormalities in memory, abstraction, mood, and motor reflexes (Savage, Keefe, et al., 1988), EMG changes (Grob and Harvey, 1953), paralysis (Drenth, Ensberg, et al., 1972), or chronic neuropsychiatric sequelae (Gershon and Shaw, 1961; Dille and Smith, 1964) in OP exposed individuals. There have also been reports of abnormal EEGs on long-term follow-up (Stoller, Krupinsky, et al., 1965; Metcalf and Holmes, 1969; Brown, 1971; Duffy, Burchfiel, et al., 1979), and of aggressive behavior following exposure to cholinesterase inhibitors in four individuals with no history of violence (Devinsky, Kernan, et al., 1992). Meanwhile, others have failed to observe defects in memory or language abilities (Rodnitzky, Levine, et al., 1975) or defects in more overt long-term psychiatric (Tabershaw and Cooper, 1966) and/or neurological (Clark, 1971) measures in man or experimental animals. Because the sample size is small in many of these studies, individual differences could play a role in generation of discrepant findings. However, other factors, such as study design and subject selection, most likely play a major role.

Atypical BChE Is Unlikely to Account for Illnesses in Persian Gulf Veterans. Other polymorphisms and quantitative differences in BChE activity have not been excluded as a participating factor. Homozygous BChE atypia is rare, occurring in less than 1 percent of the population. It has been said that heterozygous individuals "almost never" have a problem with PB or succinylcholine, as the amount of wild-type BChE in their plasma is "adequate" to handle the "standard" dose (Gentry, Bitsko, et al., 1996). Nonetheless, it is possible that this 4–5 percent of the population (homozygotes plus heterozygotes) could be at heightened risk for adverse effects from PB—and that, therefore, atypical BChE genotype, heterozygous or homozygous, could play a role in selected cases. The more common "K variant" of BChE that has reduced scavenging activity provide a more promising avenue for evaluation of genetic differences. Moreover, variation in BChE *levels* in persons with the "usual" phenotype have not been excluded as a source of differential susceptibility to PB or to illnesses in PGW veterans.

Other Esterases

AChE, which also interacts with esterase inhibitors such as PB (and indeed shows stronger affinity for PB) does not appear to be subject to mutations to the degree that BChE is. Records of phenotypically relevant variants in the AChE gene (that is, variants that actually affect the structure) are limited to a single point mutation (histidine 322 to asparagine 322). This change has been identified as the basis of the Yt[h] blood group, with an incidence of 5 percent in the "general Caucasian population" and a substantially higher incidence in Israel. However, the functional effects of this mutation have not been described (Soreq, Ehrlich, 1994).

Others esterases (enzymes, such as AChE and BChE, involved in breakdown of chemicals such as ACh and PB) also involved in detoxification, have been evaluated and found to have moderate to striking individual variability. Table 8.2 illustrates individual variability in esterases for several enzymes involved in OP toxicity in a group of Caucasian males aged 17–62. OPs, like PB, are AChE inhibitors. Some veterans report exposure to OP pesticides; moreover recent estimates based on plume modeling suggest that up to 100,000 veterans may have been exposed to very low levels of OP nerve agents (sarin) following demolition of the Iraqi munitions depot at Khamisiyah (Gulflink, 1997). (This may represent a substantial overestimate, because it is based on the union of several different modeling efforts in order not to understate possible effects.) Exposures to OPs may interact with PB exposure, producing synergistic toxicity. (See Chapter Nine, "Interactions Between PB and Other Exposures.") Not all listed enzymes play a role in PB binding detoxification. For example, paraoxonase does not (Furlong, Richter, et al., 1989), although it may influence levels of sarin and of pesticides, thus influencing synergistic toxicity of PB. (However, it is unlikely that personnel would have continued to receive PB at the time of the Khamisiyah demolition, so that synergistic toxicity with sarin from this event is unlikely.) Moreover, carbamates may play a frankly protective role for the enzyme neurotoxic esterase (NTE). Differences in paraoxonase and other enzymes are discussed below. There may exist qualitative or quantitative individual variation in other unlisted enzymes that influence the metabolism of PB or its interactants.

Paraoxonase and Other Enzymes. Paraoxonase (PON) is an HDL-cholesterol associated enzyme that contributes significantly to the metabolism of certain cholinesterase inhibitors; individual variability in this enzyme could contribute to differences in susceptibility to AChE-inhibitor combinations, such as PB with a nerve agent or with a pesticide. PON contributes to the metabolism of such nerve agents as sarin and soman, as well as insecticides. Parathion, chlorpyrifos, and Diazinon are bioactivated by "cytochrome P-450" systems in the liver to become potent cholinesterase inhibitors; the resulting toxic oxon forms can be hydrolyzed by PON1 (Davies, Richter, et al., 1996). Injecting PON protects against OP poisoning in rodent model systems (Li, Costa, et al., 1993; Costa et al., 1990), andinterspecies differences in PON activity correlate well with observed median lethal dose (LD_{50}) values (Costa et al., 1987), so that PON is believed to have a physiologically significant role in OP detoxification.

Table 8.2

Individual Variation in Esterases in Humans

Enzyme	Sample Size	Measure	Range	Median/ Mean	Deviation from Normality[a]
RBC AChE	127	Acetylthiocholine (nmol/mg Hb/min):	22.7–49.3 (2.2-fold)	36 (median)	$p > .05$
Cholinesterase	127	Benzoylcholine (nmol/ml/min)	659–1,628 (2.5-fold)	1,085 (median)	$p < .05$
NTE	113	Phenylvalerate (nmol/mg/min)	2.5–6.2 (6.0-fold)	7.0 (median)	$p < .001$
PON	127	Paraoxon (nmol/ml/min)	38–237 (6.2-fold)	116 (median)	$p > .05$
NaCl-stimulated PON	123	Paraoxon + 1 M NaCl (nmol/ml/min)	67–468 (7.0-fold)	176.4 (mean)	$p < .001$
Arylesterase	124	Phenylacetate (μmol/ml/min)	38–126 (3.3-fold)	1.41 (mean)	$p > .05$
PON:arylesterase ratio	123		0.8–2.2 (2.8-fold)	1.41 (mean)	$p > .05$
NaCl-stimulated PON:arylesterase ratio	123		0.9–4.4 (4.9-fold)	2.03 (mean)	$p < .001$

[a]$p < .05$ signifies a significant deviation from a normal or Gaussian distribution, using the Shapiro Wilks W test.
SOURCE: Adapted from Mutch, Blain, et al., 1992.

PON is polymorphic in human populations. Moreover, in addition to qualitative (amino acid structure) differences in PON, people express wide quantitative variation in this enzyme or in its activity (Davies, Richter, et al., 1996). While one isoform, the Arg_{192} (R_{192}) isoform, hydrolyzes paraoxon rapidly, the Gln_{192} (Q_{192}) isoform hydrolyzes paraoxon slowly. This difference suggests a greater protective effect for the former. However, this enhanced protection is chemical-specific: the enzyme isoforms hydrolyze some chemicals at approximately the same rate (such as chlorpyrifos-oxon and phenylacetate); the apparently less protective isoform (Gln_{192} or Q_{192} isoform) hydrolyzes nerve agents sarin and soman *more* rapidly, actually conferring greater protection against these nerve agents and reversing the perspective on which isoform is considered more protective (Davies, Richter, et al., 1996). This finding serves as a caution that persons relatively robust to one exposure may be relatively susceptible to another and that susceptibility to a specific agent does not imply an implicitly "weaker" or more vulnerable trait. Different populations have different frequencies of these isoforms, with Hispanic persons showing a frequency of 0.41 for the R_{192} allele and those of Northern European origin showing a 0.31 frequency (corresponding to around 16 percent versus 9 percent homozygotes, respectively) (Furlong, Richter, et al., 1989; Geldmacher-von

Mallinckrodt and Diepgen, 1988). The mean value for sarin hydrolysis for the R_{192} homozygotes was only 38 ± 47 U/l, compared to 355 U/l for the Q_{192} homozygotes (Davies, Richter, et al., 1996)[4] (see Table 8.3).

While average differences in detoxification ability between PON alleles are marked, actual ability to hydrolyze substrates varies substantially for persons with a given isoform, dictating the need to identify phenotype as well as genotype, by enzymatic analysis, to determine the level of risk (Davies, Richter, et al., 1996). (See Table 8.3 for mean values and range for different isoforms.) Of note, exposures to OPs themselves may result in reduced levels of PON (Dwyer, 1998), which may be important not only for detoxification but also because PON may determine whether HDL-cholesterol confers protection or harm for atherosclerosis. Thus it may be instructive to follow exposed veterans and controls for atherosclerotic development.

Polymorphisms that influence susceptibility to nerve agents and pesticides modify the effect of PB, potentially rendering it more toxic; and PB administration may enhance the neurotoxicity of the other agents, an effect that could interact with PON type and quantity. Thus far the influence of PON isoforms has been discussed, not in regard to PB but in relation to susceptibility to pesticide and nerve agent effects. In fact, there is no role for PON in breakdown of PB (Furlong, Richter, et al., 1989). However, "chemical stress" in the form of nerve agent exposure may, in animal models, lead to enhanced ability of PB to penetrate the blood-brain barrier (see Chapter Seven, "Blood-Brain Barrier Passage"; and Chapter Nine, "Interactions Between PB and Other Exposures"). Moreover, the toxicity of PB has been shown to be synergistic with pesticides in

Table 8.3

PON Isoforms: Substrate Activities in Human Sera for Sarin, Soman, and PON[a]

	Sarin		Soman		PON	
	Mean±SD	Range	Mean±SD	Range	Mean±SD	Range
All	230±191	0–758	1,658±660	616–2,982	924±603	121–2,786
QQ isoform	355±183	0–758	2,143±576	870–2,982	328±79	121–532
QR isoform	198±161	0–541	1,518±558	616–2,815	977±171	653–1.418
RR isoform	38±47	0–144	992±263	754–1,616	1,769±354	1,237–2,786

SOURCE: Davies, Richter, et al., 1996. Note that the isoforms that are most active against PON are least active against sarin and soman.

[a]Sample sizes range from 26–33 (QQ), 38–41 (QR), 11–18 (RR), 75–92 (all).

---

[4]Of peripheral relevance, the Q_{192} allele destroys biologically oxidized phospholipids, which contribute to heart disease, while the R_{192} allele represents instead a risk factor for CAD, so that PON polymorphism is associated with other health-related effects.

animal studies (see Chapter Nine). Many veterans report exposure to personal pesticides; and the degree of exposure to nerve agents in the PGW is a matter of continued investigation. For this and other reasons, PON polymorphisms could contribute to neurotoxic effects of exposures in ill PGW veterans, and this effect could be amplified by administration of PB. Additionally, PON is acutely reduced following exposure to OPs (Dwyer, 1998), and this could additionally burden nonspecific scavengers, contributing to interactive toxicity.

Other Enzymes. While no literature suggesting a specific role for other enzymes has been evaluated in the present literature review, there are likely ("almost certainly") other enzymes not yet known that have a role in metabolism of PB, which may contribute to individual differences in response to PB (Patrick, 1997).

Effects of Native Differences in Brain Chemistry

PB is used by scientists to assess function of growth hormone. Ordinarily, administration of PB leads to a growth hormone surge. However, the influence of PB on growth hormones is altered in a variety of conditions, conditions that are presumed to differ in cholinergic responsiveness for reasons that, in many cases, have not been elucidated. Among the variables and conditions known to modify the growth hormone response to PB are: age (Arvat, Gianotti, et al., 1996; Corsello, Tofani, et al., 1991); sex (Corsello, Tofani, et al., 1991), perhaps mediated through effects of sex steroids estrogen and testosterone (O'Keane, O'Flynn, et al., 1992; Eakman, Dallas, et al., 1996); dementia (Arvat, Gianotti, et al., 1996; Ghigo, Goffi, et al., 1993; Murialdo, Fonzi, et al., 1993); obsessive compulsive disorder (Lucey, Butcher, et al., 1993); affective disorder including depression (Thakore and Dinan, 1995) and mania (Dinan, O'Keane, et al., 1994); obesity (Procopio, Invitti, et al., 1995); hypercortisolism (Procopio, Invitti, et al., 1995; Borges, Castro, et al., 1993); and cognitive disorders (such as schizophrenia) (O'Keane, Abel, et al., 1994).

Thus, identified individual differences alter the effect of PB on one outcome—growth hormone response—that is commonly measured. Differences in cholinergic responsiveness as measured by a growth hormone response may or may not reflect more general differences in cholinergic responsiveness.

Concurrent, Antecedent, and Subsequent Exposures

Exposures to chemicals with which PB interacts, such as pesticides (use of personal pesticides was reported by 17 of the 20 CCEP-registered PGW cases in the BChE trial cited above (Gentry, Bitsko, et al., 1996)), nerve agents, cocaine (Loewenstein-Lichtenstein, Schwarz, et al., 1996; Kaufer, Friedman, et al., 1998), and other medications such as antihistamines, may provide a basis for apparent individual differences in response to PB, even in the absence of native differences in biochemistry or susceptibility. (See also Chapter Nine.) Moreover, differences in biochemical susceptibility to these exposures may amplify the potential for individual differences in response to PB. Nonetheless, the role of such differences in biochemical susceptibility to PB and subsequent development of chronic illness, such as that seen in PGW veterans, remains undefined.

Circadian Effects

Circadian differences may play a role in individual differences, since individuals may have received PB at different times of day.

The role of circadian variation in drug effects is increasingly appreciated: "In humans, variations during the 24 h day in pharmacokinetics (chronopharmacokinetics) have been shown for cardiovascularly active drugs (propranolol, nifedipine, verapamil, enalapril, isosorbide 5-mononitrate and digoxin), antiasthmatics (theophylline and terbutaline), anticancer drugs, psychotropics, analgesics, local anesthetics and antibiotics, to mention but a few. Even more drugs have been shown to display significant variations in their effects throughout the day (chronopharmacodynamics and chronotoxicology) even after chronic application or constant infusion. Moreover, there is clear evidence that even dose/concentration-response relationships can be significantly modified by the time of day. Thus, circadian time has to be taken into account as an important variable influencing a drug's pharmacokinetics and its effects or side-effects" (Lemmer, 1995). Susceptibility to illness is also influenced by time of day (Lemmer, 1995).

These effects have been capitalized on in treatment protocols. For example, one European multicenter randomized trial found the a chemotherapy regimen for colorectal cancer that was sensitive to circadian timing of delivery resulted in "2 to 10 times fewer" severe toxic effects and a 70 percent increase in objective response rate compared to non-circadian-sensitive treatment (51 percent response with "chono" treatment and 30 percent with other treatment; $p < 0.001$) (Levi, Giacchetti, et al., 1995). Otherwise phrased, wrongly timed drug delivery could result in 2 to 10 times more toxic effects (or more, if the "bad" delivery was not selected to be worst-case) and a 41 percent reduction in efficacy for these cancer chemotherapeutic agents.

Circadian effects have also been shown for drugs that influence the cholinergic system. In mice, the lethality of the drug lithium depends on what time of day the injection is given (Hawkins, Kripke, et al., 1978). Lithium appears to antagonize cholinergic effects in rodents, including effects on behavior (Janowsky, Abrams, et al., 1979) and on REM sleep (Campbell, Gillin, et al., 1989), and may do so by acting on the central cholinergic system (Janowsky, Abrams, et al., 1979).) More directly pertinent is evidence that the effects of ACh inhibitors, such as soman and OP pesticides, are modified in a circadian fashion (von Mayersbach, 1974; Fatranska, Vargova, et al., 1978; Elsmore, 1981; Augerson, 1986). Moreover, the cholinergic system itself modulates circadian variation of hypothalamic pituitary adrenal activity (Llorente, Lizcano, et al., 1996), suggesting the possibility that PB effects may modify or amplify stress hormone (and other hormone) responses depending on circadian timing of drug delivery.

Indirect evidence further suggests circadian-related effects on response to acetylcholinergic drugs. Bright light prevents the development of super-sensitivity to an anticholinesterase (oxotremorine) occurring as a result of forced stress or treatment with a muscarinic receptor antagonist in the rat (Overstreet, Dilsaver, et al., 1990). Treatment with bright light during the regular photoperiod (a time that does not produce a phase-shift or free-running) differentially affects the hypothermic response and activity suppressing effect of both Flinders Sensitive Line (FSL), sensitive to an anticholinesterase) and the Flinders Resistant Line (FRL) rats (Overstreet, Dilsaver, et al., 1990). Both lines exhibit decreased hypothermia without reduction in motor activity in response to oxotremorine following six days of treatment with bright light. The magnitude of blunting of the hypothermic response was greater in the FSL than the FRL rats (Overstreet, Dilsaver, et al., 1990). Thus, the effects of bright light are contingent on the endpoint measured, and the capacity of bright light to blunt the hypothermic response to a muscarinic agonist is greater in animals with a endogenously hyperactive muscarinic cholinergic system (Overstreet, Dilsaver, et al., 1990). Thus, cholinergic stimulation appears to have less of at least some effects when there is exposure to bright light. The possibility cannot be excluded that this factor could have contributed to relatively greater susceptibility to effects of PB in security personnel who worked at night.

Age, Sex, and Weight

Sex differences in mean AChE and BChE have been reported in a case control study of 20 veterans and 20 "normal volunteers." Spontaneous reactivation half-times, in minutes, were 45.2±5.6 minutes in men, and 38.6±5.0 minutes in women (p < .05). The effect on the population as a whole was attributed largely to the difference seen between male and female veterans (Gentry, Bitsko, et al., 1996).

Although one study failed to find sex or weight differences in AChE inhibition with PB (Lasseter and Garg, 1996), large individual differences in AChE inhibition were present; the variability due to individual differences from other factors is likely to have obscured statistical differences based on weight and perhaps sex. Alternatively, if one accepts that weight truly has no bearing on the effect of the drug, then it becomes unnecessary to correct doses when extrapolating from animal studies using smaller species, such as rodents. "High" doses of PB given in animal studies are generally higher than PGW doses on a per-weight basis—but not necessarily higher in terms of actual mg given. Thus, if one credits the view that weight is immaterial, toxicity findings from such animal studies might be more directly extrapolated to what might be expected in PGW veterans. It is far more likely however, that inability to show differences in AChE inhibition as a function of weight merely reflects the many other sources of individual variation that add to the variance. In that case, a large sample size would be needed to show the independent effect of weight.

SUMMARY ANALYSIS

Likelihood of "Exposure" (i.e., of PGW Veterans Experiencing Individual Differences in PB Susceptibility)

Individual differences occur in response to administration of any chemical agent. For example, for virtually any chemical an "LD_{50}" can be identified—a dose at which 50 percent of the animals will die while 50 percent will not—even in highly genetically inbred strains, although the animals are presumed genetically homogeneous and the exposure was the same for all. Moreover, small differences in susceptibility can lead to large differences in clinical outcome in selected instances. For instance, a study examining the effect of the breach of the blood-brain barrier on penetration to the CNS by a virus found that those animals that did not die were entirely healthy, though all received the same dose (see Chapter Seven, "Blood-Brain Barrier Passage"). Therefore, "exposure" to individual differences in susceptibility to PB was certainly present in PGW veterans. Data demonstrating major differences in absorption of PB and rate of choline inhibition for a given blood level of PB (Chapter Three) further support the certainty that individual differences in effective exposure (gauged by measures of PB in the blood, or by consequences of PB in the body), and in response to PB, occurred.

Symptoms Consistent With "Exposure" (Individual Differences)

Individual differences in acute response to PB are reflected in differences in side effects to PB that have been reported (Chapter Three). Character and severity of chronic symptoms in PGW veterans differ from one individual to the another, compatible with (though not persuasive for, or even necessarily suggestive of) individual differences in susceptibility to PB.

Evidence Relating Symptoms to Individual Differences

One relatively weak line of evidence suggests a relationship between chronic illnesses in PGW veterans and individual differences in acute response to PB—differences that might be presumed to reflect differences in susceptibility to toxic effects of PB, including chronic effects if any exist. This stems from the previously cited study that found a relationship between two of three factor-analysis derived syndromes in ill PGW veterans and self-reported adverse response to administration of PB during the PGW (Haley and Kurt, 1997).

No evidence has demonstrated a correlation between identified biochemical differences and chronic illnesses. (Although evidence has failed to show a relation between atypical BChE and CCEP registration in a small sample, a role for atypical BChE appears unlikely in any case, based on its very low prevalence in the population.)

Scientific Recommendations

1. An attempt should be made to replicate the syndromes identified by Haley, et al. (1997a), and particularly to determine whether self-reported adverse response to administration of PB is linked to chronic illnesses in PGW veterans in a second, preferably larger, sample of ill PGW veterans. Moreover, an attempt should be made to replicate the results using different techniques such as unsupervised neural networks, and/or employing cross validation, on the same pool of veterans. Potential confounding factors will be an issue because subjects may be concerned about long-term effects of PB, and recall bias remains an issue. Nonetheless, the information provided will add or lessen support for a connection between individual adverse response to PB and illnesses.[5]

2. Consideration should be given to testing for mutations—such as the K variant of BChE-that occur more commonly than atypical BChE, and that have also been shown to be less active.

3. Studies should be performed to assess the impact of phenotype (quantity and activity, as well as type of enzyme), rather than exclusively for genotype, for BChE, PON, and possibly for other esterases. Phenotypes should be compared in PGW veterans with and without illness. Phenotype (amount and activity and consequent ability to hydrolyze PB) varies greatly

---

[5]Since the draft of this report was originally circulated, other factor analyses have been published, as has another study linking self-reported PB to illness in PGW veterans (Unwin, Blatchley, et al., 1999). These findings are discussed in limited fashion elsewhere in the report.

within those with a normal genotype, and could contribute (along with other factors, such as pesticide and possible nerve agent exposure) to individual differences in response to PB. (If a highly susceptible group is identified by genotype or phenotype, future testing of military personnel might be performed to identify susceptible individuals, who might be debarred from deployment to high chemical warfare threat areas in which military use of PB might occur.)

4. Prior to future deployment, it would be prudent to ascertain the effect of phenotypic differences in AChE and BChE on the effect of PB measured by AChE inhibition.

5. A sample of PGW veterans with and without illnesses, of adequate size to permit testing for modest effect sizes with high power, should be developed as a study group. Careful delineation of symptoms should be made, and blood should be collected and processed for storage for future genetic and blood analyses as new candidate explanatory factors are uncovered.

Chapter Nine

INTERACTIONS BETWEEN PB AND OTHER EXPOSURES

DO INTERACTIONS BETWEEN PB AND OTHER EXPOSURES ENHANCE THE TOXICITY OF EFFECTS?

It is possible that PB may act synergistically with other exposures to lead to adverse or toxic effects that may relate to illnesses in PGW veterans. Some have referred to a putative "toxic cocktail" (Shays, 1997), or to "cumulative health consequences of exposure to multiple risk factors" (Metcalf, 1997) including PB, vaccines, chemical weapons, pesticides, depleted uranium, infection, and smoke from oil fires.

Many ambiguities exist regarding drug-drug and drug-chemical interactions. We know that they are common and often not predicted by the effects of individual drugs given separately; moreover, no FDA regulations require testing of drug combinations for individually approved or licensed agents. While personnel involved in the PGW experienced many drug and chemical exposures, it is not known with certainty whether interactions between these exposures contributed to illnesses in PGW veterans.

However, common mechanisms of effect among certain exposures (such as AChE inhibition by PB, nerve agents, and pesticides), and common side effects of certain exposures (such as enhanced permeability of the blood-brain barrier with chemical mixtures, stress, and aluminum used in vaccine adjuvants) make an effect of drug-chemical interactions possible. These may have contributed to reported illnesses in PGW veterans. Additional research is needed to evaluate the possible impact on reported illnesses of combinations of agents and exposures experienced in the PGW.

This chapter addresses the evidence available regarding the possible role of interactions and illnesses in PGW veterans. It will

- Briefly cite some findings of the Institute of Medicine (IOM) report, *Interactions of Drugs, Biologics, and Chemicals in US Military Forces*

- Review and extend the concept, introduced by the IOM, of matrices of toxicity as a source of investigation for interactions

- Inquire what can be learned from other populations with multiple drug exposures

- Address the evidence regarding interactions between PB and other drug and chemical exposures in the PGW

- Suggest a strategy for investigating PGW drug interactions.

IOM APPROACH TO DRUG/VACCINE INTERACTIONS

The Committee to Study the Interactions of Drugs, Biologics, and Chemicals in U.S. Military Forces, from the Medical Follow-Up Agency of the Institute of Medicine (IOM), drafted a report entitled *Interactions of Drugs, Biologics, and Chemicals in US Military Forces* (Committee to Study the Interactions of Drugs, 1996), to which the interested reader is referred. This 80-page report describes one general approach to investigating interactions, which will not be reprised in detail here. This report correctly identifies drug interactions as a potential problem when multiple drug or chemical exposures are present, notes the paucity of evidence regarding the scale of the problem with drug interactions, and observes that it is difficult to obtain such data. It identifies difficulties with studying toxic interactions among drugs, due to the rapid growth of possible interactions as more exposures are added. (With n exposures there are on the order of 2^n potential interactions—not counting the need to study different dosage ranges.) And it formulates recommendations for surveillance and testing for interactions in the military.

Relevant points from the IOM report include the following:

- Whereas adverse effects of most single products have been relatively well studied (for instance in data submitted to the FDA for approval of a new drug), for most drugs it is largely unknown whether their combined use may provoke unanticipated reactions.

- The epidemiology of drug interactions is poorly understood, because very little of the literature on drug interactions has resulted from epidemiological investigations. Data derive instead from pharmacokinetic or pharmacodynamic studies, case reports, review articles, and animal and in vitro studies. Consequently, little is known about how often drug interactions actually occur and how often they produce clinically meaningful adverse effects.

- The published scientific literature on the interactions of militarily relevant drugs, biologics, and chemicals does not provide an adequate basis for assessing the degree of safety; however, no basis was found for extraordinary concern.

- Vaccines have been shown to affect the metabolism of other drugs, possibly by interfering with human liver cytochrome P450 isozymes.

- Newly discovered interactions are not likely to exactly mimic previously described disease and may indeed have unique presentations.

- The process of coding medical information can change that information. Often sentinel events are more difficult to recover from a system once they have been coded.

- Unpredictable interactive toxicities are certain to occur. Thalidomide, benoxaprofen, and other instances are cited. Even less predictable toxicities should be expected when complex mixtures of agents are used together.

To these the following comments may be added:

- Drug interactions are common.

- Typically, adverse effects of drugs (such as rash or GI symptoms) terminate when the drug is discontinued, but many known exceptions exist. For example, dexfenfluramine was recently removed from the market followed discovery of frequent heart valve abnormalities associated with use of fenfluramine (often in combination with phentermine) as a diet agent. This, and the finding of pulmonary hypertension with fenfluramine, represents recently identified instances of effects that persist beyond drug discontinuation.

- The mechanism of adverse effects is often not understood.

MATRICES OF TOXICITY

The IOM provides a table of sites of action and toxicity for certain agents and suggests that such a table can direct research to sites of common effects between agents. The rationale is that sites of common action or toxicity might more likely be sites at which interactive toxicity may take place.

This approach has value, but also limitations. It is limited conceptually—since interactions may occur from effects on *different* systems that themselves interact. More practically, the approach is limited by the depth of inquiry used to ascertain the actions of the drug in question. Thus, it is constrained both by *available* knowledge (information available in the scientific literature) and perhaps equally by *accessed* knowledge (the subset of the available literature accessed for use in the matrix).

PB was included in the IOM matrix and provides one example pertinent to the present discussion. Using this matrix, we would not be concerned about inter-active toxicities related to, for instance, the gastrointestinal or cardiac system. In the IOM report, the nervous system was the sole cited locus of action or of toxicity for PB. However, PB should have also been noted for toxicity or for site of action in virtually all of the other categories named, and more (Table 9.1). For example, *mucous membranes* are influenced by PB to produce increased secretions, or to reduce mucociliary clearance if ACh downregulation occurs. This latter response could potentially enhance pharyngeal sensitivity to chemi-cal or infectious exposures (see Chapter Eleven, "Multiple Chemical Sensitiv-ity," section on nasopharyngeal factors). The *airways and lungs* are affected by the muscarinic and nicotinic properties of PB, producing bronchorrhea and airway constriction (see Chapter Three's section on muscarinic effects). Indeed, severe exacerbations of asthma in response to PB led some asthmatic PGW personnel to be flown from the theater. *Cardiac* effects not only exist but are expected; generally, relative bradycardia is produced with routine PB administration, with an average five beat per minute reduction in heart rate in persons (see Chapter Three, section on "Side Effects"). Tachycardia may also be produced if the nicotinic effects exceed the muscarinic influences on heart rate. *Hepatic* effects in the form of competition for the hepatic cytochrome P450 system, may be responsible for part of the synergistic toxicity seen with PB and pesticides. *Musculoskeletal* effects are well known; indeed, PB is used ther-apeutically in myasthenia gravis with the intent of influencing the neuromuscu-lar junction, and motor endplate toxicity with PB is well described (see Chapter Twelve, "Neuromuscular Junction Effects"). Musculotendinous junctions and sarcolemma and sarcoplasm are other sites with cholinergic involvement. ACh receptors exist on *hematologic* (Sastry and Sadavongvivad, 1979) *and immune* cells, so that PB has a potential site of action for these systems (Chapter Four-teen, "Other Considerations"). *Gastrointestinal* effects are common (including cramping, increased intestinal secretions and diarrhea), due to muscarinic effects of PB (see Chapter Three). (The "enteric nervous system has more neu-rons than the brain" (Patrick, 1997)). *Urologic* effects can occur due to ureteral spasm from muscarinic effects (see Chapter Three). *Endocrine* effects are widely known; indeed, PB is used in testing procedures to induce growth hor-mone secretion (see Chapter Fifteen). Effects on the *reproductive* system might be anticipated based on evidence that cholinergic signaling is involved in chorionic villi, which express the BChE gene; in the placenta; and in sperm motility, in which ACh, AChE, ChAT (choline acetyltransferase, the enzyme catalyzing production of ACh), and BChE are present (Sastry and Sadavong-vivad, 1979; Schwarz, Glick, et al., 1995) (see also Chapter Fifteen).

Table 9.1

**Sites of Action of PB; Possible Sites at Which Interaction
May Occur with Other Drugs and Chemicals**

Site Of Toxicity	IOM Version	Expanded Version
Nervous system	X	X
Mucous membrane		X
Heart		X
Liver		X
Lung/airway		X
Musculoskeletal		X
GI		X
Reproductive		X
Urinary		X
Hematologic		X
Immune		X

It is possible—perhaps likely—that similar in-depth knowledge of effects of the other identified drugs used in the PGW would lead to identification of effects on many systems rather than the one or two noted in the report. Thus, the strategy of concentrating on interactions in tissues and systems for which there is known toxicity or site of action may be useful in understanding the reason for interaction but less useful in restricting which interactions warrant concern and further study. The prospect of studying all those interactions suspected by commonality of sites of action, using the more complete PB matrix (and more complete matrices for other agents) could be understandably daunting. An alternative approach to evaluating interactive toxicity will be suggested below, although this approach has its own limitations. See Table 9.2 for a summary of known binary interactions.

WHAT CAN WE LEARN FROM OTHER POPULATIONS WITH MULTIPLE DRUG EXPOSURES?

The elderly constitute one population at risk for multiple drug exposures. In this population, as in medically ill populations on multiple medications, it is widely understood that medication effects and interactions represent a common source of morbidity and that drug effects and drug interactions must be considered when new unexplained problems arise. The problem arises in part from the multiplicity of agents and in part from reduced capacity to metabolize administered drugs.

Deployed troops represent another group that may be, in some instances, exposed to multiple medications and other chemicals. Although deployed troops are younger and more likely to have robust liver and kidney function and

Table 9.2

Data Matrix: Interactions Between PB and Selected Exposures

	PB	Nerve Agent	Pesticide	Insect Repellent	Stress	Adrenergic agents	Caffeine	Cipro	Anti-histamines	Vaccines	DU
Demonstrated interaction	NA	+	+	+	+	+	+	–	±	–	–
Closest Model		Primate	Rodent; hen; cockroach	Rodent; hen; cockroach	Rodent	Rodent	Rodent				
Evidence Theory		(R)CT[a] ACh action	(R)CT ACh action; common metabolism	(R)CT Enhanced absorption of PB; common metabolism	(R)CT Enhanced penetration of PB into NS	CT Enhanced penetration of PB into CNS	(R)CT Enhanced penetration of PB into NS	Indirect GABA; musculoskeletal; liver	Indirect ACh	Indirect Liver metabolism; blood-brain barrier	No theory

[a] (R)CT = (Randomized) Control Trial

are therefore more likely to metabolize foreign products expeditiously, here, too, exposures to multiple drugs and chemicals should be considered for their possible role if untoward health effects occur. This is especially true in light of evidence that some of these drug interactions may influence the metabolic systems that normally allow younger persons to tolerate medications with relative facility.

Populations with multiple vaccine exposures will be discussed separately (see *A Review of the Scientific Literature As It Pertains to Gulf War Illnesses*, Vol. 8: *Immunizations* (Golomb, forthcoming)).

SPECIFIC INTERACTIONS OF PB WITH OTHER FACTORS

Interactions with Pesticides and Insect Repellents

Much of the interest in interactions related to PB has concentrated on interactions with pesticides and insect repellents. Several pertinent studies will be reviewed here. Studies have demonstrated additive or synergistic effects of PB with the insect repellent DEET, and with the pesticides permethrin and chlorpyrifos. To date, such studies have been performed in cockroaches, hens, and rats. Further work in this area is ongoing.

Interactant: DEET. DEET (*N,N*-diethyl-*m*-toluamide), an aromatic amide, is an EPA-approved personal insect repellent widely used commercially, though it is known to produce mammalian CNS effects at high exposures by an unknown mechanism. Cases of acute toxicity and death in humans (primarily in children (Osimitz and Murphy 1997)) have been reported following dermal application (De Garbino and Laborde, 1983; Heick, Shipman, et al., 1980; Roland, Jan, et al., 1985; Edwards and Johnson, 1987; Gryboski, Weinstein, et al., 1961; Zadikoff, 1979). Symptoms of DEET toxicity include tremor, restlessness, slurred speech, seizures, impaired cognition, and coma (McConnell, Fidler, et al., 1986). Near lethal doses in rats produce spongiform myelinopathy in cerebellar roof nuclei (Verschoyle, Brown, et al., 1990). The nervous system may not be a selective target for DEET (Schoenig, Hartnagel, et al., 1993; Osimitz and Grothaus 1995; Schoenig, Hartnagel, et al., 1996), and possibly some of the apparent neurotoxicity may be mediated by DEET's postulated ability to allow penetration to the CNS by other agents. (DEET is known for its permeability enhancing effects (Windheuser, Haslam, et al., 1982; Kondo, Mizuno, et al., 1988); however one study found that DEET did not enhance, and in some preparations reduced, absorption of carbaryl and permethrin (Baynes, Halling, et al., 1997).)

Several formulations, including 75 percent DEET in ethanol formulation, a 33 percent extended-duration formulation, and 19 percent in stick were prepared for the U.S. Army. Low usage of insect repellent was reported during the conflict. The cool climate at the time of the war (January and February 1991) resulted in few biting insects, though exposure may have been higher at other times during the deployment. However, these instances would probably not have coincided with PB use. (See also Geschwind and Golomb, forthcoming).

Interactant: Permethrin. Permethrin is a third-generation synthetic (Type 1) pyrethroid insecticide with four stereoisomers (that is, chemicals with the same constituents but different configurations; they may be "cis" or "trans" and "+" or "–"), that often provides insecticidal activity for several weeks following a single application. Permethrin has some esterase-inhibiting activity, as well as other mechanisms of toxicity.[1] Symptoms include hyperactivity, tremor, ataxia, convulsion, and paralysis; peripheral nerve damage has been produced by a near-lethal dose in rats (Abou-Donia, Wilmarth, et al., 1996b) (Rose and Dewar, 1983). Permethrin is metabolized by enzymes termed "hydrolases" and "oxidases"; both esterase and oxidase inhibitors may enhance toxicity in mammals (Pelligrini and Santi, 1972; Casida, Gamman, et al., 1983; Abou-Donia, Wilmarth, et al., 1996b).

Permethrin is EPA approved and commercially available. Aerosol spray cans with 0.5 percent aerosol in a two-gallon compressed air sprayer were available to fewer than 5 percent of deployed units, for impregnation of battle dress uniforms (McCain, 1997). The aerosol spray can method is thought to provide protection for about six washings, or six weeks of use (McCain, 1997). Data in rabbits suggest that permethrin may be resistant to removal with laundering, and may continue to be absorbed into the skin at a constant rate after many washings (Snodgrass, 1992). These data were also noteworthy for one animal that persistently absorbed markedly more than the others, suggesting that dermal absorption differences may constitute yet another of many sources of possible individual differences (see previous Chapter Eight, "Individual Differences in Reactions to PB").

Interactions among pesticides are not always potentiating. For instance, in one study in rats, the addition of 380 mg/kg and 464 mg/kg of methyl parathion reduced the LD_{50} of permethrin by 9 percent (NS) and 37 percent (p < 0.001) respectively (Ortiz, Yanez, et al., 1995). Permethrin reduced the cholinesterase inhibition of parathion by 50 percent. (These doses are extremely high and bear no relation to exposures that could have occurred in PGW veterans.) (See also Geschwind and Colomb, forthcoming).

---

[1]Other mechanism of permethrin toxicity include delayed closure of sodium channels during a depolarizing pulse, evoking repetitive after-discharges by a single stimulus, inhibition of calcium-magnesium ATPase, and inhibition of calmodulin (Narahashi, 1985) (Abou-Donia, Wilmarth, et al., 1996b).

Interactant: Chlorpyrifos (Abou-Donia, Wilmarth, et al., 1996b). Chlorpyrifos (*O,O*-diethyl *O*-3,5,6-trichloropyridinyl phosphorothioate) is a phosphorothioate insecticide used in the PGW that undergoes first pass metabolism to chlorpyrifos oxon, which in turn inhibits rat brain AChE in vitro (that is, in studies in rat brain preparations not performed in a living animal). Chlorpyrifos toxicity results in muscarinic, nicotinic, and CNS symptoms (see Chapter Three, "Characteristics of PB"), and sensory and CNS toxicity may ensue (Kaplan, Kessler, et al., 1993; Moretto and Lotti, 1998). Moreover, near-lethal doses may produce OPIDN (OP-induced delayed neurotoxicity—also called "OPIDP," or OP-induced delayed polyneuropathy—see Chapter Fourteen, "Chronic Effects") in humans (Abou-Donia, Wilmarth, et al., 1996b; Lotti and Moretto, 1986). Doses equivalent to two to three times the LD_{50}, with protection from lethality, produce OPIDN in the hen, suggesting that some humans may be more sensitive relative to the lethal dose than hens. OPIDN consists of delayed protracted ataxia (gait incoordination) and paralysis accompanied by a "Wallerian-type" degeneration of the central and peripheral nervous system. Concurrent exposure to other agents, including an organophosphorus insecticide that does not produce OPIDN, may reduce the threshold dose of chlorpyrifos that produces OPIDN (Abou-Donia, Wilmarth, et al., 1996a). Chlorpyrifos produces an unusually prolonged dose-dependent fall in the activity of brain AChE, lasting for weeks after treatment ends (Chiappa, Padilla et al., 1995), and therefore it might participate in interactions with other agents well after the time of administration.

PB Interaction Studies

Cockroach Study. (PB, lambda-cyhalothrin, permethrin) (Moss, 1996). Synergism of DEET with lambda-cyhalothrin, permethrin, and PB. Studies in adult male German cockroaches demonstrated that DEET toxicity was increased by lambda-cyhalothrin and permethrin as well as by PB. Specifically, the LD_{50} for DEET, in μg/g, was reduced from 2,711 to 404 with addition of PB at a dose of 2,049 μg/g, an effect that was highly statistically significant. DEET, in turn, at a dose of 7.003 μg/g, contributed synergistically to the toxicity of pyridostigmine, changing the LD_{50} from 7.003 to 1,868, an effect that was statistically significant. Synergism was also produced by DEET for malathion and carbaryl, but not bendiocarb or chlorpyrifos.

Hen Studies (Abou-Donia, Wilmarth, et al., 1996c). Hens are used as a model of human anticholinesterase effects because hens, like people (and unlike many mammals) are susceptible to anticholinesterase effects, including OPIDN.

Doses of PB (5 mg/kg in water—about 12 times the PB dose, unadjusted for route), DEET (500 mg/kg, "neat"—that is, undiluted), and chlorpyrifos (10 mg/kg in oil) were given parenterally five days a week for two months to hens. Individually these doses produced no deaths (although they produced clinical illness). In combination they led to mortality (or euthanization due to severe ill-ness) in approximately 20 percent with PB and chlorpyrifos, 35 percent for PB and DEET, 65 percent for all three; and 75 percent for DEET plus chlorpyrifos. Significant reductions in body weight (up to 20 percent) were seen for chlor-pyrifos alone and for all combinations.

A measure of severity of clinical signs, as well as locomotor dysfunction (abnormal walking), histopathological changes in the cervical and thoracic spinal cord, and the mean of ranked scores of these tests were all increased in hens given drug combinations compared to hens given any drug individually. These abnormalities were greatest in those hens given all three agents. Histopathological alterations were increased with all combinations but were greatest with PB plus chlorpyrifos.

Plasma BChE (see Chapter Eight, "Individual Differences in Reactions to PB") was significantly reduced with each drug individually, and with all combinations. (This reduction was maximal with PB and combinations including PB; and values were as low as 10 percent of control with PB and DEET; however, these employ levels that produce significant immediate toxicity.) Brain AChE was reduced with chlorpyrifos (to about 70 percent of control) and to a greater extent with all combinations, including chlorpyrifos (to approximately 30 percent of control with DEET, 55 percent of control with PB, and 25 percent of control with all three). Neuropathy target esterase was significantly reduced with all combinations containing chlorpyrifos (to about 75 percent of control in all cases) but not with chlorpyrifos alone.

Similar findings were produced in another study in hens, by the same research group, involving PB, DEET, and permethrin (Abou-Donia, Wilmarth, et al., 1996c). Doses that resulted in minimal toxicity when given individually produced more significant toxicity when given in combination. Measures used included clinical evaluation (of walking, flying, tremor, leg movement, ability to enter home cage, weight loss, and death), histopathological assessment of spinal cord and sciatic nerve, BChE and AChE determination, and a neurotoxicity score using the above factors. No mortality was seen in the control hens or with those given a single drug (PB, permethrin, or DEET), but combinations produced about 20 percent (PB+P), 40 percent (D+P, or D+PB), or 80 percent mortality (PB+D+P). Days to onset of clinical signs were affected with all single drugs except permethrin alone, and with all drug combinations. (All three drugs in combination led to clinical signs within several days; this compares to no signs by 60 days—the end of the experiment—in control and in permethrin animals.) Locomotor dysfunction (problems walking) resulted from all drug combinations but not from single drugs, and the same results were found with tremor (Abou-Donia, Wilmarth, et al., 1996b, 1996c). Neuropathic changes were nonexistent in PB+P, mild in D+P, mild to moderate in PB+D, and mild to severe in PB+D+P.[2] Plasma BChE activity was markedly reduced to 83 percent of that of the control group in D+P (p < 0.05), to 26 percent with PB+D+P, to 20 percent with PB+P, and to 8 percent with PB+D (all p < 0.01). No changes were seen in brain AChE with any treatment. A "Mean Rank" score, based on ranking in the above categories, was significantly greater for two than for one agent, and for three than any combination of two agents in all cases except one: PB+P results did not differ significantly from P alone. It must be emphasized that these studies used extremely high doses of P, PB, and D.

Rats (McCain, 1997). Studies have sought to evaluate potential toxic interactions of PB, DEET, and permethrin given by gastric lavage (that is, by tube through the mouth to the stomach) to male rats. Rats are more closely related to humans than are hens or cockroaches, though they are not susceptible to certain adverse effects of cholinesterase inhibitors that have been identified in humans and hens (such as OPIDN). An oral route for PB more closely mimics the PB route of administration to veterans in the PGW. DEET and permethrin were also administered orally, in contradistinction to the probable route of delivery in PGW veterans, who would most likely have been exposed through skin contact or perhaps by inhalation. However, the oral route allows more control over dosing than the dermal and inhalational routes.

This study determined the LD_{16} (dose that was lethal in 16 percent of rats) for all three agents individually, then determined what happened to rats when two of the three were given at the respective LD_{16}, and the third was varied in dose. A clear synergistic effect (more than additive toxicity) was demonstrated. While only about 10 percent of animals died when given permethrin and DEET each at its respective LD_{16} (compared to 32 percent predicted, or 16 percent for each drug), when the LD_{16} of PB was added (45.76 mg/kg or 107 times the PGW dose) mortality rose to approximately 90 percent—far more than the 26 percent expected on top of the dual drug effect or the 48 percent expected if the three drugs behaved independently. (Actually, the predicted deaths should be slightly less than 26 percent and 48 percent assuming independence of effect, because some of the animals that would have been killed with the first drug, or a pair of drugs, might be the same that would have been killed with the second; therefore, the actual predicted rates would have been 24 percent and 41 percent. Consequently, the synergism is more striking.) Similar studies were con-

---

[2]These results reinforce the idea that individual variation in the development of illness is the rule, even in genetically homogeneous animals with highly similar exposures. Such variation would be expected a fortiori in genetically heterogeneous humans with highly diverse exposures (see Chapter Eight).

ducted holding PB and DEET at their LD_{16}s and adding different doses of permethrin; or holding PB and permethrin at their LD_{16}s and adding different doses of DEET. In each case, toxicity—gauged by lethality—exceeded that expected by independence.

Mice Studies. One study in ICR mice, to date published only in abstract form, found that combinations of PB (2.3 mg/kg, or 5.2 times the PGW dose, intra-peritoneally) and DEET (200, 300, 400, 550 mg/kg intraperitoneally contra-laterally) resulted in a significant increase in lethality compared to either agent alone (Chaney, Moss, et al., 1997). Moreover, caffeine (5 mg/kg) given 15 minutes prior to one or both led to increased PB but not PB/DEET lethality in mice. Selected adrenergically active agents enhanced lethality of PB alone (α blockers, including phentolamine (mixed $\alpha1/\alpha2$) 1 mg/kg; prazosin (α 1) 2 mg/kg; yohimbine ($\alpha2$) 1 mg/kg). Several enhanced PB and PB/DEET lethality (α- and ß-agonist epinephrine 5 mg/kg; ß1 and ß2 agonist isoproterenol 3 mg/kg; and a ß2 agonist salmeterol 0.4 mg/kg). Several other agents did not significantly increase either PB- or PB/DEET-induced lethality ($\alpha2$ agonist clonidine, 1 mg/kg; ß1 antagonist acebutolol 1, 5 mg/kg; ß1ß2 antagonists propranolol 1.5, 3 mg/kg and nadolol 1, 5 mg/kg; and ß2 agonist terbutaline 1 mg/kg) (Chaney, Moss, et al., 1997; Hardman, Limbird, et al., 1996).

Suggested mechanisms. Several possible mechanisms for an interaction have been proposed (McCain, 1997; Abou-Donia, Wilmarth, et al., 1996b, 1996c).

First, it has been suggested that DEET (and perhaps permethrin) may act as a permeability-enhancing agent for PB and pesticides; or more generally that concurrent exposure to chemicals may increase their absorption. PB is poorly absorbed by the gut and has a steep dose-response curve, so that enhanced absorption leading to increased bioavailability of PB could lead to increased toxicity or lethality (McCain, 1997). It has further been suggested that the epidermis may serve as a depot site for DEET, resulting in its slow release into the circulation (Blomquist and Thorsell, 1977; Spencer, Hill, et al., 1979; Snodgrass, Nelson, et al., 1982), so that exposures need not be concurrent for synergistic interaction to occur. (Similarly, DEET could enhance the dermal absorption of such pesticides as chlorpyrifos, which are known to produce OPIDN). DEET has been used to increase permeability of other agents dermally (Windheuser, Haslam, et al., 1982; Hussain and Ritschel, 1988).

Second, enzymes including plasma esterases, hydrolases, and amidases are involved in metabolism of these compounds, enhancing their removal from the circulation by scavenging or breakdown into water-soluble metabolites (Abou-Donia, 1995). PB may bind to and inhibit nonspecific esterases (such as BChE) preventing detoxification of other chemicals, such as permethrin (an ester). More generally, the compounds may compete for metabolizing enzymes, leading to decreased breakdown and increased delivery of toxic compounds to nervous tissues (Abou-Donia, Wilmarth, et al., 1996b, 1996c; McCain, 1997).

Third, pyrethroids, like carbamates, are also metabolized by cytochrome P-450 in the liver (Kostka, Palut, et al., 1997). Once again, there may be competition for degradation leading to decreased breakdown and increased circulating levels of these agents (McCain, 1997). A mechanism in which there is an increased effective dose of the agents caused by competition for metabolizing enzymes is consistent with the result that inhibition of brain AChE and NTE was greatly amplified after combined exposures of PB and/or DEET with chlorpyrifos, possibly causing increased chlorpyrifos oxon in the brain tissue (Abou-Donia, Wilmarth, et al., 1996c).

Fourth, PB in concert with other agents may increase permeability of the blood-brain barrier, leading to enhanced access of toxins into the brain (see Chapter Seven, "Blood-Brain Barrier Passage"), including access of normally excluded PB to the CNS. Increased permeability of the blood-brain barrier may occur through vascular damage or trauma (perhaps including chemical trauma or alterations of membrane lipids by lipid-soluble pesticides and nerve agents), or it may relate to inhibition of BChE and AChE in the capillary wall and in astrocytes (supporting cells in the nervous system). Increased permeability of the blood-brain barrier has been reported with physostigmine (a centrally penetrating analog of PB) and with ACh (Greig and Holland, 1949), suggesting that AChE inhibition, or increased ACh activity, may itself enhance permeability of the blood-brain barrier, leading to increased access by toxins. Further evidence for a mechanism involving the blood-brain barrier is suggested by findings that "stress" (at least of certain types), has been reported to increase blood-brain barrier permeability in animal studies (see Chapter Seven); in other studies, adrenergic agents enhance PB- and PB/DEET-induced lethality (in mice) (Chaney, Moss, et al., 1997). These findings suggest that a stress-induced adrenergic surge, or heightened adrenergic tone, may play a role in the breach of the blood-brain barrier caused by stress.

Limitations. First, these studies are limited by the use of nonhuman animal models. Insects are phylogenetically distant from humans; hens are not mammals, though they share with humans a susceptibility to at least one long-term consequence of OP toxicity that most evaluated mammals do not, namely OPIDN; and mice and rats, although mammals, are neither close mammalian relatives nor ones that experience OPIDN. Animals differ in susceptibility to adverse outcomes from chemicals and chemical combinations compared to humans. Nonetheless, preservation of the finding of synergism between PB and other chemicals across such diverse species strongly suggests that such synergism, if not its particulars, is conserved and may occur in humans.

Second, these studies assume concurrent exposure. As previously noted, insect biting was viewed as infrequent in January and February, the times of the air and ground wars (PGW, 1997) when PB use is believed to have predominantly occurred. (However, some veterans report having taken PB for prolonged periods (Zeller, 1997; Hamden, 1997).) Insect biting did not increase until March, and pesticide use may have occurred predominantly starting in March, after most PB use is believed to have ceased. (Nonetheless, it is not possible to exclude significant use of pesticides in the theater before that time.) The effects of exposures staggered in time would likely differ, though it has been suggested that DEET, for one, may be stored in the epidermis for slow release into the circulation (Blomquist and Thorsell, 1977; Snodgrass, Nelson, et al., 1982; Spencer, Hill, et al., 1979), and permethrin, if uniforms are impregnated, may remain in the material and continue to be absorbed slowly through the dermis at a constant rate despite many launderings (Snodgrass, 1992).

Third, these studies employ different routes of exposure than those experienced by PGW veterans and employ doses (per kg of body weight) markedly in excess of doses that might conceivably have been experienced by PGW veterans. For instance, for the rat study, corresponding per-kg oral doses in a 70 kg person would be: 107 30-mg PB tablets; 23 6-oz cans of 0.5 percent permethrin; and six two-ounce tubes of 33 percent DEET. In the hen studies, the corresponding doses are 467 PB tablets, 1,667 permethrin cans, and 76 DEET tubes (Young, undated). However, while these doses vastly exceed those that might have been experienced by PGW veterans, the outcome measures—e.g., lethality—are also greatly in excess of the more subtle effects on sleep, energy, cognition, and joint pain experienced by many veterans. Thus, while these studies by no means confirm a connection between PB-chemical interactions and illnesses in PGW veterans, they are mutually consistent and clearly do not exclude such a connection. The persistence of additive or synergistic toxicity across species suggests that interaction studies need to be done in more physiologically plausible dose ranges—but also perhaps with more-sensitive outcome measures. In addition, none of these studies discontinued the exposures and performed long-term follow-up to determine whether persistent neurological problems were evident.

PB and Nerve Agents

Although PB is used in the military for *protection* against the effects of the nerve agent soman, in some instances no effect (Kerenyi, Murphy, et al., 1990) or potentiation of a toxic effect (Shiloff and Clement, 1986) for soman has been reported. (The studies finding no effects took place in rats. Moreover, PB doses in studies demonstrating a toxic effect are much higher than those used in the PGW.) PB confers protection against soman if given in advance of soman exposure; however, additive toxicity, rather than protection, may occur if PB is administered following nerve agent exposure. (This is because PB will bind to, and inhibit, additional AChE, without "blocking" nerve agent from binding, since the nerve agent has already had the opportunity to bind AChE and undergo aging.) PB may lower the PR for some nerve agents (for lethality), but protection against lethality using standard postexposure protocols remains quite good despite addition of PB, at least in nonprimate mammals (see Chapter Three, section on "Military Uses"). Further work is needed on sublethal exposures and on primates. DoD reports that up to 100,000 troops may have been exposed to low levels of sarin in association with the Khamisiyah ammunitions depot demolition which occurred particularly on March 10, 1991 (U.S. troops are believed to have destroyed chemical weapons at Khamisiyah on March 4, 10, and 12 1991, but primarily March 10) (PGW, 1997; OSAGWI, 1997). The exposures, based on modeling of data guided by simulations, were to very low doses—below those needed to produce "first effects" (such as runny nose or tearing) but above the exposure limit considered safe for long-term exposure for the public. Most administered PB is believed to have been given in association with the air and ground wars, which began respectively on January 17, 1991, and February 24, 1991, with cease-fire declared February 28, 1991 (PGW, 1997). Thus, it would be expected that most personnel would have terminated use of PB prior to any exposure to sarin associated with the Khamisiyah incident.

PB and Combat Anesthesia

It has been noted that the presence of a chemical threat (with a consequent decision to administer PB) does not preclude injury by conventional weapons, with a subsequent need for surgery and concomitant anesthesia. Some agents used during anesthesia may interact with PB through cholinergic or anticholinergic effects, or through end-organ effects, and these interactions have been reviewed (Keeler, 1990). However, conventional casualties were rare in the PGW and need for surgery during use of PB was not common; PB-anesthetic agent interactions cannot be responsible for the illnesses currently seen in PGW veterans who did not have surgery.

PB and Stress; PB and Heat

Chapter Seven describes one possible interaction between stress and PB—enhanced access of PB to the CNS through increased permeability of the blood-brain barrier due to stress.

This study used a "forced swim" test in rodents as the encountered "stress." It should be reinforced that the different classes of events that to which the term "stress" may be applied do not produce uniform consequences. Rather, the many different forms of "stress" (heat stress, cold stress, grief, embarrassment, acute threat to safety, chronic threat to safety, sleep deprivation, hunger, exposure to a given toxin, exertion stress, illness stress, etc.) may have some effects in common but also have distinct biochemical signatures. As one example of differing effects, serum cholesterol typically rises sharply, with a time-course of hours, after certain types of emotional stress, an effect mediated by catecholamine-induced hemoconcentration (Wertlake, Wilcox, et al., 1958; McCabe, Hammarsten, et al., 1959; Dimsdale and Herd, 1982; Muldoon, Bachen, et al., 1992; Patterson, Gottdiener, et al., 1993); on the other hand, serum cholesterol typically plummets, with a time-course of days, after some kinds of major physical stressors such as surgery, childbirth, myocardial infarction, or severe illness (Goodman, Kellogg, et al., 1962; Ryder, Hayes, et al., 1984; Brugada, Wenger, et al., 1996; Ploeckinger, Dantendorfer, et al., 1996), perhaps because cholesterol from the blood may be used to repair membranes in injured tissues. Thus, in the absence of detailed knowledge about the mechanisms of an effect, it cannot be presumed that consequences of stress from one type of stressor also occur with a distinct type of stressor (even if both can be broadly described as "physical," or both as "emotional"). Specifically, it remains to be determined which forms of "stress," in addition to forced swim, restraint stress, or exposure to heat (the latter two serve a facilitatory role), produce or enhance permeability of the blood-brain barrier.

A second possible interaction may occur through activation of nicotinic receptors on chromaffin cells in the adrenal medulla; increased ACh binding (from increased ACh availability due to PB) may enhance secretion of catecholamines or perhaps potentiate the ability of stress to do so.

Third, the heightened toxicity reported with interactions between PB and adrenergic agents, noted above, may result in part or in whole from effects of PB distinct from those on the adrenal medulla. Studies discussed in Chapter Fourteen report that physostigmine, a carbamate related to PB that readily crosses the blood-brain barrier even in the absence of stress, produces catecholamine surges by a central rather than peripheral mechanism.

A fourth, perhaps speculative mechanism by which PB could interact with stress, leading to death of cells in a region of the brain, is discussed in the footnote.[3]

---

[3]PB could interact with stress to produce chronic neurological change in an area of the brain termed the hippocampus, thought to be involved in memory. Stress produces release of corticosteroids. The hippocampus is uniquely rich in receptors for corticosteroids, and that provides negative feedback regulation for corticosteroids—which holds stress responses in check (Sapolsky, 1992). (Many receptors are also found in an area termed the amygdala that is mentioned in Chapter Eleven, "Multiple Chemical Sensitivity"; this area is also rich in receptors for corticosteroids but

PB and Caffeine

A study previously discussed also examined the effect of caffeine on toxicity from PB and DEET in mice (Chaney, Moss, et al., 1997); see the section on PB and pesticides, above.

PB and Fluoroquinolones

Fluoroquinolones, such as ciprofloxacin (used as an antidiarrheal agent in the PGW), are GABA inhibitors (Committee to Study the Interactions of Drugs, 1996). GABA is the major inhibitory neurotransmitter of the vertebrate nervous system (Saleh, Zied, et al., 1993; Allen and Albuquerque, 1987). GABA released from "interneurons" in the brain activates chloride ion channels in the receiving cell, changing their voltage to make them more resistant to "firing" or sending a signal to other cells. Bromide in PB may influence these chloride channels (see Chapter Ten, "Bromism"); PB may influence the GABA system by this means. Moreover, ACh modulates release of GABA presynaptically (Albuquerque, Boyne, et al., 1995; Lena, Changeux, et al., 1993) (see section on GABA in Chapter Three), so that PB and fluoroquinolones could interact through joint modulation of ACh. (This may be a subtractive interaction, however.)

Fluoroquinolones may also have musculoskeletal and liver effects (Committee to Study the Interactions of Drugs, 1996), offering additional potential sites of interaction.

PB and Nicotine

Interactions with nicotine have played little role in existing investigations into chemical interactions with PB. Because nicotine is a drug well known to affect the acetylcholinergic function—specifically, to amplify action at nicotinic receptors (discussed further in Chapter Thirteen, "Neurotransmitter Dysreg-

---

provides positive rather than negative feedback regulation to the corticosteroid system.) Particularly in an area of the hippocampus termed "CA1," it has been shown that corticosteroids may lead to cell death under certain circumstances—for instance, when there is reduced blood flow or reduced oxygen (Sapolsky and Pulsinelli, 1985; Morse and Davids, 1990; Sapolsky, 1992). But if PB successfully enters the brain, it would engender excessive activity of ACh neurons (as it has been shown to do in studies using mice (Friedman, Kaufer, et al., 1996)), which would be expected to result in increased need for oxygen and bloodflow. If the needs for blood and oxygen exceed the ability to supply it, death of hippocampal neurons may ensue, potentially leading to problems with memory—and perhaps with other functions to which the hippocampus contributes—as well as increased subsequent stress responses. However, this speculation hinges on the supposition first that PB is able to access the brain; and second that the resulting need for blood and oxygen in this region is exceeded. At present these assumptions have not been assessed empirically, although studies in other species could be done. (Exertion, via exercise, might be anticipated to further divert flow of blood.)

ulation")—it is imperative that future research related to PB interactions include potential interactions with nicotine.

PB and Vaccines

Anthrax vaccine was given to an estimated 150,000 individuals in the PGW, while botulinum toxoid vaccine was given to an estimated 8,000. There is evidence that some personnel, particularly special forces and perhaps some on the front lines, received both (see Golomb, forthcoming).

PB and vaccines might interact to increase permeability of the blood-brain barrier. Aluminum, contained in vaccine adjuvants for botulinum toxoid and anthrax vaccines, and cholinergic effects such as those anticipated with PB have both been demonstrated to enhance permeability of the blood-brain barrier (see Chapter Seven, "Blood-Brain Barrier Passage"). Whether this effect of aluminum takes place at the low doses employed in vaccines is not known. Moreover, other exposures may further interact with PB and vaccines to enhance permeability and promote breach of the protection of the blood-brain barrier. These include chemical cocktails involving PB, stress, and pesticides or nerve agent chemical combinations, all of which have also been implicated in increases in blood-brain barrier permeability in animal models (Chapter Seven).

It has also been suggested that at least some vaccines may influence the metabolism of other drugs, perhaps by interfering with the liver cytochrome P450 metabolizing system (Committee to Study the Interactions of Drugs, 1996; Kramer and McClain, 1981). Since the P450 system has been implicated in the metabolism of several drugs that interact with PB (see Chapter Eight, "Individual Differences in Reactions to PB"), the addition of vaccines could amplify the effects of drug interactions among agents that compete for metabolism through this system and through other systems, such as BChE. Finally, aluminum (in vaccines) may reduce the activity of both choline acetyltransferase and AChE, thus affecting the ACh system, another avenue for possible interaction with PB.

There is no direct evidence for an interaction between PB and vaccines used in the PGW. However, there are common sites at which both PB and vaccines may exert an effect, such as the blood-brain barrier and drug-metabolizing systems. Thus, interactions between PB and vaccines are "possible" in accordance with the IOM model, which recognizes possible interactions when there are common sites of effect. However, the presence of such interactions is purely speculative.

PB and Antihistamines

Antihistamines might be speculated to influence central effects of PB by several mechanisms. First, histamine modulates heat-stress-induced increases in blood-brain barrier permeability in animals (resulting from exposure to four hours at 38° C) (Sharma, Nyberg, et al., 1992): H-2 receptor blocker appear to protect against the increase in permeability, while H-1 receptor blockers may enhance it. Second, antihistamines may increase central ACh, possibly potentiating any central effects of PB. Histamine H-2 receptor blockers have been shown to have AChE-inhibiting effects, stronger for ranitidine and nizatidine than for cimetidine (Laine-Cessac, Turcant, et al., 1993); and histamine H-1 receptor blockers have been shown to increase central ACh and ACh action in animal studies (Dringenberg, De Souza-Silva, et al., 1998). The net effect for H-2 blockers is unclear; they may be protective if given before heat is encountered. However histamine H-1 receptor blockers might be expected to doubly heighten the effect of PB, both enhancing PB penetration in conditions of heat and further increasing the excess ACh available centrally. Personnel may have received H-2 blockers for GI complaints and H-1 blockers for allergic problems and perhaps sleep complaints.

PB's Effect on the Immune System

There is no direct evidence for an influence of PB on susceptibility to infection. However, several characteristics of PB would make such an interaction possible. During acute PB administration, enhanced mucociliary clearance due to ACh might be experienced. This acute effect might be reversed on discontinuation of PB if cholinergic downregulation occurs (see Chapter Thirteen). It is thus conceivable that infections transmitted through the "respiratory" route might be facilitated by prior administration of PB. Whether this effect occurs (and if so, what duration of treatment is required and for what duration the downregulation would occur) is not known, but is amenable to scientific inquiry.

The existence of ACh receptors located on immune cells (Schwarz, Glick, et al., 1995; Sastry and Sadavongvivad, 1979) suggests a role for cholinergic activity in the immune system. But the role of the these receptors is not known. Heightened cholinergic activity with active treatment, and suppressed cholinergic activity due to downregulation following treatment, could influence these cells. The nature of the effect, and the consequences of a putative effect, are not known. Rates of infectious diseases (indeed, of all disease and nonbattle injury) among U.S. military personnel in Operation Desert Storm/Operation Desert Shield were quite low relative to wartime expectation (Hyams, Wignall, et al., 1995). Improved data on who received PB might allow evaluation of infectious illness requiring hospitalization in those who did and those who did not receive PB. However, if an unidentified infectious agent were responsible for symptoms that do not lead to hospitalization in PGW veterans (see *A Review of the Scientific Literature As It Pertains to Gulf War Illnesses*, Vol. 1: *Infectious Diseases* (Hilborne and Golomb, 1998)), this approach might not uncover a connection.

In combination with other agents, PB may affect the blood-brain barrier (through its cholinergic effect and possibly through other effects) so that it more readily allows passage of infectious agents (see "Interactions," below). Cholinergic action is believed to enhance the permeability of the blood-brain barrier; and studies have demonstrated that neuropathic viruses that are normally denied access to the CNS may cause fatal disease in animals when the blood-brain barrier is breached by administration of PB; aluminum in vaccines could, theoretically, participate in enhancing the permeability of the blood-brain barrier (see Chapter Seven). However, such neurovirulent but non-neuroinvasive viruses are rare, and there is no evidence of increased CNS infection in PGW veterans.

In summary, there are theoretical reasons PB could affect the immune system or enhance susceptibility to selected infectious diseases. However, there is no evidence that enhanced susceptibility to any class of infection was present in PGW veterans (but see Golomb, forthcoming, chapter on "Mycoplasma.")

Interactions and Individual Differences

Individual differences occur in the properties of enzymes used to metabolize certain drugs, in the levels of such enzymes, in past exposures, and in other endogenous and exogenous factors. These differences might control which individuals experience effects with drug combinations, just as these factors influence which individuals experience benefit and adverse effects with individual drugs. Thus, for instance, individual differences in the enzyme "PON" may influence the rate at which certain cholinesterase inhibitors (other than PB) are broken down—such as certain pesticides and nerve agents. The resulting differences in amount of nerve agent or pesticide in the body may in turn influence the degree to which synergistic toxicity may be produced with the "same" dose of PB. (See Chapter Eight.)[4]

---

[4]For instance, one form of PON is relatively good at metabolizing sarin but relatively bad at metabolizing protein pesticides (Davies, Richter, et al., 1996). For the other form, the reverse is true. Thus, which form of PON is present will determine relative susceptibility to pesticide exposures (that is, levels of pesticide after a given exposure); and pesticide levels in turn condition the degree of synergistic toxicity seen with PB. Thus, individual differences determine differences in sensitivity to other exposures, which in turn influence response to PB.

Unidentified Interactions

PB appears to have many possible interactions. Many such interactions have only recently been identified, as scientific work has just begun to approach this issue. It is likely that as such work continues, additional potential interactions will be identified. Identification of interactions becomes more complex when multiple exposures are considered together, and the full effects of PB interactions may never be known. (This is particularly true because high-quality work on such interactions cannot readily be done in humans, so that data from animal studies must be relied upon.)

STRATEGY FOR TESTING DRUG INTERACTIONS

There is no ideal strategy for testing of long-term effects of PB with other chemicals, for reasons including the following:

1. The number of possible combinations increases rapidly with the number of agents considered, and there are many agents to be considered. (There are $2^n - 1$ interactions when n interacting drugs are considered, counting the effect of each drug given individually.) This effectively eliminates the option of testing all possible interactions. (Even more combinations are obtained when possible timing of interactions is taken into account. For instance, PB may enhance the toxicity of soman if given after soman, but protect against its toxicity if given in advance.)

2. Some agents may protect against the effects of others (or counteract their toxicity), rather than producing synergistic or additive toxicity. Because some agents could mask interactions among others, the strategy of testing all possible interacting agents together and weeding down to a smaller number if an effect is seen, could in theory miss important interactions, interactions that would be seen if the "correct" subset of chemicals were examined. Nonetheless, this may be a reasonable first approach.

3. Human studies designed exclusively to identify adverse effects, such as those from interactions among possible toxins, are usually unacceptable for ethical reasons; however, no animal model can accurately reflect the human physiology and the constants and the diversity that will influence toxic interactions.

Bearing in mind these significant limitations, it is necessary to accept some approach to systematically evaluating drug interactions as possible causes of illnesses in PGW veterans. One approach might consist of conducting a first-step screen for interactions by starting with multiple agents and paring down contributing factors, as follows:

- Select the set of exposures of interest. This set may include PB, low-level nerve agent, the anthrax and botulinum vaccines, caffeine, nicotine, petrochemical products, and some form of stress. Use per-kg doses somewhat higher than those employed in humans, to take into account differences in native sensitivity and differences in the sensitivity of available outcome measures (animals cannot be queried regarding whether they feel fatigue or experience discomfort). Employ routes of exposure similar to those experienced by PGW veterans, or justify the use of other routes.

- Select several animal models that have desirable characteristics: No model will be ideal, and interactions uncovered in any suitable model may merit further evaluation. For example, the hen might be selected for the sensitivity to OPIDN that it shares with primates, but mammals should also be tested.

- Select the outcome variables of interest. These should, where possible, include variables that reflect systems prominent in complaints of PGW veterans, who commonly report joint symptoms, cognitive symptoms, sleep symptoms, and reduced energy and/or fatigue. Thus, one might choose a complex learning task, a test of movement strength, sleep studies (including circadian rhythms of endogenous hormones), and measures of activity.

- Test a set of animals with all exposures concurrently. Note that this approach will not be effective if some exposures negate the side effects of others. Where such instances can be identified, additional testing might be performed excluding each such exposure.

- If a relevant effect is seen, undertake binary partitioning of exposures for repeat testing. (That is, test half the exposures, then the other half. If one "daughter" half maintains the adverse interaction, repartition that set. If neither does, recombine exposures and select a different partition.) If at any point the effect is lost, perform a repartition, recombining elements that have been separated in the partitioning. PB might, for instance, reduce the side effects of soman.

This approach, like others, has significant limitations, and other approaches may be preferred.

CONCLUSION

Drug-drug and drug-chemical interactions involving PB cannot be excluded as a contributor to illnesses in PGW veterans: The effect of PB may be enhanced by the presence of other agents. For instance, if metabolism of PB is interfered with or if PB is assisted in gaining access to the brain, PB may, analogously, enhance the effect or toxicity of other agents; PB and chemically similar agents, or those affecting similar processes, may affect those processes additively or synergistically; or new effects may occur that would not be predicted from each drug individually. Thus, toxic effects of PB could be enhanced through interactions with other drugs or exposures, toxic effects of other drugs could be enhanced through interactions with PB; or new unexpected effects could ensue.

SCIENTIFIC RECOMMENDATIONS

- Current information on exposure to PB in individual veterans is weak, making it difficult to use epidemiological evidence to assess the possibility that PB, alone or in concert with other agents, is tied to illnesses in PGW veterans. Self-report information may be the best information available. Further attempts should be made to evaluate the presence of other exposures in ill and well PGW veterans. Where objective or record information is available, it should be used, but information on these exposures may be gauged, if necessary, by self-report. This exposure data should be evaluated against outcome information. Thus, an effort should be made to evaluate whether PB exposure in the PGW is associated with symptoms in PGW veterans and whether co-administration of PB with other agents, exposures, or individual factors was associated with heightened risk. (Some such efforts have been made; see Chapter Fourteen, "Chronic Effects.")

- Continued efforts should be made to evaluate the interaction among PB, pesticides, and insect repellents used in the PGW. Evidence is now available in widely divergent species to suggest interactions between PB and (high doses of) DEET, chlorpyrifos, and permethrin. Further work should be performed to examine interactions using dosing schedules and routes of delivery closer to what may have been experienced by veterans and outcome measures more reflective of complaints of PGW veterans (along with physiologic measures). This includes long-term follow-up data after exposure is discontinued. Because nicotine also influences (heightens) activity at (nicotinic) ACh receptors, consideration should be given to testing interactions that include nicotine.

- Further effort should be made to examine, using controlled experimental studies in animals, the effects of various exposures, alone and in combination, that might be hypothesized to compromise the blood-brain barrier, enhancing its permeability to PB and other substances. These exposures include PB itself, stress, heat, caffeine, antihistamines, pesticides and insect repellents, nerve agents, and aluminum from vaccines.

- Consideration should be given to testing a "cocktail" of PGW exposures against a set of carefully devised outcomes. If outcomes are positive, the test should be repeated following successive binary splitting. (Clearly, the split need not be exactly binary and will not be unless the number of candidate exposures is a power of two.) If no effect is found in either split even though an effect was seen in the parent, then an adding-back process can be initiated until the effect is reconstituted. This process may be iterated to identify the pertinent interaction(s).

Chapter Ten

BROMISM

DOES ACCUMULATION OF THE BROMIDE FROM PB PRODUCE BROMISM?

Intake of excessive bromide can induce a condition termed *bromism*, with neurological, psychiatric, dermatological, and possibly endocrine effects. It has been suggested that intake of PB by PGW veterans may have induced symptoms of bromism, which may account for some illnesses in PGW veterans (Allan, 1997). This chapter evaluates the evidence for this hypothesis, briefly reviewing the symptoms, diagnosis, treatment, and mechanism of bromism and the possible relationship of illnesses in PGW veterans to bromism from PB ingestion.

It is concluded that the relatively low doses and short duration of bromide administration in PGW veterans, and the usually self-limiting nature of bromism, which normally abates following discontinuation of bromide-containing substances, suggest against bromism as a significant cause of ongoing illnesses in PGW veterans.

SYMPTOMS OF BROMISM

Bromide intoxication, from prolonged consumption of excessive doses of bromide, may cause protean symptoms, particularly psychiatric, cognitive, neurological, and dermatologic. Symptoms may be incorrectly perceived as "psychosomatic" (Pelckmans, Verdickt, et al., 1983), or may lead falsely to other diagnoses.

Psychiatric symptoms may include, in the earlier stages, disinhibition, self-neglect, fatigue, sluggishness, impairment of memory and concentration, irritability or emotional instability, and depression. Symptoms of more advanced disease may include confusion but occasionally schizophrenic-like psychotic behavior or hallucinations in clear consciousness. Behavior may become violent, especially at night. There may be severe auditory or visual hallucinations, or both. There may be clouding of consciousness, including stupor and coma

(Horowitz, 1997; Fried and Malek-Ahmadi, 1975; Wacks, Oster, et al., 1990; Carney, 1973).

Neurological abnormalities of "all kinds" occur, including headache, tremor, slurred speech, spontaneous movements, incoordination, ataxia (abnormal gait), tendon reflex changes (increased or decreased reflexes), and extensor plantar responses (abnormal reflexes that signify "upper motor neuron" disease, disease in the brain or spinal cord that affects nerve signaling to the muscles) (Horowitz, 1997; Fried and Malek-Ahmadi, 1975; Wacks, Oster, et al., 1990; Carney, 1973). Vision changes have included decreased visual acuity often in conjunction with enlarged and poorly reacting pupils; disturbances of color perception, photophobia (abnormal sensitivity to light), micropsia and macropsia (perception of things as smaller or larger than they are), blurring of vision, and the quite characteristic mydriasis (enlarged pupils) (Levin, 1960; Kunze, 1976).

EEG: Generalized slowing of the EEG has been reported (Carney, 1973).

Dermatologic: Some patients will develop "bromoderma," an acne-like "papular" (raised) eruption of the face and hands (Horowitz, 1997; Wacks, Oster, et al., 1990); a "macular" (nonraised) rash may also be seen (Carney, 1973). In one case series, four of six bromism patients had abnormal pigmentation, usually of the sun-exposed areas (Carney, 1973).

Acute bromism is seldom seen because the bromide ion is irritating to the GI tract and produces vomiting before sufficient blood levels can be reached to cause bromism from short-term use. However, chronic bromism may develop—bromide is excreted slowly through the kidney, giving it the opportunity to build up in the body through ongoing ingestion (Morgan and Weaver, 1969).

DIAGNOSIS OF BROMISM

Diagnosis of bromism is often difficult due to the protean manifestations of bromism, and physicians' failure to consider bromism as a cause of illness. Above all, diagnosis requires "clinical suspicion"—that is, the physician must *consider* the diagnosis or it will be missed.

Bromism was substantially more common prior to removal from the market of certain over-the-counter remedies high in bromide, such as Bromo-Seltzer and Miles Nervine (Wacks, Oster, et al., 1990); it was particularly common in the 1930s and 1940s but is substantially less so since the 1970s. Because of its relative rarity, physicians are less likely to consider bromism in the differential diagnosis, so that many cases may remain undiagnosed or misdiagnosed

(Horowitz, 1997). One report observes that in almost every case report in the literature, including their own, the diagnosis of bromism was delayed while other causes of illness, including acute psychiatric or neurological illness, were considered (Horowitz, 1997). Another observes that "Perhaps because he regards it as extinct, the family doctor almost invariably fails to recognize bromism, even when, as in four of my (six) cases, he was the source of the supply" (Carney, 1973).

In the presence of clinical suspicion (typically arising from signs or symptoms of neurological or psychiatric disturbance without other identified cause), (1) a careful review of prescription and over-the-counter medications should be undertaken to elicit use of medications that may contain bromide. A dietary history may also be helpful; one report has implicated excessive consumption of colas containing brominated vegetable oil (Horowitz, 1997). Absence of identification of bromide-containing agents should not thwart further inquiry, as in some instances the source of bromide is never determined (Battin and Varkey, 1982); for this reason it has been suggested that bromide intoxication be considered "in the differential diagnosis of obscure, unusual, or refractory psychiatric symptomatology" (Battin and Varkey, 1982). (2) A chemistry panel should be obtained to evaluate presence of hyperchloremia, which may occur in the absence of a negative anion gap (Horowitz, 1997), and to allow calculation of the anion gap (Wacks, Oster, et al., 1990; Horowitz, 1997). Where suspicion directs, (3) serum bromide level should be secured (Wacks, Oster, et al., 1990). A serum bromide concentration above 50 mg/dL is considered confirmatory (Carney, 1973), and significant symptoms usually do not occur below this level (but see section on "Low-Level Bromism," below).

TREATMENT OF BROMISM

The most important element of treatment is cessation of bromide exposure. Additional treatment of bromide toxicity has traditionally involved saline loading (administration of large quantities of sodium chloride in water, typically by vein), which enhances kidney excretion of bromide. The chloride ion from sodium chloride competes with and replaces the bromide ion throughout the body. While the usual half-life of bromide (the time for half the body's complement of bromide to be eliminated) is 12 to 14 days (Horowitz, 1997), a half-life of 65 hours has been calculated with saline loading. Cases failing to respond to saline loading have been successfully treated with mannitol or "loop" diuretics (a type of diuretic, or water-excretion enhancing agent, that acts on a specific part of the kidney), and one report calculated a half-life of 1.65 hours with "diuresis," using the agents mannitol and ethacrynic acid (Horowitz, 1997). Hemodialysis has been used to treat bromism. Calculated bromide half-lives with hemodialysis in different case reports have been 1.78 hours (in a case report from 1951) (Merrill and Weller, 1952), 0.9 hours, and 1.38 hours in a more recent case report (Horowitz, 1997). Hemodialysis led to prompt resolution of focal neurological signs in a patient who failed to respond to saline (sodium chloride solution) (Horowitz, 1997). Patients with a depressed mental status due to bromism, or with bromide levels in excess of 200 mg/dL (25 mmol/L) may not achieve nontoxic levels (without treatment) for almost a month and would require five days of saline loading to achieve levels below 50 mg/dL (6.3 mmol/L), the threshold of what is normally construed as the toxic level (Horowitz, 1997). Therefore, in these cases it may be appropriate to use hemodialysis to remove the bromide ion from the blood rather than relying on the kidney (Horowitz, 1997).

CAUSES OF BROMISM

Causes of bromism are reviewed here to allow the reader to evaluate the likelihood of interactions between PB and other agents that may contribute to bromism.

Cases of bromism have been reported with consumption of bromide-containing prescription and nonprescription medications, including PB in one reported case (in a patient with myasthenia gravis, receiving longer duration and higher-dose treatment than PGW veterans) (Wacks, Oster, et al., 1990), sleeping medications, and tonics; with consumption of cola that contains brominated vegetable oil; and with consumption of bromide-tainted well water (Fried and Malek-Ahmadi, 1975).

Most cases represent one of three groups: organic bromides, bromoureides, and biotransformation of bromide compounds (Horowitz, 1997). "Organic bromides" include the salts of sodium, potassium, and ammonium bromide; these salts have been available since 1857, with wide use during the 1930s and 1940s as sleep aids and antiepilepsy drugs (Horowitz, 1997). In 1938, bromide sales in the United States were surpassed only by sales of aspirin (Horowitz, 1997). However, many patients admitted to psychiatric institutions were found to suffer from bromism from overuse of these products, rather than from the psychiatric illnesses for which they had been incorrectly diagnosed, and the use of these products thereafter decreased until they were withdrawn from the market in 1975. Widely cited culprits included the sedative Nervine, produced by Miles Laboratory, which contained all three bromide salts; and Bromo-Seltzer, which contained 3.2 milliequivalents per teaspoon (mEq/tsp) of sodium bromide (Horowitz, 1997). Since these agents were withdrawn from the market, bromism has been far less frequent. "Bromoureides" are sedative-hypnotics available primarily in Europe, including Bromisovalum (Bromural) and carbromal (Carbitral) (Horowitz, 1997). Occasional reports of bromism from long-term overuse have been reported (Maes, Huyghens, et al., 1985). Finally, of particular relevance here, bromide released through the "biotransformation" of medications containing the bromide ion is an infrequent cause of bromism. PB and dextromethorphan bromide (used in cough medicine) have been reported to cause bromism. Anesthesia with the agent "halothane" will increase bromide levels, peaking at two to three days postanesthesia. Pesticide residues from common agricultural fumigants, such as "methyl bromide" and "ethylene dibromide," may elevate the bromide content of vegetables, but bromide toxicity has not been reported from this source (Horowitz, 1997).

MECHANISM OF BROMISM

It is assumed that bromide acts by replacing part of the chloride in the body (Blumberg and Nelp, 1966). In spite of the use of bromides for their anti-epileptic action for more than a century, we know little about the action of bromide on the cellular level in the CNS other than that it may influence synaptic processes by its action on the transport systems (Kunze, 1976), or by substituting for chloride ions in actions of neurotransmitters. (Neurotransmitters classically communicate by producing membrane voltage changes through the movement of ions, including chloride, through specialized ion channels associated with neurotransmitter receptors on the signal-receiving cell. For instance GABA, or gamma amino butyric acid, the chief inhibitory neurotransmitter in the brain, functions through specialized chloride ion channels (Allen and Albuquerque, 1987).)

Regional cerebral blood flow, that is, blood flow to different parts of the brain, may also be altered with bromism. Regional cerebral blood flow was assessed in a case of bromide psychosis using radioactive xenon (^{133}Xe) inhalation (Berglund, Nielsen, et al., 1977). On the first exam, when the serum bromide level was 45 mEq/L (extremely high, within the potentially lethal range), the cerebral blood flow was reduced to approximately one-third of normal, with abnormal regional flow characterized by low flow in regions of the cortex, including frontal and parieto-occipital regions. Dialysis led to improvement in the clinical condition, and restoration of regional cerebral blood flow (Berglund, Nielsen, et al., 1977). Changes in regional cerebral blood flow—reflecting or perhaps influencing altered regional neuronal activity in the brain—could relate to symptoms of bromism.

BROMIDE LEVELS THAT RESULT IN BROMISM

Serum bromide levels at which toxic symptoms appear are extremely variable (see Table 10.1); nonetheless, symptoms are seldom seen at plasma concen-

Table 10.1

Bromide Blood Concentration and Toxicity

mg/dL	mEq/L = mmol/L	Toxicity
< 50	<6.3	"Therapeutic"
50–100	6.3–12.5	Possible toxicity
100–200	12.5–25	Usually serious toxicity
200–300	25–37.5	Possible coma
>300	>37.5	Possibly fatal

SOURCE: Ellenhorn, Schonwald, et al., 1997.

trations under 50 mg/dl (6.3 mEq/L); symptoms are commonly seen at concentrations between 50 and 100 mg/dl (6.3–12.5 mEq/L); and symptoms are almost invariable when the serum concentration exceeds 100 mg/dl (Ellenhorn, Schonwald, et al., 1997; Gaff, Rand, et al., 1969). At 200–300 mg/dl (25–37.5 mEq/L) coma may occur, and levels exceeding 300 mg/dl (37.5 mEq/L) may be lethal (Morgan and Weaver, 1969; Ellenhorn, Schonwald, et al., 1997), although mortality from bromism is low (Morgan and Weaver, 1969).

Of note, chronic use of bromide-containing drugs may result in serum bromide levels capable of interfering with chloride measurements without causing signs or symptoms of overt bromide toxicity. In one reported case of a myasthenic patient taking a total daily dose of 360 mg of PB (four times the daily PGW dose, and 110.4 mg bromide per day) (Wacks, Oster, et al., 1990), this measurement problem occurred. The patient was admitted with symptoms of myasthenia (but no symptoms of bromism). The abnormal anion gap was noticed in the course of evaluation of the patient for symptoms of reduced muscle strength, facial weakness, and slurred speech, compatible with myasthenia undertreatment or overtreatment. Serum bromide was 8.1 mEq/L (64.8 mg/dL).

A double-blind study has been performed in which several subjective and objective outcomes were evaluated following three months of bromide administration. Men and women receiving 0, 4, or 9 mg/kg/d of bromide (seven subjects in each group) for 12 weeks reported decreased ability to concentrate and increased sleepiness (among men only) who received bromide; and a statistically significant increase in several measures of thyroid function (among women only) (Sangster, Blom, et al., 1983). Mean plasma bromide at the end of treatment was 0.08, 2.14, and 4.30 mEq/liter in males; and 0.07, 3.05, and 4.93 mEq/liter for females, for the 0, 4, and 9 mg/kg/d groups, respectively. (The conversion is 8 mg/dL for 1 mmol/L, or 1 mEq/L). No changes were observed in measurements of hormones produced in the adrenals, the gonads, and the pituitary gland (Sangster, Blom, et al., 1983).

Of note: A study in rats found a significant decrease in thyroid function among female rats. Other rodent studies have reported (1) that bromide behaves more like iodine than like chlorine in the thyroid (iodine administration can induce hypo- or hyperthyroidism); and (2) that bromide can produce changes in thyroid hormones T4 and T3, in the absence of changes in thyroid-stimulating hormone (Vobecky and Babicky 1994; Vobecky, Babicky, et al., 1996a; Vobecky, Babicky, et al. 1996b; Velicky, Titlbach, et al., 1997a; Velicky, Titlbach, et al., 1997b; Velicky, Titlbach, et al., 1998). In humans, the action of PB in particular on thyroid-related hormones is well known, and PB is used in testing of certain thyroid hormone responses. It ordinarily enhances the release of a pituitary hormone, thyroid-stimulating hormone, in response to administration of a hypothalamic hormone, thyrotropin-releasing hormone (Coiro, Volpi, et al., 1998).

LOW-LEVEL BROMISM

It is said that bromism seldom produces symptoms at blood levels below 50 mg/dL (Ellenhorn, Schonwald, et al., 1997). Most reports note dramatic neuropsychiatric symptoms associated with markedly high serum levels of bromide. Only the Sangster study, described above systematically evaluated the dose of bromide at which more subtle symptoms may become manifest in a double-blind trial. This study suggested the possibility, requiring confirmation, that men may be subject to mild sleep abnormalities and concentration difficulties and women may develop thyroid abnormalities at serum levels slightly below this 50 mg/dL (Sangster, Blom, et al., 1983; however, these levels remain substantially higher than levels of bromide that would be expected from doses of PB given to PGW veterans.

Several studies have cited instances of bromide toxicity at doses of serum bromide under those usually viewed as toxic (Sayed, 1976; Gerner, 1978), as low as 25 mg/dL (Battin and Varkey, 1982). Individual susceptibility varies greatly and it has been suggested that following prolonged intoxication serum levels may not accurately reflect nervous system involvement. (However, prolonged intoxication was quite unlikely to have characterized the PGW experience.) Moreover, toxic states may depend more on other factors. Suggested factors include the "general mental state," "premorbid personality" (both may be reflections of prior neurochemical state), duration of ingestion, state of hydration, and electrolyte balance of the patient (Battin and Varkey, 1982; Whybrow and Ewing, 1966; Freedman, Kaplan, et al., 1978)).

TIME-COURSE OF RESOLUTION OF BROMISM

The untreated half-life of bromide (time for half the initial blood amount to be excreted) administered orally is approximately 12 days (Vaiseman, Koren, et al., 1986); the half-life with saline is several days (about 65 hours), and a half-life as low as one hour has been reported with hemodialysis (see section on "Treatment"). Evidently there is no "slowly exchangeable" pool of bromide (bromide sequestered somewhere in the body where it is not readily eliminated); rather all bromide appeared to be "easily exchangeable" because adding a small amount of radiolabeled bromide (Br^{82}) in a case of severe chronic bromide intoxication showed rapid and apparently complete equilibration of the stable and radioactive bromide (Blumberg and Nelp, 1966). The plasma-specific activity (radiolabeled bromide in counts per minute, or "cpm," divided by fraction of unlabeled bromide in mEq) remained constant as the plasma bromide decreased, and the bromide space (volume of distribution in liters) remained approximately constant).

Most reported cases resolve promptly with treatment of bromism through saline diuresis (sodium chloride delivery with enhanced urination) or hemodialysis. However, several reports indicate instances of partial resolution with long-lasting sequelae (see section on "Long-Term Symptoms").

BROMISM DUE TO PB

In one report, PB at doses of 60 mg three times daily plus 180 mg at bedtime (four times the daily PGW dose) was associated with a negative anion gap[1] and a bromide level of 65.1 mg/dl (8.1 mEq/L) (Wacks, Oster, et al., 1990); although this bromide level is compatible with symptoms of bromism, no such symptoms were reported. Another report implicates PB in generation of bromism (Rothenberg, Berns, et al., 1990). However doses of PB administered in these

---

[1]The "anion gap" (or difference between measured cations and measured anions) is calculated by subtracting the sum of anions (negatively charged ions of chloride and bicarbonate, in mEq/L, that are measured in the blood in a routine chemistry panel) from the major cation (positively charged ions of sodium, in mEq/L). The normal anion gap ranges from about 12 to 16 mEq/L. (An alternative strategy adds the potassium to the sodium prior to subtracting the chloride and bicarbonate, leading to a slightly different normal range). Because the anions and cations in the body are balanced—that is, total anions are equal in number to total cations in the blood—therefore measured anions ("MA") plus unmeasured anions ("UA") equals measured cations ("MC") plus unmeasured cations ("UC"). Rearranging the equation, measured cations minus measured anions (the anion gap) is equal to unmeasured anions minus unmeasured cations: (MC–MA) = (UA–UC). Bromide might be thought to be an unmeasured anion, and is increased—so one might suppose that the anion gap would be increased compared to usual. However, bromide interferes with many or all existing measures of chloride and produces a (spurious) increase in the measured chloride. (Thus, bromide is in a sense actually measured, though as chloride, and not necessarily in 1:1 proportion to its presence.) The "ion selective method" for chloride evaluation ("potentiometry") exhibits the greatest interference, while "colorimetry" (also called "photometry," or the "thiocyanate method") produces a lesser elevation of the reported chloride, and "coulometry" produces the least. Potentiometry may reveal a strongly negative anion gap, while a positive, normal or nearly normal anion gap may appear with the coulometry method (Wacks, Oster, et al., 1990). However, most major methods of chloride determination are affected by bromide (Elin, Robertson, et al., 1981).

reports were substantially higher than in PGW veterans, and such reports are rare.

LONG-TERM SYMPTOMS

Persistent Symptoms Following Bromism

Several case reports of bromism have noted the presence of persistent symptoms attributed to bromism that lasted beyond the time of elevated blood bromide levels.[2]

Such case reports are rare, and it is difficult to exclude the possibility of concurrent pathology leading to persistent symptoms. That is, the residual symptoms, associated with observed cerebral atrophy, a seizure disorder, and a history of head trauma in the second case, could have had an independent cause. Neither can one exclude an effect or interaction of bromide with other drugs given prior to or during treatment, including in these instances the treatment agents clomethiazol or mercaptomerin. However, persistent effects resulting from bromism must be considered a possibility. Long-term effects from chronic regional cerebral blood flow abnormalities or from chronic chloride ion channel alterations (see "Causes of Bromism," above) could be hypothesized to relate to persisting effects. It is conceivable, but certainly not demonstrated, that prolonged hypoperfusion of selected brain regions with ongoing bromide

---

[2]Cases of persistent symptoms attributed to bromism: In one case, a 40-year-old woman initially showed "typical symptoms and signs of chronic bromide intoxication," including psychiatric symptoms, such as irritability and lethargy, a 30-pound weight loss, hand tremor, and minor gait difficulties while taking about 5 gm per day of bromdiathylacetylcarbamid as a sedative (Kunze, 1976). She developed a delirious state (fluctuating mental function) when the bromide-containing drug was stopped by a physician. (Such transient delirium has been not infrequently reported with bromide discontinuation.) Although the psychiatric symptoms cleared rapidly, the neurological state deteriorated; the most severe neurological state appeared 8 to 10 days after the drug was stopped, including a resting tremor of the head and upper extremities and a marked cerebellar dysfunction with severe generalized incoordination (ataxia) but without nystagmus. (Nystagmus is a rhythmic oscillation of the eyeballs that occurs, for a few cycles, with gaze far to one side, but is prolonged with some kinds of nervous system dysfunction.) The patient received a drug called Clomethiazol during this period, but no other CNS-toxic drugs, and all neuropsychiatric symptoms were assumed to result from bromism and the cessation of the bromide containing agent. A year after discharge from the hospital, despite some initial improvement, the patient was left with a mild dysarthric speech (altered speech production caused by difficulty performing the muscle movement involved in speech), a mild gait ataxia, and a moderate ataxia of her upper extremities so that writing was almost impossible. She had a marked constriction of her visual fields (that is, a loss of peripheral vision) which could be verified by formal testing (Kunze, 1976).

In the second case, a 60-year-old woman who had taken at least four teaspoons daily of triple bromide elixir for seven years, prescribed for a post-head-injury seizure condition, was hospitalized with bizarre behavior and hallucinations and a serum bromide concentration of 44.6 mEq/l. She was treated with isotonic saline and daily injections of mercaptomerin sodium (Thiomeri), but even after serum bromide levels fell to below 4 mEq/L and her mental state improved considerably, a significant deficit in orientation and memory remained. A pneumoencephalogram showed bilateral cerebral atrophy, which was presumed responsible for the residual abnormalities.

intoxication could engender permanent changes, perhaps with frank loss of neurons or supporting glia, or reduction in synaptic contacts. It is also possible that chronic substitution of bromide for chloride could affect chloride channel behavior in the CNS, with consequent altered neurotransmission, leading to compensatory changes in neurotransmitter regulation. Still, such changes would be unlikely to be produced with short-term use of relatively low doses of bromide, such as occurred in PGW veterans taking PB.

Persistent Symptoms Following Bromisovalum

Bromisovalum has been reported to cause toxic symptoms, which in some instances are prolonged or permanent. In one series of eight cases with persistent symptoms, initial bromide levels were 105–169 mg/dl (with a mean of 140 mg/dl) (Harenko, 1967). The principal symptom was gait ataxia in all cases, with difficulty maintaining balance and staggering (8/8); then dysarthria (difficulty producing the muscle actions of speech) (6/8), exaggerated deep tendon reflexes of lower limbs (4/8), nystagmus (1/8), positive Babinski reflex (a pathological reflex) (1/8), tongue deviation to one side (1/8), and auditory impairment (Harenko, 1967). Changes in the eye, as seen with an ophthalmoscope ("fundal" changes), and impaired vision had been previously reported as irreversible lesions caused by bromisovalum, but were not encountered in these cases. Compared to patients who achieved complete recovery from bromisovalum poisoning, no differences were established in age, sex, duration and degree of abuse, prior illness, serum bromide level, symptoms, and severity of the subacute phase. Factors speculated to predispose individuals to persistent symptoms were recurrence of severe intoxication states, poor nutritional and general condition, and overlong continuance of the toxic condition (Harenko, 1967). It has been suggested that persisting symptoms with bromisovalum may result not from bromide ion or bromisovalum itself, but from 3-methylbutyrylurea (a breakdown product) or its metabolites (Harenko, 1967). Nonetheless, similarities between symptoms with bromisovalum toxicity and with bromide intoxication are sufficient for a common mechanism to be operative.

It is not possible to exclude a role for bromide in the two cases with symptoms that persisted long after elevated blood bromide levels would be presumed to be normal (or in the cases of prolonged symptoms with bromisovalum); nonetheless, these reports are rare and occurred in patients who ingested bromide at high doses for prolonged periods. Therefore, their experiences cannot be presumed to extend to PGW veterans who experienced low doses of bromide for brief periods.

BROMIDE INTERACTIONS

There is wide variation in the level of blood bromide at which symptoms of bromism begin. Arteriosclerosis, alcoholism, dehydration, malnutrition, psychosis, or heart disease may reportedly cause an earlier onset of symptoms with lower blood levels (Morgan and Weaver, 1969). There is little information to assess whether other conditions or exposures occurring concurrently may cause bromide to induce a chronic condition, persisting beyond the time of high blood bromide levels.

AMOUNT OF BROMIDE IN PB GIVEN TO PGW VETERANS

60 mg of PB as Mestinon (the commercially available form of PB in the United States) contains 18.4 mg (30.6 percent) of bromide (Wacks, Oster, et al., 1990). Therefore, the expected daily dose of bromide in PGW veterans receiving PB as a pretreatment adjunct, at 30 mg three times daily, is 27.6 mg/day of bromide. As the prior section indicates, even far higher doses (9 mg/kg/day, or about 630 mg/day—about 23 times the PGW dose) administered for much longer time (12 weeks, compared to usually under two weeks for PGW veterans) produce bromide levels of 4.3 mmol/L, or about 34.4 mg/dL, still well under the 50 mg/dL that is generally viewed as the lower bound for toxic effects. Thus doses and durations of treatment with PB in PGW personnel would be highly unlikely to reach toxic levels. Although there are reports of chronic bromide ingestion on the range of four times the PGW dose leading to potentially toxic bromide levels, because PGW veterans received lower doses of PB and seldom for more than very short periods, it is highly unlikely that bromism from PB was a substantial contributor to illness in most veterans. It is conceivable that some veterans may have received higher and/or more prolonged doses of PB (some report durations of PB usage as long as six months or report taking two pills with each dose) and also had especially high native susceptibility; even so this would imply development of bromism at lower doses of PB than have been reported, and this is unlikely to be a significant contributor to illnesses in PGW veterans.

BROMISM AS A CAUSE OF PGW ILLNESSES

Neurological and psychiatric symptoms, including memory loss, as well as dermatological symptoms, including rashes, are common to bromism and to illnesses in PGW veterans. Nonetheless, short-term use of PB, at 30 mg three times daily for periods seldom exceeding two weeks, would appear to be an unlikely cause of long-term illness due to bromism in PGW veterans, because the low daily dose of bromide administered and the short time period of administration make it exceedingly unlikely that toxic bromide levels would be reached unless unknown interactions with other exposures are at play.

In clinical reports of bromism, symptoms have generally cleared quickly with clearance of bromide; exceptions have typically involved chronic use with high doses and perhaps repeated toxicity. The relatively long half-life of bromide in the absence of treatment for bromism (approximately 12 to 14 days) remains quite short in comparison to duration of symptoms reported by many veterans. Even extreme bromism would be expected to resolve spontaneously in a month or two after bromide-containing agents are discontinued; and myasthenics taking substantially higher doses of PB (e.g., 12 times as high) for much longer times have seldom been reported to experience bromism, even when serum bromide levels were elevated and anion gaps modified. In contradistinction to the acetylcholinergic effects of PB, which might be expected to differ for myasthenics and PGW veterans, no reason has been identified that would suggest that bromide metabolism should differ systematically between myasthenics and PGW service personnel. Thus, although it is conceivable that experience with a much larger population, as seen in the PGW, would unveil a hitherto unrecognized longer-term syndrome at low doses, it would be expected to affect a relative minority of subjects reporting continued illnesses following participation in the PGW.

SCIENTIFIC RECOMMENDATIONS

There is insufficient evidence to warrant placing a high priority on additional testing of bromism as a cause of long-term illnesses in PGW veterans.

If studies on drug-drug or drug-chemical interactions are undertaken, using drug and chemical exposures in the PGW, addition of bromide to study regimens may be considered. (This may assist in unraveling relative contributions of AChE inhibition and bromide, if effects appear to involve PB as an interactant.)

SUMMARY ANALYSIS

Compatible exposure? Bromide exposure occurred in all veterans receiving PB; the cumulative bromide dose, however, appears too low to be consistent with bromism, based on a best reading of present literature.

Compatible symptoms? Some ill veterans report some neuropsychiatric symptoms crudely compatible with symptoms of bromism

Compatible relation of exposure to symptoms? Exposure to PB for longer durations and at higher doses would be more likely to produce bromism; however, seldom was the cumulative dose of PB received sufficient for production of bromism by our current understanding of bromism from decades of former use of bromide-containing agents. Disappearance of symptoms with a defined time-course after discontinuation of PB would be expected if bromism were the cause. This resolution of symptoms has not been widely reported. Thus, dose and time-course of exposure, and the relation to existence and time-course of illnesses, do not favor bromism as a cause.

Chapter Eleven

MULTIPLE CHEMICAL SENSITIVITY

DOES PB LEAD TO MCS?

Multiple chemical sensitivity (MCS) is a putative condition without a widely accepted clinical case definition, in which persons report new subjective sensitivity to low-level exposures to multiple chemicals and foods, typically following a (self-reported) environmental exposure to pesticides, organic solvents, or building remodeling. The condition has also recently been termed "toxicant-induced loss of tolerance" (TILT) (Miller, 1997; Miller, Ashford, et al., 1997). Symptoms referable to multiple organ systems are reported by subjects with MCS; these include ear-nose-and-throat, CNS, GI, genitourinary, skin, and musculoskeletal symptoms, among others (Davidoff and Keyl, 1996; Miller and Mitzel, 1995).

Many ill veterans report new intolerances to chemicals (Gordon 1997), and some studies are underway to further assess chemical sensitivity in ill PGW veterans (Fiedler, Kipen, et al., 1996).

The lack of a clinical case definition for either MCS or illnesses in PGW veterans complicates examination of a connection between these two phenomena. Nonetheless, several factors are consistent with a connection between illnesses in some PGW veterans, and "toxicant-induced loss of tolerance," or MCS. Similar exposures, namely to acetylcholinesterase-inhibiting agents, characterize ill PGW veterans and many MCS patients. Some work is beginning to *suggest* mechanisms by which cholinergic exposures, experienced by some PGW veterans, could induce chemical sensitivity. These mechanisms include partial kindling of the limbic system and alteration of nasopharyngeal mucosal function. Studies have found that similar EEG abnormalities may characterize persons with selected AChE inhibition exposures seen during the PGW (sarin, OP pesticides) and persons with MCS, though it has not been shown that ill PGW veterans with consistent symptoms share these EEG abnormalities (neither has it been shown that they do not). SPECT studies (single photon emission computerized tomography, which evaluates regional cerebral blood flow) in a small segment of PGW veterans with chemical sensitivities have reportedly been abnormal, as have SPECT scans in individuals exposed to pesticides (see Chapter Fourteen, "Chronic Effects"), although larger samples of all veterans and controls should be evaluated using blinded testing. At present, it is premature to accept a connection between illnesses in PGW veterans and MCS; however, it is premature to reject the possibility of such a connection. Further study is warranted. The following text explores these issues in greater detail.

MCS CASE DEFINITION

While no case definition is universally accepted, several attempts at a case definition for MCS have been made (See review in Miller, 1994). According to one researcher, "MCS is an acquired disorder characterized by recurrent symptoms, referable to multiple organ systems, occurring in response to demonstrable exposure to many chemically unrelated compounds at doses far below those established in the general population to cause harmful effects. No single widely accepted test of physiologic function can be shown to correlate with symptoms" (Cullen, 1987). Although exposures that produce symptoms are far below legal exposure levels, it has been stated that no-effect levels for chemical exposures from chronic animal studies are often orders of magnitude below current legal exposure limits (Ziem, 1992). Another researcher suggests five criteria for MCS: Symptoms are reproducible with exposure; condition is chronic; low levels of exposure result in manifestations of the syndrome; symptoms resolve with removal of the incitants; and responses occur to multiple chemically unrelated substances (Nethercott, Davidoff et al., 1993).

MCS ETIOLOGY

No objective correlate has been identified for MCS. Not surprisingly, then, many theories of causation have been advanced (Rest, 1992), including immune dysfunction (Levin and Byers, 1992; Albright and Goldstein, 1992) (not confirmed, see Simon, Daniell, et al., 1993), respiratory epithelium dysfunction (Bascom, 1992), behavioral or biological conditioning (see "Limbic Kindling," below), psychiatric illness (Staudenmayer, Selner, et al., 1993; Gots, Hamoosh, et al., 1993) and cultural suggestion or "overvalued beliefs" (Staudenmayer, Selner, et al., 1993). For a cogent review of some of these theories, see Sparks, et al. (1994). The present text will concentrate on theories and mechanisms that may relate use of PB and other PGW exposures to development of an MCS-like condition.

MCS AND ILLNESSES IN PGW VETERANS

MCS and illnesses in PGW veterans have several characteristics in common, some of which support a comparison whereas others complicate it.

For each condition, the following is true:

- There is no clear case definition.

- There are no identified objective measures that distinguish persons with and without the condition.

- Persons with a common or similar (self-reported) exposure report common or similar subsequent symptoms of debilitating disease. In the case of MCS, typical AChE-inhibiting OPs or carbamate exposures are to pesticides, solvents, or remodeled buildings (with presumed mixed solvent exposures); organic solvents have been shown to inhibit AChE in vitro (Korpela and Tahti, 1986; Korpela, Tahti, et al., 1986). For PGW veterans AChE-inhibiting exposures that may have attended Gulf War participation include PB, pesticides, and low-level nerve agents. (Again, current modeling efforts supported by DoD estimate that over a three-day period up to 100,000 U.S. veterans, as a result of allied forces destruction of an Iraqi ammunitions depot at Khamisiyah, may have been exposed to levels of sarin and cyclosarin above the general population limit—the level presumed safe for indefinite exposure but below the level at which first symptoms would be identified (Gulflink, 1997))—although this estimate is likely high.

- Chronic multisystem complaints follow the exposure.

- Many persons with apparently similar exposures fail to report similar symptoms of disease.

- Patients, as well as some physicians and researchers, are firmly convinced the condition is organic. Other physicians and researchers believe the origin is psychological.

Because the MCS condition is itself not well understood or even universally accepted, this condition is poorly positioned to serve as an "explanation" of illnesses in PGW veterans. Nonetheless, parallels between these conditions may allow cross-fertilization of ideas in exploration of the cause of illness in persons labeled with each of the two conditions.

This chapter will consider the following topics: parallels in exposures and symptoms in ill PGW veterans and patients with MCS; incidence of chemical sensitivities in PGW veterans; results of a SPECT study in a sample of PGW veterans with chemical sensitivities; and points of contact between MCS and PB.

Parallels in Exposures and Symptoms in Ill PGW Veterans and in MCS

Many patients with MCS and ill PGW veterans have in common prior exposures to AChE–inhibiting agents. Subgroups of MCS patients have self-reported exposures to carbamate or OP pesticides or chlorpyrifos (Ziem, 1997), to solvents in industry, or to mixed solvents associated with building remodeling. Carbamate and OP pesticides are AChE inhibitors, and, as previously noted, organic solvents have been shown to inhibit AChE in vitro (Korpela and Tahti, 1986; Korpela, Tahti, et al., 1986). Many PGW veterans experienced exposures to PB, to low levels of nerve agents, pesticides, and solvents, as well as oil fires, vaccines, and perhaps infectious disease.

MCS and PGW patients both report prominent alterations in concentration and memory (Miller, 1994; Fukuda, Nisenbaum, et al., 1998; Iowa Persian Gulf Study Group, 1997). Moreover, MCS and PGW subjects share other categories of symptoms, including musculoskeletal, respiratory, and dermatological. Moreover, as previously mentioned, many ill PGW veterans report new chemical sensitivities (Gordon, 1997).

The ten most frequent complaints of PGW veterans enrolled in the Persian Gulf Health Registry with complaint data available are shown in Table 11.1. Symptoms in MCS patients are shown in Table 11.2. These tables are not directly comparable because the mode of questioning influences the symptoms reported. Nonetheless, both lists share fatigue (systemic complaints), headache,

Table 11.1

Complaints of PGW Veterans Enrolled in Persian Gulf Health Registry (%)

Complaint	Men	Women
Fatigue	23.3	20.7
Headache	23.0	17.7
Skin rash	18.2	18.5
Muscle or joint pain	14.5	16.5
Loss of memory or "other general symptoms"	13.9	14.2
Shortness of breath	7.6	8.0
Sleep disturbances	5.3	5.9
Abdominal pain	3.9	2.5
Other symptoms involving skin and integument	3.8	3.2
Diarrhea and other GI symptoms	3.6	4.5

SOURCES: IOM report (Committee to Review the Health Consequences of Service During the Persian Gulf War; IOM, 1996); Persian Gulf Health Registry data provided to IOM Committee to Review the Health Consequences of Service During the Persian Gulf War.

Table 11.2

Symptoms in MCS Patients

Symptom	Percentage[a]
Ear-nose-throat	90–100
GI	40–95
Systemic	60–90
Musculoskeletal	80–100
CNS, excluding headache	80–85
Headache	65–100
Dermatologic	60–80
Lower respiratory	75–100
Genitourinary	20–65
Circulatory	25–80

[a]Percentage ranges reflect prevalence for four MCS subgroups.
SOURCE: Miller and Mitzel, 1995; Davidoff and Keyl, 1996.

skin rash, musculoskeletal complaints, CNS complaints, GI complaints, and respiratory complaints. But ear, nose and throat symptoms, sleep disturbances (unless that is included in systemic complaints), genitourinary, and circulatory symptoms are distinct. MCS subjects report higher levels of these complaints—a difference that could reflect true differences in subjective symptom patterns, differences in exposure levels, or differences in referral and self-referral patterns for the two conditions. Moreover, both similarities and discrepancies in listed symptoms could be artifacts of the methods of questioning. Indeed, one investigator reported, in testimony, quite similar rates of various symptoms in ill PGW veterans and MCS subjects, presumably employing a common mode of questioning (Miller, 1996b). However, these findings have not been published in a peer-reviewed source.

EEG abnormalities have been reported in MCS subjects (Miller, 1992) and in persons exposed to AChE inhibitors, such as OPs (Duffy, Burchfiel, et al., 1979; Duffy and Burchfiel, 1980). (Such changes include increased beta and decreased alpha activity.) How similar these changes are in those with different exposures, and whether the EEG changes seen in pesticide-exposed persons with MCS also occur in ill Gulf War veterans with PB exposure, is unknown.

Incidence of Chemical Sensitivities in PGW Veterans

No peer-reviewed data are available regarding the incidence of new chemical sensitivities in PGW veterans. Testimony from many veterans has included comments about new sensitivities to foods, cigarettes, alcohol, and chemicals (Subcommittee on Human Resources, 1997a, 1997b), and in one report, many of 549 PGW veterans evaluated reported "high intolerance" to chemicals in the environment (Gordon, 1997). Moreover, according to evidence presented in testimony, of 59 consecutive PGW veterans seen at the Houston VAMC Regional Referral Center, 78 percent reported new intolerances (Miller, 1996b) (see Table 11.3).[1] While this analysis is severely limited by the absence of a control population, it does suggest possible development of new chemical and food sensitivities in some ill PGW veterans, at a rate that may exceed that in the general population. Consequently, it favors efforts to examine PGW illnesses in the context of efforts to study putative MCS.

SPECT Study in PGW Veterans with Chemical Sensitivities

One small study (six cases, six controls) performed SPECT scanning (a method for looking at regional cerebral blood flow) on six male PGW veterans "with chemical sensitivities" and six controls reportedly determined not to have toxic exposures. Abnormalities were reported in all six SPECT reports from PGW veterans with sensitivities (abnormalities were classified as mild in one, moderate in two, and severe in three), while all six reports from controls were read as normal. Soft tissue diversion was noted in three cases (but no controls), lobar discrepancies in three cases (and one control), focal findings in five cases (and one control), and phase mismatching in four cases (and one control). Findings in all PGW veterans were noted to be similar to those seen in patients with

Table 11.3

New Onset Intolerances Reported by Gulf War
Veterans: n = 59 Veterans Seen at Houston
VAMC Regional Referral Center

Food or Chemical	Percentage with New Intolerances
Chemical inhalants	78
Medications	40% of those taking drugs
Alcohol	66% of alcohol users
Caffeine	25% of caffeine users
Tobacco use	74
Foods	78
Specific foods	64
Illness after meals	49

SOURCE: Non–peer reviewed testimony (Miller, 1996b).

---

[1]Anecdotal stories from some PGW veterans suggested striking changes in sensitivity: One veteran reported that his idea of the perfect perfume had been WD-40, whereas since the PGW that and many other low-level chemical exposures made him feel ill. Other mechanics stated they used to "bathe" in solvents, or enjoy the smell of engine exhaust before the war, while afterwards they reported severe symptoms with these exposures (Miller, 1996b).

known exposure to widely recognized neurotoxins "including petroleum distillates and pesticides" (Simon, Hickey, et al., 1994). (Indeed, qualitative and quantitative SPECT performed on patients with OP pesticide and solvent exposures have demonstrated abnormalities despite nondiagnostic MRI brain scans—abnormalities that are reportedly distinct from the findings seen with depression and "late-life chronic fatigue syndrome." (Heuser, Mena, et al., 1994).) SPECT is regarded by some as a "sensitive and potent" indicator of CNS function impairment after neurotoxic exposure (Heuser, Mena, et al., 1994). However, specificity remains an issue, because SPECT abnormalities may occur in many conditions, including depression. Of note, it has been suggested that focal cortical hypoperfusion with limited temporal lobe involvement may suggest a direct cortical effect of neurotoxins, rather than a limbic effect suggested in the kindling hypothesis.

The reported SPECT findings in PGW veterans may have important implications if they can be replicated in a larger, more carefully controlled study, but the present study has significant limitations. The sample was extremely small; subject selection procedures, including criteria for "chemical sensitivity," were not clearly delineated; the SPECT readings were qualitative and not stated to be blinded; no primary outcome variable was identified; and no statistics were offered. Moreover, results in all veterans with chemical sensitivities might not be reflective of results in other ill veterans; the estimate of 78 percent of ill veterans with new sensitivities, cited previously, might not reflect values in larger samples of veterans or ill veterans, and criteria for chemical sensitivity may differ from those in the present study. Therefore, these findings, while intriguing, must be viewed as preliminary. Nonetheless, attempts should be made to replicate the finding of SPECT abnormalities in the form of focal hypoperfusion and to extend this work by ascertaining if these defects are selectively enhanced when patients are symptomatic following reexposure to an offending chemical, to determine whether SPECT scanning could offer a much needed, if costly, objective marker for chemical sensitivity.

Points of Contact Between MCS and PB

Because a clinical case definition has not been accepted for either MCS or PGW illnesses, any discussion of common etiology must be regarded as hypothesis-generating rather than hypothesis-supporting. Nonetheless, there are points of contact between cholinergic function (which is influenced by PB) and the putative MCS syndrome, and these points of contact merit review:

1. AChE Inhibitor Exposure: Several defined MCS subgroups have self-reported exposure to AChE inhibitors. Exposure to OP or carbamate pesticides (all AChE inhibitors) reportedly produces particularly severe MCS

symptoms. Exposure to organic solvents (shown in vitro to inhibit AChE (Korpela and Tahti, 1986; Korpela, Tahti, et al., 1986)) is also reportedly linked to MCS; and exposure to recent building remodeling (or "tight buildings") has been postulated to occur through solvent exposure.

At least 250,000 PGW veterans were exposed to AChE inhibition through PB. An estimated 100,000 may have been exposed to low levels of nerve agent following the demolition of the Iraqi Khamisiyah ammunitions depot (Gulflink, 1997), and many additional veterans were exposed to pesticides, solvents, and petroleum products. Thus, AChE exposure is common to many PGW veterans and to many or most MCS subjects.

2. Cholinergic hypothesis: It has been reported that reduced AChE parallels the increase in hypersensitivity to stimuli (Girgis, 1986), that the limbic system is especially rich in AChE, and that AChE may play a protective role by maintaining ACh concentrations within safe bounds and protecting susceptible limbic neurons from developing "bizarre sensitivity" (see "Limbic Kindling," below). Indeed, AChE inhibitors including OP pesticides and organic solvents (from industrial exposure or exposure following building remodeling) are common reported "incitants" of putative MCS. If this cholinergic hypothesis is correct, then administration of PB during stress (leading to PB crossing the blood-brain barrier), or administration of PB in concert with exposure to AChE inhibitors that cross the blood-brain barrier, could promote heightened susceptibility to chemical sensitivities. At present this is speculative.

3. Nasopharyngeal factors and the respiratory mucosa: The airway epithelium (the outermost layer of cells that make up the "mucosa" or lining of the respiratory tract) and the fluid it produces and regulates are the first line of defense against constituents in the air inhaled each day; moreover, the nasal cavity contains enzymes that help to metabolize foreign substances (Bascom, 1992). It has been suggested that patients with MCS have altered function of the respiratory mucosa (Sparks, Daniell, et al., 1994; Bascom, 1992), perhaps through alteration of "c-fiber neurons,"[2] altered function of the respiratory epithelium per se, or an altered interaction between the nerve cells and the epithelium (Bascom, 1992). Increased vascular permeability of the respiratory tract has occurred with some chemical irritants, through activation of the c-fiber neurons (Bascom, 1992); and certain "cytokines" (another form of chemical signal in the body involved in such functions as inflammation) are released by epithelial cells in response to

---

[2]C-fiber neurons are nerve cells that branch extensively in the mucosa and contain neuropeptides, or small proteins that serve to convey signals, such as "vasoactive intestinal peptide," "substance P," which is involved in perception of pain and production of inflammation, and calcitonin gene–related peptide.

chemical exposures. Moreover, some alteration in properties of the mucosa in MCS patients is indicated by the finding that these individuals have increased nasal resistance (Doty et al., 1988).[3] Study of airway epithelial "neutral endopeptidase" has been suggested, as reduction in this enzyme could result in amplified response to subsequent c-fiber stimulation by other inhaled irritants (Bascom, 1992).

In one study, 10 of 10 MCS subjects were found to have abnormal rhino-laryngoscopic findings including edema, excess mucus, "cobblestoning" (an alteration in the appearance of the mucosa), mucosal injection (redness of the mucosa from surface capillaries), and blanching around vessels (Meggs and Cleveland, 1993). However, there were no controls and no blinding in evaluation.

A relation to PB could conceivably occur, since cholinergic function is involved in nasopharyngeal mucociliary action (Sastry and Sadavongvivad, 1979). Therefore dysregulation of cholinergic function (which may be influenced by PB alone or in concert with other exposures influencing the cholinergic system) could prolong nasal exposure to chemicals and perhaps participate in altering nasal resistance and contributing to symptoms. As a related or independent mechanism, some lipophilic pesticides and other agents could partition into membranes of the respiratory mucosa, altering their properties (Moya-Quiles, Munoz-Delgado, et al., 1995).[4] This mechanism would not require central exposure to AChE inhibition.

4. EEG abnormalities: EEGs from 58 "universal reactors" (MCS patients) were compared with EEGs from 55 healthy controls. The MCS positives were shown to have evidence of increased beta and reduced alpha activity (Staudenmayer, 1990), similar to EEG abnormalities demonstrated following exposure to AChE inhibitors, including OP pesticide or sarin (Duffy, Burchfiel, et al., 1979; Duffy and Burchfiel, 1980). PB is an AChE inhibitor and may also potentiate the effects of other AChE inhibitors (see "Interactions"); one could speculate that PB could contribute to development of EEG abnormalities in some PGW veterans. Some studies have reported EEGs to be "normal" in PGW veterans. Others maintain that specific abnormalities are present and must be specifically sought, but have

---

[3]One cross-sectional survey, cited in a review only as "personal communication," reportedly found a relationship between self-reported mucosal symptoms in the workplace, such as eye, nose, throat, and respiratory irritation, and self-described heightened chemical sensitivity to such workplace elements as tobacco, fumes from a photocopying machine, new carpet, pesticides, new furniture, or paint (Bascom, 1994).

[4]Of anecdotal interest, some patients with self-described chemical sensitivities report noticeable symptom abatement with behaviors that increase salivation such as chewing gum; however, abatement of symptoms through this means does not necessarily imply that the pathology involved is nasopharyngeal.

not been examined in published negative studies (Baumsweiger, 1998). Blinded studies involving sleep and waking EEGs in ill PGW veterans and matched controls, including examination of beta activity, are currently under way (Haley, 1998, citing work with R. Armitage and R. Hoffman).

LIMBIC KINDLING: ONE PROPOSED MECHANISM FOR MCS

Kindling refers to a condition in which potent or repeated electrical or chemical stimuli permanently augment the tendency for neurons to "fire" (send a signal) in response to future excitatory inputs, even in response to much lower level signals than those originally involved. The amygdala, an area of the brain involved in emotion and aversive conditioning, is particularly susceptible to kindling, as are the olfactory pathways (Sato, Racine, et al., 1990).

Animal studies suggest that priming an animal with high or repeated concentrations of any of various chemicals, including pesticides (Bell, Miller, et al., 1992), and subsequently reexposing the animal to low concentrations of the same or different chemicals may produce increased likelihood of paroxysmal electrical discharge in the amygdala. Though the agents used to sensitize animals may differ chemically, the effects on the limbic system are quite similar. Bokina (1976) has suggested that these findings parallel clinical observations in MCS and that kindling could amplify reactivity to low-level inhaled and ingested chemicals and initiate persistent affective, cognitive, and somatic symptomatology (Bell, Miller, et al., 1992). Partial kindling (kindling leading to levels of paroxysmal electrical discharge below those resulting in seizure activity) has been shown to increase avoidant behavior in animals, including cats (Bell, Schwartz, et al., 1993a). One could speculate that MCS results from entrainment of strong aversive signaling in response to chemical exposures. (Of note, vagal stimulation has been approved by the FDA for treatment for intractable partial seizures (Zoler, 1998), potentially consistent with a connection between the ACh system and seizures, but the nature of the relationship remains confusing.)

The amygdala is closely connected to the hippocampus, another brain area involved in limbic functioning that is also felt to play an important role in learning and memory (in which many MCS and PGW subjects report impairments). Hippocampal damage may affect production, storage, or release of excitatory and inhibitory neurotransmitters, and small perturbations in hippocampal function can have lasting effects on behavior and cognition. The hypothalamus, part of the brain with rich limbic input that controls many autonomic and somatic functions, has also been postulated to play a role in development of symptoms in patients with subjective sensitivities (Miller, 1992).

Factors that lower the seizure threshold (that is, factors that facilitate the development of seizures in response to potentially seizure-producing stimuli), such as estrogen in women, might be expected to facilitate kindling sensitization (Bell, Schwartz, et al., 1993a).[5]

Indeed, studies in rats have found a greater susceptibility to sensitization in female than male rats (Antelman, 1988); and sex differences have been found for other, analogous neuronal effects (such as long-term facilitation following a single exposure to amphetamine) (Robinson, Becker, et al., 1982). This finding may have a clinical correlation in that predominantly females report symptoms of MCS (Miller and Mitzel, 1995), though the MCS cases that follow certain incitants are more commonly male (such as exposure to industrial solvents), reflecting the predominantly male group that is exposed. Self-reported illness from foods and chemicals in young adults (ascertained with no attempt to meet MCS "criteria") also occurs predominantly in females (Bell, Schwartz, et al., 1993b). Meanwhile, although 93 percent of PGW veterans were male, and while there may be a slight trend toward higher reported incidences of symptoms in female veterans, differences, if any, are not marked. Among those veterans in the VA Persian Gulf Health Registry, 69 percent of women reported their health as all right, good, or very good compared with 73 percent of men (Committee to Review the Health Consequences of Service During the Persian Gulf War; IOM, 1996). These subjects were self-selected to participate in the registry, and the generalizability to all PGW veterans is uncertain. (Of note, exposures for male and female veterans may have differed. If male veterans experienced more exposures then females, then symptom rates may underrepresent differences in response to exposures. No data regarding differences in exposures between males and females have been identified.)

INDIVIDUAL DIFFERENCES AND INTERACTIONS

Self-reported chemical sensitivities following exposures to pesticides, solvents, or building remodeling affect some but not all exposed persons. Since there are no experimental dose-response studies (and perhaps such studies cannot be

---

[5]Consistent with the identified effect of estrogen on seizures in animals, recent studies in humans have found that epileptic women have fewer seizures after menopause, and hormone replacement treatment may worsen seizures (Harden, 1997). The effect of estrogen on enhancing ACh function or action is suggested by postmenopausal estrogen's ability to delay onset of dementia (Jacobs, Tang, et al., 1998)—Alzheimer's-type dementia involves ACh dysfunction and is treated by drugs that increase ACh action. However, complicating the question of how ACh influences seizures, evidence has recently shown that stimulation of the vagus nerve—which produces ACh action in the periphery—has been shown to significantly reduce the number of seizures (Handforth, 1998). Of incidental note, headache may occur as a preseizure event (French 1997), suggesting a possible role for increased ACh action in some headaches. Headaches are a prominent symptom in many ill PGW veterans.

ethically performed), it cannot be established whether the fraction of persons affected varies smoothly with degree of exposure to an agent. No organic markers have been identified to predict which subjects will be affected, and no organic markers are known that correlate strongly with who reports subjective symptoms. Some small studies report alterations in lymphocyte subsets, activated T lymphocytes, or autoimmune antibodies; however, these differences require replication and are of unknown significance (Miller, 1992).

Genetic polymorphism and quantitative variability in many enzymes involved in detoxification of xenobiotics offer a possible mechanism by which individual differences in susceptibility could be examined (see Chapter Eight, "Individual Differences in Reactions to PB"). Moreover, interactions with other drugs, exposures, or stresses may influence the effective dose received by an individual (see Chapter Nine, "Interactions Between PB and Other Exposures"). Interactions between chemicals may produce an effect in other ways, perhaps by targeting the same or different elements of the nervous system. It has been observed that less than 10 percent of the 70,000 commercially available chemicals have been evaluated for neurotoxicity. Furthermore, data regarding effects of such chemicals are almost universally deficient in information about chronic or long-latency effects (Landrigan, Graham, et al., 1994).

INTERACTIONS AND TIME-DEPENDENT SENSITIZATION

A putative phenomenon termed "time-dependent sensitization" refers to the progressive amplification of behavioral, neurochemical, hormonal, and/or immunological responses to a single or to multiple exposures to an exogenous agent (Antelman, Eichler, et al., 1980; Antelman, 1988; Antelman, Knopf, et al., 1988; Antelman, Kocan, et al., 1992). It has been reported that nonpharmacological stress can accentuate pharmacological kindling (Cain and Corcoran, 1985) and that the hypothalamic stress hormone, CRF, can facilitate the acquisition of sensitization and kindling while CRF antagonists may inhibit development of sensitization (Karler, Finnegan, et al., 1993). (Of note: the amygdala and hippocampus, noted earlier to be key participants in the limbic system, are the brain areas with greatest density of receptors for corticosteroids.) Additional work must be done to confirm these observations. Moreover, the relevance of these observations to MCS and to illnesses in PGW veterans remains to be defined.

PSYCHOSOMATIC VERSUS ORGANIC DISEASE: ONE PERSPECTIVE

For both MCS and illnesses in PGW veterans, there is active debate about the relative roles of psychological and organic factors.

Cacosmia (abnormal perception of smells as bad) is found to be at best weakly related to such psychological variables as trait shyness (r = 0.18), anxiety (r = 0.08), and depression (r = 0.16) (Bell, Schwartz, et al., 1993b). Moreover, MCS subjects do not differ significantly from controls in factors thought to predict psychiatric illness, such as family psychiatric history, treatment of a psychiatric condition not linked to illness, or unusually intense or long-lasting stress during childhood (Davidoff and Keyl, 1996). Though overall psychiatric symptoms are greater in MCS patients than in controls (correlating significantly with the presence of illness) (Simon, Daniell, et al., 1993; Davidoff and Keyl, 1996), this may reflect effect rather than cause. Similar studies could profitably be undertaken in PGW veterans: a negative result in a well-designed study would reduce the likelihood that illness is of "psychological" origin. A positive result would not necessarily discriminate between organic and "psychological" origin.

It must be remembered that some mood disorders (for instance) are linked to abnormalities in ACh system function. Persons with altered ACh function could have different susceptibility to effects from drugs like PB that act on the ACh system: thus, if a relation between development of illnesses in PGW veterans and prior mood disorder (or other conditions known to be associated with altered ACh function) were found, this would not necessarily imply increased likelihood of a "psychosomatic" origin to disease (if such a concept has any meaning at all); rather, if susceptibility to illnesses in PGW veterans is found to be differential according to psychiatric predisposing factors and existing conditions, the relevant neurochemistry of those conditions should be assessed for clues to the biological basis of illnesses in PGW veterans (see Chapter Thirteen, "Neurotransmitter Dysregulation").

Several observations have been cited to suggest that MCS and illnesses in PGW veterans could have an organic basis. These include the following:

- The groups reporting similar symptoms and intolerances following an exposure event are demographically diverse (Miller, 1996b).

- Temporal cohesiveness exists between the onset of multiple intolerances and an exposure event (Miller, 1996a and 1996b). (In fact, temporal cohesiveness is present in at best a loose sense in ill PGW veterans; for many, symptoms began significantly after PGW exposures.)

- There is internal consistency in these patients' reporting not only intolerances to common airborne chemicals, but also to various foods, drugs, caffeine, and alcoholic beverages (Miller, 1996b).

- Many MCS patients who have avoided problem chemicals and foods report marked improvement or resolution of their symptoms (Miller, 1996b).

- Psychological "overlay" occurs in many chronic illnesses such as diabetes, atherosclerotic heart disease, or lupus; presence, if any, of psychological symptoms is a common consequence of illness and in no way precludes an organic cause (Levin and Byers, 1992).

Labeling either MCS or illnesses in PGW veterans as psychogenic or as primarily stress-related is both unsubstantiated and potentially counterproductive. At present, no solid evidence indicates that illness in either MCS patients or in PGW veterans is psychogenic; rather, the cause of symptoms is unknown.[6]

METHODS OF STUDY

Blinded attempts to replicate MCS symptoms following selective exposures have not been successful (Staudenmayer, Selner, et al., 1993), but testing strategies used have been criticized. Improved empirical approaches to the study of MCS have been suggested. These recommend using carefully controlled double-blind testing, employing people of a similar background, and in particular they recommend a period of "unmasking" (Miller, 1992, 1997; Miller, Ashford, et al., 1997) involving an expensive Environmental Medical Unit. Unmasking entails removing the subject from interfering exposures for a period so the effect of a target exposure can be identified, isolated from interfering recent exposures. This method sounds promising but would be expensive and fraught with difficulty. (How can subjects be challenged without infringing on the environmental properties of the proposed unit? How can one be certain that potentially problematic exposures have been extinguished from the unit? How can one "blind" chemicals with identifiable smells, since addition of a "blinding" smell may block olfactory receptors required for action of the exposure?) Moreover, unmasking has yet to be validated as a technique for discriminating subjects who report and who fail to report symptoms of sensitivity to multiple chemicals or for distinguishing chemicals to which subjects are and are not sensitive. Nonetheless, if obvious problems can be overcome, such a unit might be useful in demonstrating or refuting blinded reproducibility of MCS symptoms in response to selected exposure in MCS patients and PGW veterans who report new sensitivities. This may provide a basis for objective testing for MCS that could be a foundation for future research.

---

[6]Distress at being labeled with psychogenic illness has been voiced by both MCS patients (Miller, 1994) and by PGW veterans (Subcommittee on Human Resources, 1997a, 1997b; Zeller, 1997). Such characterizations have engendered alienation among veterans, who have referred to them as degrading and have correctly described them as unfounded (Sumpter-Loebig, 1997).

QUANTITATIVE VALIDATION

MCS remains to be uniformly accepted as a medical condition. Nonetheless, two studies have compared the frequency of different symptoms in persons with putative MCS resulting from different exposures. In one study, the frequency of reported symptoms in MCS patients with self-reported pesticide exposure was compared to the frequency of reported symptoms in persons with MCS following building remodeling. Frequencies of symptoms resulting from a long list of inhalants and food were similar in the two groups, though severity of symptoms for all organ systems affected was higher for the pesticide group (see Figure 11.1) (Miller and Mitzel, 1995). Similarly, comparing four groups of MCS subjects (patients with sick-building syndrome, chlorine dioxide exposure, OP pesticide exposure, and exposure to individual organic solvents) resulted in health and illness status reports and specific organ system symptom reports that were similar within MCS groups and different between MCS groups and controls for 11 of 12 symptom categories (the twelfth was diagnosed autoimmune conditions) (Davidoff and Keyl, 1996). These similarities occurred despite the fact that the four groups had remarkably diverse demographics. Demonstration of similar symptom frequencies for these groups enhances validity of the MCS symptom complex. Evidence for a possible link between illnesses in PGW veterans and the MCS complex would be strengthened or weakened to the extent that rankings of symptoms reported by ill PGW veterans agreed or disagreed with symptom rankings in those with the presumed MCS symptom complex.

(Claims that stress or "psychogenic illness" is substantially responsible for illnesses in PGW veterans can and should be subjected to the same minimal scrutiny. That is, the fraction of ill subjects who have various symptoms following other stressful circumstances would be expected to be similar to the fractions with the same symptoms among PGW veterans for the stress hypothesis to be supported. To the extent this is untrue, the stress hypothesis is weakened. No attempt to verify quantitative comparability of symptom frequencies in illness following major stressors has been identified.)

As noted previously, Miller (1996b) reported quantitatively similar ordering of symptoms (using eight symptom scales derived by factor analysis) in 59 consecutive ill PGW veterans (of whom 78 percent reported new onset chemical sensitivities since the war) as in 37 pesticide-exposed civilians with chemical sensitivities, in non–peer reviewed testimony (Miller, 1996b). These results were quite different from those in normal controls. If ranking of symptoms referable to different organ systems are indeed confirmed to be similar in PGW veterans and MCS patients, this strengthens the case for operation of a similar mechanism for illnesses in some PGW veterans.

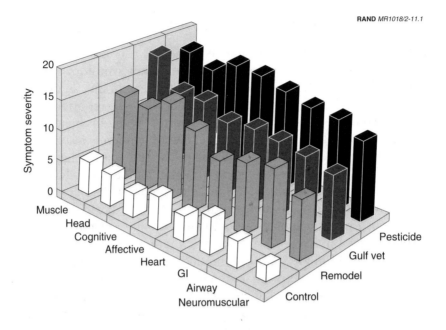

SOURCE: Miller (1996a)

Figure 11.1—Comparison of Symptom Severity

SUMMARY

The lack of a clinical case definition for either MCS or illness in PGW veterans complicates the examination of a connection. Therefore and predictably, any connection between MCS and illnesses in PGW veterans is based on weak and indirect evidence. One unpublished study finds a high rate of new chemical sensitivities in ill PGW veterans. The same investigator reports evidence of similar symptom frequencies for the two conditions (Miller, 1996a). These findings require confirmation and replication in peer-reviewed sources. One postulated mechanism for MCS involves cholinergic system activity, perhaps linked to limbic system kindling. PB with stress or chemical combinations might be expected to facilitate development of MCS if this mechanism is sub-stantiated. Other postulated mechanisms for, or contributors to, MCS (such as nasopharyngeal mucosal dysfunction) could also be linked to cholinergic dys-function. Evidence of brain SPECT abnormalities in PGW veterans with chem-ical sensitivities needs to be confirmed in a larger sample, with blinded reading of SPECT images. SPECT abnormalities have also been reported in subjects exposed to pesticides and may suggest that chemical exposures underlie symptoms in PGW veterans with chemical sensitivities. Whether similar SPECT abnormalities will be seen in larger samples of ill PGW veterans with subjective chemical sensitivities, or in those without subjective chemical sensitivities, remains to be determined. EEG findings in MCS parallel those in pesticide-exposed individuals, providing some internal consistency for toxin-induced illness in MCS. Moreover, similar EEG abnormalities have been observed with exposure to other AChE inhibitors including sarin, which is an AChE inhibitor to which some PGW veterans may have been exposed. Therefore, careful EEG and SPECT studies may be warranted in ill PGW veterans with and without reported chemical sensitivities and in controls to evaluate whether chronic abnormalities in brain activity are present by this measure. However, a cogent interpretation of a positive finding may be complicated by the presence of EEG and SPECT abnormalities in some psychiatric conditions.

Although the connection between MCS and illnesses in PGW veterans is supported only by limited evidence, enough suggestive evidence is present to warrant further scientific study.

SCIENTIFIC RECOMMENDATIONS

Future work should concentrate on the following:

- Ascertain (replicate in a larger sample) the fraction of PGW veterans, ill PGW veterans, and controls reporting new chemical sensitivities.

- Ascertain (replicate in a larger sample) whether (rank-ordered) symptoms in ill PGW veterans (and/or in PGW veterans reporting chemical sensitivities) occur with similar rank and at frequencies consistent with those of patients with putative MCS.

- Ascertain whether ill PGW veterans with chemical sensitivities share similar EEG abnormalities with subjects exposed to pesticides and with MCS patients.

- Evaluate whether enzyme polymorphisms or low enzyme levels (e.g., paraoxon, BChE) partially discriminate OP-exposed subjects who develop MCS versus similarly OP-exposed subjects who do not and PGW veterans who develop illnesses and those who do not.

- Evaluate whether respiratory mucosal epithelial abnormalities (perhaps including measures of nasal resistance and of neutral endopeptidase) are present in ill PGW veterans with chemical sensitivities compared to controls and replicate the presence or absence of these abnormalities in MCS.

- Evaluate (replicate in a larger sample, using blinded qualitative readings supplemented by quantitative SPECT) whether SPECT abnormalities characterize ill PGW veterans with and without chemical sensitivities, compared to matched controls.

- Evaluate whether quantitative SPECT shows differences in cerebral perfusion before exposure to a target chemical (after a period of "unmasking") and after exposure, and whether these findings differ for those complaining of new sensitivities compared with those not complaining of such sensitivities and in ill PGW veterans compared with healthy controls, in an effort to develop an objective marker for chemical sensitivity and for illness in some PGW veterans.

SUMMARY ANALYSIS

Compatible Exposures

Many veterans are known to have been exposed to AChE-inhibiting chemicals (including PB, pesticides, and low-level nerve agents), which some feel may predispose to subjective chemical sensitivities.

Compatible Illness

Unpublished, non–peer reviewed research reports new chemical sensitivities in a high fraction (78 percent) of a small number (59) of tested ill veterans. Unpublished, non–peer reviewed research finds that ranking and frequency of symptoms is similar in these veterans and in non-PGW patients with subjective chemical sensitivities following self-reported exposures. No peer-reviewed evidence is yet available to support or refute these findings.

Compatible Link Between Exposure and Illness

No published effort has been made to link presence of "compatible" exposures to new subjective chemical sensitivities in PGW veterans.

Chapter Twelve

NEUROMUSCULAR JUNCTION EFFECTS

DOES PB PRODUCE NEUROMUSCULAR JUNCTION CHANGES?

Acetylcholinesterase (AChE) inhibitors, including PB, produce acute destructive changes at the neuromuscular junction, the site of connection between nerve cells and muscle fibers, at which nerve cells signal muscles to contract. Because studies of the neuromuscular junction require microscopic inspection of muscle tissue and tests of electrical and chemical properties of the neuromuscular junction at a fine level, studies investigating these alterations have not been performed in living humans but primarily in muscle preparations from rats and frogs exposed to PB or other AChE inhibitors (also called "anticholinesterases"). These studies have examined the effects of PB and other "carbamate" AChE inhibitors, sarin and other OP nerve-agent AChE inhibitors, and nonnerve-agent OP (e.g., pesticide) AChE inhibitors on the muscle and neuromuscular junction.

These observed alterations fall into several classes.

"Histopathological" and "ultrastructural" changes are changes in structure and fine structure of the muscle and nerve muscle junction observed by light and electron microscopy. Some of the muscle changes are referred to as "AChE inhibitor myopathy."

"Prejunctional" changes refer to changes that occur on the nerve or signaling side of the neuromuscular junction. Prejunctional or "presynaptic" changes include changes in production and release of the neurotransmitter acetylcholine (ACh); or withdrawal of nerve branches from the motor endplate (muscle side).

"Postjunctional" or "postsynaptic" changes refer to changes that occur on the muscle or signal-receiving side of the neuromuscular junction. Since the signal is "received" by binding of ACh to receptors on the postjunctional side, changes in receptor sensitivity or density are examples of postjunctional changes. These changes are reflected in alterations in currents and voltages produced, for instance, by binding the ACh to the receptor; and changes in time constants of electrical response measured at the "motor endplate."

Clinical or behavioral changes are changes in muscle function or strength believed to result from alterations at the neuromuscular junction.

Many of the alterations observed are similar regardless of which AChE inhibitor is used. However, specific drugs differ to some degree in their effect even within a class of anticholinesterase chemicals (for instance, different carbamates, or different organophosphorus nerve agents may produce effects that differ in detail) (Albuquerque, 1986). For example, differences may occur in how extensive certain changes are, in which specific muscles are affected and to what degree, in the time-course of the effect, and in the response to a change in dosage. Differences are not only quantitative but may also be qualitative, and a drug that produces a more profound change than another when examined by one technique (for instance, by examining receptor blocking) may produce a less pronounced change when viewed through the lens of another technique (for instance, AChE inhibition, or "MEPP rise time").

The existence of marked, and in some instances long-lasting, changes at the neuromuscular junction is unequivocal. (These findings derive primarily from animal studies using high doses of AChE inhibitors.) The clinical significance these changes may have is less clear. Some have suggested that they may be responsible for a putative reduction in the rate of cure of myasthenics with thymectomy since the onset of treatment with PB (Rockefeller, 1997; Phillips and Torner, 1996). Others have suggested that these alterations may be responsible for symptoms in ill PGW veterans (Tiedt, 1994). In fact, current information is sufficient neither to confirm nor exclude long-lasting structural and/or functional effects at the motor endplate in humans with the doses and durations of PB treatment used in PGW veterans. Current information is also insufficient to confirm or exclude a role for changes in symptoms, such as fatigue or joint pain, reported by PGW veterans. ("Joint" pain might or might not be produced by abnormal regulation of signals to opposing muscle groups during rest or activity. Abnormal strength or timing of signals could result in alterations in the pattern of highly coordinated contraction of some muscles with relaxation of others that occurs during normal activity and at rest.) Concomitant exposure to other AChE-inhibiting drugs, such as sarin or organophosphorus pesticides, could conceivably cause, modify, or amplify effects on the motor endplate. Again, while existing evidence does not exclude long-lasting biological and clinical effects on the motor endplate with PB use, neither is there persuasive evidence favoring such effects. Data to address the clinical significance and time-course of such changes as those seen in animal studies remain inadequate.

This chapter does not purport to contain a wholly comprehensive review of the literature regarding AChE inhibitors and motor endplate alterations. Rather, a sample of available information is provided to impart the nature of changes seen, the similarity and variation of alterations observed with different types of AChE inhibitors, and some of what is known regarding the time-course of these changes. Effects not only of PB but of other AChE inhibitors are reviewed. Because not all measures have been performed with PB, including assessments of long-term effects, it is useful to describe effects both for PB and for other AChE inhibitors.

STUDIES WITH AChE INHIBITORS

Animal Studies

Animal studies (largely using muscle from rats given AChE inhibitors, such as PB; occasionally from frogs and other species treated with cholinesterase inhibitors) constitute the bulk of the evidence indicating changes in the neuromuscular junction that occur with use of PB and other anticholinesterases.

Histopathological and Ultrastructural Changes: Postsynaptic and Myopathic Changes. PB has been shown to lead to light and electron microscopic changes in rats. These changes are primarily postsynaptic (causing alterations at the muscle side of the nerve-muscle junction), and myopathic (destructive to muscle tissue). Some investigators find the presynaptic region (the nerve side of the nerve muscle junction) to be less affected. The nature of the changes in the muscle of rats given high-dose PB (98 mg/kg/day orally in feed—76 times the Gulf War daily dose and 228 times the per-dose Gulf War dose) include alteration in the striped appearance of muscle filaments and changes in the appearance of subcellular structures like mitochondria and sarcoplasmic reticulum. Some evidence of regeneration appears by 15 days, partially reversing the destructive changes.[1]

---

[1]In rats given high-dose PB (98 mg/kg/day administered orally in feed), unlike control animals, degenerative changes in muscle are seen with light and electron microscopy. Under the light microscope, approximately 1 percent of muscle fibers (or "myofibers") from the diaphragm were damaged. (Such damage is made evident by loss of "striation" or stripe pattern of "myofilament" architecture and presence of many centralized, highly convoluted cell nuclei in the muscle cells (Bowman, Schuschereba, et al., 1989).) On electron microscopy, myofibers were seen to contain swollen mitochondria (mitochondria are energy-producing "organelles" or subcellular structures) with accumulation of internal inclusions and numerous inflammatory cells (Bowman, Schuschereba, et al., 1989).

By two days of PB administration, degenerative changes were seen in the postsynaptic region of the neuromuscular junction. By seven days, myofibers had additional changes. Myofibers were still damaged, with centralized nuclei, dilated sarcoplasmic reticulum, and disruption of "Z bands"; and myofibers had increased glycogen. By 15 days, damaged fibers appeared to be in the process of regeneration, evidenced by large nuclei with dispersed chromatin and prominent nucleoli with

It has been suggested that some adaptive mechanism may be responsible for the partial reversal of early myopathy even in the presence of continued treatment. Seventy-four percent or more inhibition of AChE was observed throughout the study (Bowman, Schuschereba, et al., 1989), so that the reversal of myopathy cannot be the result of lessened cholinesterase inhibition, for instance from heightened metabolism of PB.

A second study of rats with somewhat lower doses of PB (20 and 40 mg/kg—47 and 93 PGW dose-equivalents, respectively) but still greater than 50 percent AChE inhibition confirms the presence of changes on light microscopy.[2] Changes were unexpectedly more severe in the group with the lower dose of PB, for reasons that are unclear. The earliest changes could be detected immediately after the two-hour period required for complete inactivation (Gebbers, Lotscher, et al., 1986).

In a third study on rat diaphragm, PB producing 78 percent reduction in AChE activity was again seen to induce marked changes, most directly adjacent to the synapse, with damage greatly reduced a few microns away and some normal-appearing muscle filaments 12–14 microns away.[3] Stimulated muscles (in which the nerve leading to the muscle was stimulated to produce a signal) showed the same pattern of organelle damage and myofibril disorganization, but the damage was more severe and the affected area more extensive. Damage was well developed 30 minutes after PB administration and was maximal at two hours. Myopathic or destructive changes can involve the endplate region of nearly all muscle fibers, but light microscopy revealed necrosis in only about 10 percent of fibers sampled, even after nearly complete ACh inhibition. It is unclear why some nerve fibers degenerate but most are preserved in spite of marked abnormalities in the fine structure of the fibers ("ultrastructural"

---

dense chromatin rims; sarcoplasmic reticulum in the postsynaptic region appeared less dilated. The presynaptic region appeared grossly normal at all times in this study.

[2]Changes included acute focal necrosis (cell death) of disseminated single fibers and groups of fibers, mixed leukocyte infiltrates, and marked changes in motor endplates in skeletal muscle; changes were greater in diaphragm than in quadriceps muscle in this study (Gebbers, Lotscher, et al., 1986) (though another study found similar changes in three tested muscle types differing in the amount of fast- and slow-twitch muscle fibers, namely diaphragm, soleus, and extensor digitorum longus (Hudson, Foster, et al., 1985)).

[3]Changes included supercontracted sarcomeres near the endplate region, subjunctional areas marked by disorganization of the myofibrillar apparatus, streaming of the Z-bands, and mitochondrial swelling. The most severely affected mitochondria were observed proximal to the junctional folds with progressively less severe alterations away from the junction. Regions closest to the synaptic cleft had the most severely damaged organelles. Essentially all mitochondria immediately adjacent to the neuromuscular junction exhibited marked intracristal swelling and some mitochondria showed an apparent absence of matrix. Contractile filaments were supercontracted with only remnants of Z-line material visible. The ultrastructural damage was greatly reduced within a few microns from this region, and by 12–14 microns from the subjunctional membrane it was possible to detect precisely aligned sarcomeres and "normal" intracellular organelles (Adler, Hinman, et al., 1992).

abnormalities). The incidence of necrotic fibers is dose-dependent, suggesting that some muscle fibers may be especially sensitive to AChE inhibitors, perhaps related to the threshold or firing pattern of the muscle cell (or "motor unit") (Adler, Hinman, et al., 1992).

Importantly, PB administration in rats produced marked postsynaptic ultra-structural changes,[4] even when no animals displayed outward signs of anti-cholinesterase intoxication (Hudson, Foster, et al., 1985).

Presynaptic Changes. Some neuromuscular junctions of all three muscles tested in rats underwent partial denervation (withdrawal of nerve terminal branches from the muscle) following either acute injection of PB (1 mg/kg—or 2.3 times the Gulf War dose—by single injection) or subchronic delivery of PB by osmotic minipump (with constant 70 percent inhibition throughout a 14-day period) (Hudson, Foster, et al., 1985). The three tested muscles were the diaphragm, the soleus (a posterior lower leg muscle), and the extensor digitorum longus (which extends the toes). Together these muscles include fast-twitch and slow-twitch fiber types.

Withdrawal of nerve branches constitutes a presynaptic change, because the nerve branches are from the signaling side. Although recovery was "in process" and in some cases reportedly complete at the termination of the follow-up 60 days after *cessation* of treatment, some changes were still present at this time (Hudson, 1985), primarily histological changes in muscle. (This is the longest identified period of follow-up after cessation of PB treatment in these studies.

A related study using PB (0.36 mg/kg by single subcutaneous injection, or sub-acute PB by osmotic minipump—0.84 of a Gulf War dose) noted that intrusion of processes from non–nerve supporting or "glial" cells termed "Schwann cells" in the synaptic region (the synaptic "cleft") and partial withdrawal of nerve terminals acted as a type of denervation, effectively reducing the amount of synapse surface available for optimal functioning (Hudson, Foster, et al., 1985).[5]

---

[4]Postsynaptic changes with acute PB treatment (0.36 mg/kg by single subcutaneous injection) included rarefied areas in mitochondria, and occasional mitochondria were associated with membranous lamellar structures. Subjunctional myofibrillar structure was disorganized in occasional neuromuscular junctions. Subacute treatment with PB (for two days) led to highly variable changes, with swelling or rarefaction of the mitochondrial matrix, some grossly altered mitochondria with multilayered membrane structures in subjunctional regions, and similar variability within each of three tested muscle types. There was loss of myofibrillar organization in some neuromuscular junctions, with more subtle changes in Z-lines, myosin, and actin filament organization in others.

[5]Synaptic vesicles (vesicles or inpouchings of membrane that contain neurotransmitters) were so densely packed that there was no space to accommodate cytoplasm in the nerve terminal. With acute treatment, mitochondria presynaptically were either similar to the controls' or were characterized by swollen regions in neuromuscular junctions of all three muscles (Hudson, Foster, et al., 1985). With subacute treatment, there was local separation of pre- and postsynaptic components. In some regions, crests of several junctional folds lacked the typical apposing nerve terminal, and

Studies in rats, using neostigmine (a carbamate compound related to pyrido-stigmine), have also noted significant presynaptic alterations[6] including deple-tion of neurotransmitter-containing vesicles (Hudson, Rash, et al., 1978).

It has been shown that destructive ultrastructural changes such as those described require that ACh interact with its receptor. These changes were eliminated if the nerve synapsing on the neuromuscular junction was cut, if ACh receptors at the endplate were chemically inactivated (by the agent "alpha bungarotoxin"), if oxime treatment was administered promptly to pull the AChE inhibitor off the AChE, or if a receptor blocker (namely d-tubocurarine, a paralytic agent) was simultaneously administered, thus preventing spon-taneous fasciculations of the muscle (Salpeter, Kasprzak, et al., 1979; Gebbers, Lotscher, et al., 1986; Adler, Hinman, et al., 1992; Hudson, Rash, et al., 1978). Moreover, damage is promoted by nerve stimulation (Adler, Hinman, et al., 1992). These findings indicate that the destructive changes may result from increased synaptic activity because of heightened availability of ACh and that they depend on successful interaction of ACh with its receptor. It has been suggested that the diaphragm may be particularly vulnerable because of its constant activity (Gebbers, Lotscher, et al., 1986; Dettbarn, 1984).

The condition may be more pronounced in slow-twitch rather than fast-twitch muscle (Wecker and Dettbarn, 1976), or this finding may simply reflect differ-ences in muscle activity. Myopathy in in vitro muscles occurs both in the absence and presence of nerve stimulation. Although nerve stimulation facilitates this effect, so evidently does spontaneous muscle twitching or "fasciculation" (Adler, Hinman, et al., 1992), which may result when spon-taneously released or leaked neurotransmitter binds to the receptor. While the detailed mechanism of the muscle damage or "myopathy" that results when AChE inhibitors (such as PB) are given is not well understood, this damage is known to be mediated through calcium (Yamaguchi, Robson, et al., 1983; Toth, Karscu, et al., 1983; Dettbarn, 1984; Kawabuchi, 1982; Salpeter, Kaszprzak, et al., 1979; Leonard and Salpeter, 1979). Several possible mechanisms have been postulated.[7]

Schwann cells frequently occupied the position normally occupied by the nerve terminal (Hudson, Foster, et al., 1985).

[6]Presynaptic changes, in addition to synaptic vesicle depletion, included appearance of numerous coated vesicles and membrane cisternae indicating continued nerve terminal hyperactivity (Hudson, Rash, et al., 1978); degeneration and partial recovery of the nerve axon were observed with chronic treatment (Hudson, Rash, et al., 1978).

[7]For instance, membrane phospholipase may be activated by calcium, directly or through calmodulin or phosphatidylinositol; the latter is split into diacylglycerol and inositol triphosphate, with the latter activating calcium, and calcium in turn activating protein kinases. Calcium in mus-cle fibers may activate an endogenous neutral protease that can catalyze degradation of myofibrils and Z-lines. Excess depolarization of endplate receptors may enhance calcium influx. PB may also directly influence neuromuscular transmission, acting as a weak agonist, thus further increasing

Other AChE Inhibitors. Similar patterns of damage to skeletal muscle have been reported in experiments with other carbamates (e.g., neostigmine) (Osame, Kawabuchi, 1975; Kawabuchi, Osame, et al., 1976; Kawabuchi, 1982; Engel, Lambert, and Santa, 1973), with OPs (Gebbers, Lotscher, et al., 1986; Salpeter, Kasprzak, et al., 1979; Preusser, 1967; Laskowski, Olson, et al., 1975; Laskowski, Olson, et al., 1977; Fischer, 1968; Gebbers, Lotscher, et al., 1986; Dettbarn, 1984; Feng, Rogers, et al., 1973; Fenichel, Kibler, et al., 1972; Fenichel, Kibler, et al., 1974; Ariens, Meeter, et al., 1969) like paraoxon (Laskowski, Olson, et al., 1975; Laskowski, Olson, et al., 1977; Fenichel, Kibler, et al., 1974); DFP (Feng, Rogers, et al., 1973), and with the nerve agents tabun and soman (Gebbers, Lotscher, et al., 1986; Preusser, 1967). For example, one study found that paraoxon, as well as OP cholinesterase inhibitors, produced progressive myopathy in skeletal muscle (Wecker and Dettbarn, 1976).[8]

Partial reversibility of these muscle damaging effects has been commonly reported. For instance, in rats exposed to DFP for two weeks, by day 14 there was loss of sensitivity to the necrotizing actions in all the muscles tested (diaphragm, soleus, extensor digitorum longus) (Gupta, Patterson, et al., 1986). Typically, some reversal of the damage occurs even when AChE-inhibiting agents continue to be given.

As noted previously, AChE-inhibiting agents that differ substantially from one another chemically produce similar effects, supporting presence of a mechanism involving heightened acetylcholinergic activity. Moreover, direct ACh enhancement produces the same effect (Fenichel, Kibler, et al., 1974). Nonetheless, neostigmine was shown to have direct action on motor nerve endings[9] in addition to inhibiting AChE, suggesting that some mechanisms idiosyncratic to individual chemicals may also be operative (Braga, Rowan, et al., 1993).

Variability of the Effect. Some studies report differences from one muscle type to another in the "ultrastructural" (pertaining to the fine structure of tissue, seen with an electron microscope) pre- and postsynaptic alterations of the neuromuscular junction. These differences have been attributed to different amounts of fast- versus slow-twitch (red versus white) muscle fibers or to differences in muscle activity that occur with the different types of muscles.

---

intracellular calcium concentration (Gebbers, Lotscher, et al., 1986; Chang and Neumann, 1976; Yamaguchi, Robson, et al., 1983; Toth, Karscu, et al., 1983; Akaike, Ikeda, et al., 1984).

[8]Myopathic changes included presence of splitting fibers, then enlargement of central nuclei, more-intense splitting and breakdown of fiber architecture, and finally total fiber necrosis and phagocytosis (Wecker and Dettbarn, 1976). There was significant recovery of enzyme activity within 24 hours. It was suggested that there may be a critical period of cholinesterase activity to initiate the myopathic process.

[9]Direct actions included blocking delayed rectifier potassium channels and enhancing transmitter release (Braga, Rowan, et al., 1993).

In one study, alterations of the neuromuscular junction occurred in diaphragm, soleus, and extensor digitorum longus with acute PB (0.36 mg/kg sc—or 0.84 Gulf War doses) or subacute PB (two days, 10 mg/ml PB by subcutaneously implanted osmotic minipump); both doses produced 60–70 percent whole blood cholinesterase depression). Changes occurred in each muscle of every animal examined, but there was considerable variation in the extent of damage even within individual fibers. The severity varied from fiber to fiber, but variability appeared "random" and not strongly related to the specific fiber type or to the dosage regimen (though effects in diaphragm muscle may have been greater) (Hudson, Foster, et al., 1985). No information was given to allow determination of the effect of muscle fiber activity on these changes.

Mitochondrial Effects. Increased cholinergic activity induced by PB (perhaps through increased intracellular free calcium) has been reported to cause deterioration in mitochondrial function resulting in heart and muscle damage. One report suggests that this may be mediated by reductions in the mitochondrial-bound enzyme "hexokinase," which is closely linked to "oxidative metabolism" in the mitochondria. PB led to a reduction in mitochondrial hexokinase in rats' tibialis anterior muscle (a muscle in the anterior lower leg) but not in heart muscle. (30 PGW doses led to 60 percent reduction of hexokinase in tibialis anterior muscle, a reduction that was statistically significant ($p < .005$). Hexokinase was reduced by only 10 percent in the heart, a difference that was not significant (Glass-Marmor and Beitner, 1996).)

Prejunctional Effects: Changes in Neurotransmitter Production. Choline acetyltransferase is the enzyme that "catalyzes" or facilitates the final step in ACh production (Albuquerque, Boyne, et al., 1983). Choline acetyltransferase activity was increased in muscle (in intramuscular nerves) following administration of the OP DFP (Gupta, Patterson, et al., 1986) and following nerve agent administration (Albuquerque, Boyne, et al., 1983); this increased activity should lead to increased production of ACh, an effect that could potentiate the AChE-inhibiting effects of these agents. No data were supplied on the effect of PB on choline acetyltransferase activity. The relative time-course of this effect, and the relation to the time-course of multiple potentially downregulatory effects, was not elucidated.

Prejunctional Effects: Changes in Neurotransmitter Release. Most studies evaluating changes at the motor endplate employ high doses of PB, leading to at least 50 percent AChE inhibition. Data are limited on effects of lower doses of PB, doses more comparable to those employed with PGW veterans.

Studies have found marked but reversible reduction in the amount of ACh released by each nerve impulse with five to seven days of (1 mg/kg) neostigmine given to rats (Roberts and Thesleff, 1969). Also, reduction in quantal content of nerve-stimulated endplate potentials has been shown (endplate potentials are changes in voltage on the postjunctional side produced by release of multiple "quanta," or vesicles of ACh, at the presynaptic side following a signal by the postsynaptic neuron) in rat extensor digitorum muscle (Tiedt, Albuquerque, et al., 1978). It has been suggested that chronic use of carbamates in myasthenia gravis patients may depress neuromuscular transmission in part because of a low endplate potential quantal content (Roberts and Thesleff, 1969), a form of "downregulation" of the acetylcholine system in response to excessive ACh activity; however, reduced transmitter release in one study had returned almost to normal after 22–25 days of continued treatment (Tiedt, Albuquerque, et al., 1978).

Postjunctional Effects: Electrophysiological and in Receptor Changes. ACh binds to receptors at the postjunctional side of the neuromuscular junction, inducing electrical currents and changes in voltage in the motor endplate (postjunctional membrane). If these changes are adequate, they result in contraction of the muscle fiber.

A single vesicle of ACh may be randomly released; one vesicle contains one "quantum" of ACh, which comprises several thousand ACh molecules, representing the smallest amount of ACh released (Kuffler and Yoshikami, 1975). If a nerve cell is excited and "fires," producing an "action potential" to signal to the muscle, about 200 quanta are released into the synapse or neuromuscular junction (Kuffler, Nicholls, et al., 1984).

Release of a single quantum by the prejunctional nerve leads to relatively small changes in current at the motor endplate. (The current is produced when ACh binds to receptors at the motor endplate, leading ions to traverse specialized ion channels in the membrane.) This change is termed a miniature endplate current (MEPC), and the size of the current is determined by fixing the voltage at the endplate. Alternatively, the endplate current can be held constant to determine the change in voltage, or miniature endplate potential (MEPP). If a nerve cell "fires" (generates an action potential), the complement of about 200 quanta produces larger changes in current and voltage termed the endplate current and endplate potential, respectively.

Nerves that signal muscle cells may be artificially stimulated to fire, and endplate currents and potentials can then be measured. MEPCs and MEPPs may be measured when random quanta are released. Moreover, ACh or other cholinergic agonists can be directly applied to the endplate to determine receptor "sensitivity," by measuring changes in currents or voltages. Information from MEPCs and from endplate currents differs slightly; for instance, a MEPC may be reduced if there are fewer ACh molecules in a quantum, or if there is reduced sensitivity of the receptor to ACh. An endplate current may be reduced if there are fewer ACh molecules in a quantum, fewer quanta for each action potential, or reduced receptor sensitivity. Moreover, amplitude is not the only property of currents and potentials—they also have temporal properties. Studies have looked both at the electrophysiological measures with spontaneous or induced signaling of nerve to muscle and at receptor sensitivity.

In several studies of rat diaphragm, soleus, and extensor digitorum muscle, PB led to prolongation of MEPC decay (threefold to fourfold slowing), with small (23 percent) increases in MEPC amplitude (Adler, Hinman, et al., 1992); and MEPP with a slow rise-time (> 1 ms) and low frequency (Meshul, Boyne, et al., 1985). Levels of AChE inhibition were higher than in PB-treated PGW veterans, e.g., 78 percent reduction in AChE activity (Adler, Hinman, et al., 1992). This effect was seen not only with PB but with other cholinesterase inhibitors, including sarin and soman; the effect was more pronounced with sarin and PB than with soman (Meshul, Boyne, et al., 1985). Moreover, PB affected both the extensor muscle and the soleus, whereas sarin affected endplates primarily of the soleus, and soman affected neither (Meshul, Boyne, et al., 1985). (This suggests that testing of only one or two muscle groups may be inadequate to exclude an effect, and effects identified may not generalize with fidelity to other muscle groups.)

In rat extensor digitorum longus muscle, treatment with neostigmine produced decreased MEPP amplitude and frequency and decreased endplate potential amplitude (accompanied by decreased junctional ACh sensitivity and decreased quantal content of nerve-evoked endplate potentials). Although by 22–25 days of continued treatment the reduced rate of transmitter release had returned almost to normal, the alterations in the postsynaptic membrane lasted for the full 106 days of continued treatment (Tiedt, Albuquerque, et al., 1978). In rat diaphragm muscle in vitro, low concentrations of neostigmine (.0001 mmol/L) led to decrement then full recuperation of compound muscle action potential (CMAP) amplitudes on repetitive stimulation of the phrenic nerve (the nerve that supplies the diaphragm), increased MEPP amplitudes, and prolonged decay time for the MEPC. Higher concentrations led to unimodal reduction in the CMAP, endplate potential, and MEPP amplitudes and a double exponential time-course of MEPC decay (Maselli and Leung, 1993a and 1993b). It was concluded that low concentrations impair neuromuscular transmission by transient depolarization of the endplate, while higher concentrations induce desensitization and direct blockade of the endplate receptor channel, probably in its open configuration.

Studies with nerve agents have actually shown opposite effects on endplate currents with low- and high-dose treatment. Except for tabun, the other OP nerve agents (soman, sarin, and VX) at low concentrations (< 1 µM) facilitated, while high doses (> 10 µM) of all four depressed, the endplate current peak amplitude, with VX producing the greatest depression (Albuquerque, 1986). Moreover, the time constant of endplate current decay t_{EPC} was prolonged, and a maximum increase was achieved with 1 μM in the case of VX, sarin, and tabun, whereas soman produced a maximal increase at 0.1μM concentration. Doses of > 1μM of all OPs shortened t_{EPC} from an enhanced level achieved by a low dose. At the 1μM concentration, all four OPs produced near-maximal enhancement (approximately three times greater than control) of t_{EPC}, while at doses of 10 μM or greater, the t_{EPC} values appeared lower than with the 1μM dose; a greater reduction was observed with VX (Albuquerque, 1986). The enhancement of t_{EPC} can be attributed to inhibition of AChE, while reduction with higher doses appears to be due to their action on the ACh receptor ion channel complex, or on the associated ionic channels (Albuquerque, 1986).

PB also facilitates receptor desensitization (a functional form of downregulation) (Meshul, Boyne, et al., 1985); indeed, it has been suggested that PB may have its therapeutic effects against OP compounds partly because it produces a "desensitized" state of the ACh receptor (Albuquerque, Boyne, et al., 1983). Receptors desensitized by PB would be insensitive to the anticholinesterase effects of the OP compounds.

Desensitizing effects of PB on the nicotinic ACh receptor have been shown in investigations of macroscopic as well as the microscopic events. Using "fluctuation analysis" as well as the "patch clamp" technique (in which the voltage of the membrane is held constant and electrical currents, resulting from movement of ions across channels, are measured), the agent has been shown to decrease single-channel conductance (conductance of ions across a single ACh receptor following binding of two molecules). PB decreases the endplate current and MEPC peak amplitudes, and, after an initial prolongation of these events presumably due to anticholinesterase effects (that is, due to increased availability of ACh), brings the time-constant of decay back to control levels (Albuquerque, Boyne, et al., 1983).

The desensitization of the ACh receptor induced by PB has been demonstrated by ACh iontophoresis experiments (direct application of ACh onto receptors) but can also be demonstrated by a patch clamp technique.[10]

---

[10]By patch clamp one can measure the characteristics only of open channels. There are multiple closed states with different receptor configuration; specific sequences of closed states must be gone through prior to a channel's opening, but this technique does not allow distinction among them. It has been possible to demonstrate the existence of an intermediate state of channel behavior by such agents as PB that enhance desensitization. The channels in the presence of PB, for example, reveal intense "flickering," and the channel openings appear in a bursting pattern, uncharacteristic of the channels in control condition. These are the channels that are presumably about to become desensitized and fail to open at all or open with a markedly decreased conductance. Following the appearance of many channels with much flickering and successive "waves" of bursting activity,

Receptor desensitization produced by PB may contribute to reduction in benefit of PB to myasthenics over time. (Throughout this section, other mechanisms are identified that may potentially be involved in functional cholinergic downregulation and could also contribute to reduction in the benefit of PB to myasthenics with continued treatment.) Neuromuscular adaptation has also been demonstrated following administration of the OP DFP in the rat; this adaptation was found to be caused by the recovery of AChE activity due to *de novo* synthesis of AChE, and reduction in the number of nicotinic ACh receptors (Gupta, Patterson, et al., 1986).

PB's ability to facilitate receptor desensitization does not prevent the development of endplate myopathy (Meshul, Boyne, et al., 1985), though one could speculate that it may contribute to the failure of endplate myopathy to progress, and the eventual partial regression of this process. More careful characterization of the time-course of the two is needed. Desensitization rates vary for different carbamate anticholinesterases acting on the ACh receptor ion channel complex, at least in rats. The effect of neostigmine exceeds that of physostigmine, which in turn exceeds pyridostigmine (Meshul, Boyne, et al., 1985). These effects differ from certain other downregulating effects, which require continued AChE inhibition and therefore are weaker (or absent) for physostigmine than for PB, since physostigmine has a shorter time-course.

Failure of neuromuscular transmission—loss of ability of a signal from a nerve cell to produce contraction in the muscle fiber to which it connects—has been reported with anticholinesterases, but the reasons for this failure are incompletely understood. When a nerve signals to a muscle, the membrane voltage becomes less negative, a process called "depolarization," which occurs as ions (such as sodium or potassium) move through channels in the membrane. Adequate depolarization leads the muscle fiber to generate an action potential (a self-propagating electrochemical signal that produces contraction of the fiber). However, prolonged depolarization inactivates the sodium channels so that effective signaling cannot take place.

According to a study using DFP in rat diaphragm muscle, two patterns of stimulation-induced endplate depolarization have been described that may account for the impairment in neuromuscular transmission reported with anticholinesterases. One pattern exhibited progressive "staircase summation" of long decay endplate potentials resulting in maximal depolarization at the end of the stimulation period. The other had maximal endplate depolarization at the start of the stimulation period followed by progressive return to the pre-stimulation levels (Maselli and Leung, 1993a). Transient endplate depolar-

---

channel opening frequency drops drastically and channel conductance decreases (Albuquerque, Boyne, et al., 1983).

ization was proposed to underlie the decremental response followed by recuperation of CMAP amplitudes in humans at early stages of toxicity with OP compounds (Maselli and Leung, 1993a). Transient endplate depolarization was suggested to account for failure of neuromuscular transmission induced by low concentrations of anticholinesterases; while high concentrations induce additional desensitization and direct blockade of the endplate receptor, which becomes the dominant mechanism for failure of neuromuscular transmission (Maselli and Leung, 1993a and 1993b). (These are mechanisms of possible cholinergic downregulation with AChE inhibitors.)

With 14 days of DFP administration in rats, postsynaptic nicotinic receptor density (Bmax) was reduced to 44 percent without a change in the affinity constant (Gupta, Patterson, et al., 1986), another potential mechanism for at least temporary downregulation.

Changes in AChE. With DFP administration in rats, though AChE activity was initially reduced to 20 to 24 percent of control, no further inhibition of AChE occurred with continued DFP for 14 days, but there was recovery of enzyme activity, especially certain forms (the 4SD and 10S forms) (Gupta, Patterson, et al., 1986). Whether this recovery results from increased AChE production, reduced sensitivity of AChE to DFP, or other effects was not elucidated. Depending on the mechanism involved, this recovery could conceivably produce another form of downregulation. However, other studies employing PB have found persistent inhibition of AChE with continued treatment.

The effect on AChE inhibition and on ACh release following discontinuation of PB has not been well defined, and the relative contributions and time-courses of agonism and downregulation remain to be determined.

Clinical Changes. Despite marked ultrastructural damage to muscle fibers, postsynaptic elements, and perhaps presynaptic elements, some reports indicate that muscle function (in in vitro tests) is not compromised, at least according to certain tests. Diaphragm muscles underwent no significant reduction in twitch or tetanic tension during or after a two-week exposure to PB, which was proposed to be due to the confined area of ultrastructural damage. Synaptic transmission and action potential generation, based on in vitro findings, were "expected to remain functional," with decrements in tension due to abnormal properties of the myopathic regions presumably too small to detect (Adler, Hinman, et al., 1992). Other studies (using neostigmine) have shown a reduction in indirectly and directly elicited muscle contraction with three days of treatment (Tiedt, Albuquerque, et al., 1978). In another study of rats exposed to DFP for 14 days, there was initial appearance followed by disappearance of fasciculations in all muscles tested (diaphragm, soleus, extensor digitorum longus) (Gupta, Patterson, et al., 1986).

It is not known whether ultrastructural changes such as those observed in animal studies could produce apparently normal function in selected muscle function challenge tests but also lead to symptoms of subjective fatigue (perhaps corresponding to abnormalities that these particular tests do not capture).

In studies of rats demonstrating ultrastructural and electrophysiological changes, animals expressing these changes demonstrated behavior varying from no identified findings to death, with fasciculations, prostration, salivation, urination, defecation, and rhinorrhea seen (Adler, Hinman, et al., 1992). Many of these changes represent activation of the muscarinic system. Of greater interest would be careful studies of muscle function and animal activity during and after acute and chronic cessation of the agent.

Human Studies with PB: Comparison of Myasthenic Changes in Humans to PB-Induced Changes in Animals

Ultrastructural and Electrophysiological. It has been speculated that carbamates used to treat myasthenia gravis, such as PB and neostigmine, may contribute in part to the neuromuscular alterations observed in myasthenia gravis. The changes produced by PB are similar to but not identical with those seen in rabbit and human myasthenia (Tiedt, Albuquerque, et al., 1978). Similarities with myasthenia gravis include reduced MEPP amplitude and frequency, reduced junctional ACh sensitivity (see "Downregulation"), alterations in neuromuscular geometry, and disruption of synaptic folds. Dissimilarities include the frequency distribution of MEPP amplitude, variation of neuromuscular junction ACh receptor sensitivity and ACh potential time-course, muscle membrane cable properties, and state of contraction of the endplate sarcoplasm (a membrane within the neuron that contains calcium) (Tiedt, Albuquerque, et al., 1978). One study concluded that "it appears likely that neostigmine treatment in patients with myasthenia gravis does not have an important role in the pathogenesis of the disease, but that it may contribute to the observed alterations." (Tiedt, Albuquerque, et al., 1978.) Others voice concern that the ultrastructural appearance of myasthenic endplates is similar to the ion accumulation myopathy caused by PB (Meshul, Boyne, et al., 1985); they note that administration of a "therapeutic" agent that increases the desensitizing effects of ACh and can still lead to excess ion accumulation (with ion leak into muscle cytoplasm as a possible proximal cause of myasthenic myopathy) may have "complex and possibly counterproductive consequences that have not been anticipated." (Meshul, Boyne, et al., 1985.)

Clinical. Some studies suggest that clinical effects on muscle function do not occur subacutely with PB use, while others have shown modest effects. For example, muscle strength and endurance were not significantly affected by eight days of PB treatment leading to 20–30 percent cholinesterase inhibition in a group of 35 healthy male 18–20-year-old volunteers in a double-blind placebo controlled trial that tested isometric handgrip, isokinetic elbow flexor and extensor strength, and knee flexor and extensor strength (Glickson, Achiron, et al., 1991). Other studies in smaller samples failed to find differences in grip strength after one or several 30 mg tablets of PB (n = 7 and n = 5; Levine, Kolka, et al., 1991; Forster, Barber, et al., 1994) (one or several Gulf War doses). Of these, one also examined and failed to show a difference in 60 percent peak hand-grip endurance time, or peak torque for leg extension (Levine, Kolka, et al., 1991). In contrast, one small (n = 7) double-blind, placebo-controlled cross-over study did demonstrate a modest (~3 percent, p < .05) reduction in grip strength in those receiving pyridostigmine (Cook, Kolka, et al., 1992). (Subjects received PB for one week and placebo for one week and received daily focused examinations.) The possibility cannot be excluded that modest effects, delayed effects, or effects with different motor measures occurred.

One study performed evaluations of neuromuscular function in 20 PGW veterans with severe muscle fatigue, weakness, or myalgias (muscular pain) interfering with their daily activities (Amato, McVey, et al., 1997). Tests included nerve conduction, effects of repetitive nerve stimulation, quantitative single fiber electromyography, and muscle biopsies. Mild increases in CK (an enzyme released by the muscle with acute muscle damage) were seen in six of 20 patients (range 223–768 IU/l); one patient who reportedly had not received PB had mildly increased jitter on single-fiber EMG, and muscle biopsies showed abnormalities in 5 of 20 patients. Both patients with tubular aggregates reported having received PB. The abnormal findings "were not believed to be clinically significant." However this conclusion is at best problematic in the face of marked clinical symptoms in these subjects, because no testing was performed in matched controls to determine the frequencies of these abnormalities in asymptomatic individuals of similar age and training. (The authors performed no power calculations; neither did they define at the outset how many abnormal biopsies or CKs would be expected if the group were "normal.") Manually tested muscle strength was measured and was reportedly normal in all instances. Unfortunately, this is an extremely crude measure (it may supply the same score for a world champion weight lifter and a non-physically-active grandmother; it is not sensitive to even substantial differences within this "normal" range). No sensitive quantitative measures of muscle strength, and comparisons to healthy non-PGW deployed individuals of similar age and training, were performed.

In summary, clinical findings with PB on motor outcomes have used short-term trials evaluating acute effects, without long-term follow-up after discontinuation, in small samples, using limited tests of motor function. Some studies but not others have shown significant but subtle effects on measured functions. One study performed biopsies, muscle enzyme testing, and limited neuromuscular testing in symptomatic PGW veterans with muscular complaints but failed to employ a control group. A set of observed abnormalities was construed as not clinically significant and unrelated to possible toxin exposures, although no cogent justification for this position was provided.

Duration of Changes

The changes that take place pre- and postsynaptically appear to be partially or mostly reversible, even with continued treatment with anticholinesterases, including PB, with much of the reversal occurring early. However there are provisos to this reversibility. First, the reversal may not be altogether complete. One study stated that recovery of "twitch tensions" following cessation of PB was "essentially complete" by one day after cessation (Adler, Maxwell, et al., 1984), but in fact although the value was indeed stable from one to 15 days following cessation, recovery to the original baseline never occurred. Second, at least some changes appear to be long-lasting. Studies in rats (extensor digitorum longus muscle) have shown that some changes at the neuromuscular junction (alterations of the postsynaptic membrane) persisted for as long as 106 days, the duration of continued treatment (with neostigmine) (Tiedt, Albuquerque, et al., 1978). More directly relevant to the issue of PGW veterans is the question of whether changes persist beyond the cessation of treatment. The study with the longest identified follow-up after cessation of PB delivery—60 days—found that while recovery was reportedly complete 60 days after cessation of PB treatment in some rats (following a single injection of PB or 14 days of PB delivery by osmotic minipump), in other animals changes were still present 60 days after discontinuing PB, perhaps more so in specific muscles such as the soleus. Sixty days is relatively chronic in the life of a rat. (One rat week is said for some purposes to correspond to one human year. Using this crude guide, extrapolation to humans of data from the rat study would suggest continued tissue damage in some individuals extending to roughly eight years, with no further testing thereafter.) Thus, current data do not exclude the possibility that some animals never fully recover the pre-PB appearance of their muscle tissue. The clinical correlation of this finding, if any, remains to be defined.

In general, each of the changes—histological and ultrastructural, electrical and chemical, and presynaptic and postsynaptic; changes in receptor density and sensitivity, withdrawal of nerve terminals, reductions in quantal content and quantal release, alterations in AChE production, or susceptibility to inhibition—needs to be evaluated more carefully for time-course of reversal following PB discontinuation, for interactions with other changes, and for individual differences in extent and in time-course.

CONCLUSIONS

Current evidence from studies in animals suggests that toxic effects result from cholinergic excitation at the neuromuscular junction in reaction to high doses of AChE inhibitors including PB. PB and other AChE inhibitors lead to alterations in function of the neuromuscular junction as well as physical destruction. These effects are partially reversible even with continued PB administration, but they may not be completely reversed even long after PB discontinuation. AChE inhibitors lead to changes in ACh production, ACh release, receptor response to ACh administration, muscle fiber organization, and clinical symptoms. These effects appear to result at least in part from excitation at the neuromuscular junction and the interaction of ACh with its receptor (with a concomitant influx of calcium). For this reason, tonically, persistently, or highly "active" muscles or muscle sites may be more affected. Some effects vary with the individual AChE inhibitor chosen or the dose employed (effects may even be opposite in direction with low and high dose of cholinesterase-inhibiting agents) (Albuquerque, Boyne, et al., 1983; Albuquerque, 1986), although the effects of dose for the many reported changes in receptor function, ultrastructure, and electrophysiological properties have not been well characterized. Many changes—in quantal release of ACh, in current and voltage changes in response to ACh at the motor endplate, and in the sensitivity to postjunctional ACh receptors—appear to reduce cholinergic function. This reduction in function may occur in response to, and may partially offset, the heightened ACh delivery at the synapse during the period of pharmacological AChE inhibition.

Although the duration of most effects (on ACh production and release, receptor sensitivity, myopathic changes, etc.) have not been well characterized, some effects have been shown to be quite long-lasting following discontinuation of the AChE inhibitor. It is not known whether all effects eventually reverse in all or most cases. The time-course of different effects has not been well characterized, neither have the doses at which the several effects are first seen. The effects have not been well studied across species or in primates. Moreover, the clinical sequelae of these changes, if any, are not well understood. It could be postulated that one consequence of these changes—namely functional cholinergic downregulation attended by reduced cholinergic activity—may lead to subjective fatigability in humans (conceivably leading to symptoms suggestive of "chronic fatigue"), but no data directly support or refute this proposition. This hypothesis would be weakly supported if treatment with cholinergic drugs led to subjective improvement in PGW veterans who report fatigue. However,

by this same hypothesis such treatment could produce undesired consequences.

LIMITATIONS IN PRESENT EVIDENCE

As noted above, the present data have several limitations. Different studies do
not all evaluate or report findings in a similar fashion—that is, they do not
necessarily employ similar doses, muscle groups, or observations, so the extent
of agreement across studies within and between AChE-inhibiting drugs
(including PB) is difficult to characterize. Observations of different types, such
as ultrastructural changes in ACh production and release, receptor sensitivity
and density, and electrophysiological change, are not well described as a
function of dose of drug (especially of PB), of duration of treatment, of specific
drug used, or of animal species observed. The influences of potentially
important covariates also have not been identified, including age at exposure,
prior (or subsequent or contemporaneous) chemical exposures, or baseline
AChE and BChE status. Importantly, the duration of these effects at the motor
endplate following cessation of PB or other AChE inhibitory treatment is also
not well characterized.

SCIENTIFIC RECOMMENDATIONS

1. Data should be obtained on ACh production and release, AChE production,
    endplate current and potential amplitude and time-course, receptor sensi-
    tivity and density, and ultrastructural changes using low doses of PB, with
    dose and route of administration more comparable to that experienced by
    PGW veterans.

2. Data as per first recommendation should be compared when AChE inhibi-
    tion occurs with muscles at rest and with stimulation or exercise, because
    some data suggest that active muscles may be more susceptible to destruc-
    tive effects.

3. Extended recovery studies should be performed, measuring data as above
    (first recommendation) following low-dose PB in one animal model, such
    as the rat.

4. Work should be extended to other mammals to evaluate the robustness of
    the effects across species. If doubts remain regarding extrapolation of data
    to primates (such as humans), consideration could be given to evaluating
    these effects in nonhuman primates.

5. The time-course of different effects (such as those noted in the first recom-
    mendation) should be characterized and compared, evaluating effects of

dose and AChE inhibitor combinations, in different muscle groups and different animals.

6. More careful correlation of the above effects to clinical sequelae (such as quantitative muscle strength and spontaneous activity of the animal) should be performed.

7. Effects on the neuromuscular junction (peripheral nicotinic effects) should be compared to and correlated with corresponding peripheral muscarinic effects and central nicotinic or muscarinic effects (determined through in vitro studies and/or by giving PB to rats under stress, or physostigmine to rats without stress). Effects of interactions of PB with DEET and other putative interactants should also be compared in these preparations.

8. Studies of muscle function in ill PGW veterans with muscular complaints should include matched controls, preferably of similar pre–Gulf War physical ability; sensitive quantitative measures of muscle function (including strength and perhaps latency); and power calculations with adequate sample size to allow determination of whether abnormalities in muscle enzyme tests or in muscle biopsies (performed blinded and preferably in several muscle groups) occur at increased rates in ill PGW veterans.

9. Studies of the effect of PB on muscle function in healthy volunteers should include an adequate placebo control group, sensitive measures of muscle function, and extended follow-up after PB discontinuation. Consideration should be given to performing (blinded) muscle biopsies, recalling that effects may not show up in all muscle groups.

SUMMARY ANALYSIS

Evidence of Compatible Exposure

An estimated 250,000 PGW veterans were exposed to PB (Brake, 1997). Neuromuscular junction abnormalities in animals have been demonstrated with PB. However, studies have not been performed at low doses, such as those experienced by PGW veterans.

Evidence of Compatible Symptoms

Subjective fatigue and musculoskeletal complaints have been reported by many veterans. For example, in one evaluation of 263 veterans referred for complaints felt referable to their PGW service, 86 percent complained of fatigue, 84 percent of arthralgias, and 60 percent of muscular weakness (Amato, McVey, et al., 1997). These may or may not constitute symptoms "compatible" with neuromuscular junction effects.

Evidence of Connection Between Exposure and Symptoms

According to one study, the factor-analysis-derived syndrome of "arthro-myo-neuropathy" in ill PGW veterans, in which musculoskeletal symptoms are prominent (including joint and muscle pains, muscle fatigue, and difficulty lifting) (Haley, Kurt, and Hom, 1997), is significantly associated with self-reported adverse acute response to administration of PB in the PGW, as well as to amount of insect repellent applied (Haley and Kurt, 1997). No other evidence has been identified that addresses a connection between musculoskeletal symptoms and use of, or response to, PB. A recent report regarding British veterans finds a link between self-report of use of PB in the PGW and in Bosnia and subsequent "Gulf War Illness" by CDC factor-analysis derived criteria (Unwin, Blatchley, et al., 1999); musculoskeletal symptoms represent one of the three major domains, in two of which symptoms must be present for the diagnosis. (PB was not the only exposure that was associated with increased illness. This study is addressed in greater detail below.)

Chapter Thirteen

NEUROTRANSMITTER DYSREGULATION

DOES PB ALTER REGULATION OF NEUROTRANSMITTERS, PARTICULARLY ACh?

Cholinergic Dysregulation

When ACh activity is artificially raised by administration of PB, it results in a host of compensatory changes, many of which act to reduce ACh activity. Changes in regulation of nerve signaling—occurring in response to excessive ACh activity—that result in reduced delivery of ACh or reduced response to ACh will be termed "downregulation." ("Downregulation" is often used technically to refer to reduced production of receptors, but here it will be used to refer to any alteration in the system that produces low ACh activity—such as decreased production or release of ACh, reduced receptors or receptor-binding affinity or sensitivity, or increased breakdown of ACh.) More generally, regulation of ACh may be altered in ways that may not be exclusively downregulatory. For instance some elements of the system may experience abnormal heightened sensitivity to ACh. In the general case, there may be elements of the very complex ACh regulatory system that are downregulated, while other elements are upregulated, or simply abnormally regulated—and these alterations may themselves interact to produce system level changes in regulation. These changes will be referred to in the aggregate as "dysregulation." In much of this discussion, downregulation—evidence of which is in the neuromuscular junction, as noted in the prior chapter—will illustrate how dysregulation could produce symptoms of altered ACh activity (low ACh activity in the case of downregulation), perhaps resulting in chronic symptoms if the changes outlast delivery of PB.

Based on the known functions of ACh—involving, for instance, muscle action, pain, sleep, and memory—such symptoms might include alterations in muscle function or muscular fatigue, altered sensitivity to or perception of pain, abnormal sleep, and disruption of learning and memory. These symptoms appear to be compatible with symptoms prominently described by PGW veterans—the top symptoms reported by PGW veterans include fatigue, headache, muscle and joint pain, loss of memory, and sleep disturbances. Evidence favoring this hypothesis include known delivery of PB to many veterans, and demonstrated dysregulatory effects in muscle and brain in animal studies following delivery of PB and other AChE inhibitors. Most of the downregulatory effects for which a time-course has been evaluated are "mostly" reversible on discontinuation of PB (or other AChE inhibitors) in a relatively short time. Nonetheless, for many changes the time-course has not been characterized, and in some cases the normalization of function is not complete within the follow-up periods examined to date. Some changes have lasted as long following discontinuation of PB as anyone has looked.

Once again, although "downregulation" appears to occur for some elements of cholinergic function, the total picture may be more complex. For instance, reduced sensitivity of central nicotinic receptors following heightened cholinergic stimulation (a form of downregulation) may be accompanied by increased production of these receptors, perhaps as compensation to the compensation. (Although the increased production of receptors has been termed "upregulation," the net effect of the several changes may still be depression of cholinergic function—or the net effect could be "supersensitivity.") Further complicating the picture is the possibility that changes in the ACh system will engender additional changes in neurotransmitter systems regulated by, or interacting with, the ACh system.

One might suppose that the relative contributions of up- and downregulation would be easy to tease apart. This is not necessarily the case. In myasthenia gravis, symptoms of the disease—involving low ACh action at the muscles—are often difficult to distinguish from symptoms of overtreatment—involving high ACh action at the muscles. Both produce weakness. Although regulation shifted "up" and "down" may be perceived as "abnormal," the valence of the abnormality may not always be easy to discern. (Challenge tests—involving administration of pro- or anticholinergic agents—would be expected to worsen or ameliorate symptoms, depending on whether excessive or reduced ACh activity took place. Such challenge tests may be helpful if simple up- or downregulation has occurred or has predominated.)

Many limitations remain in the "downregulation" (or "dysregulation") hypothesis. For instance: Although changes consistent with downregulation (dysregulation) have been demonstrated in animal studies, most of these changes have been shown at the neuromuscular junction, which is the most studied site. PB normally is denied access to the brain, and unless PB is admitted centrally, effects on learning, memory, attention, and sleep might not be expected. Most studies have used higher doses of AChE inhibitors, leading to more substantial inhibition of AChE than that experienced by PGW veterans, and it is not known whether the relatively low dose of PB—with the accordingly lower amount reaching the brain—is compatible with downregulation (dysregulation) effects. Finally, it is not known whether such downregulation (dysregulation) effects, assuming they could be produced by such doses, could last sufficiently long (or evolve in such a manner) to account for such chronic symptoms as those described by ill PGW veterans.

WHAT IS DOWNREGULATION?

Many different mechanisms regulate signaling by chemicals in the body.

When drugs or chemicals are given that abnormally elevate (or depress) delivery of and response to signals by body chemicals, compensatory changes occur in tissues in the body to counteract the abnormally high (or low) signaling produced by these drugs. When drugs abnormally increase signaling, the compensatory effects that occur and that produce attenuation of this heightened signaling may be termed "downregulation." (At the signal-receiving side, effects—such as reduced sensitivity of receptors to ACh—may be termed "subsensitivity.") The corresponding clinical or behavioral effects reflecting the reduced response by the body to the drug are termed "tolerance." The clinical effects of reduced response by the body to the native signaling chemical after discontinuation of the drug may be termed "rebound."

"Tolerance" is familiar to physicians, including tolerance to the effects of nitrates, sleep medications, or opiates. Exposure of catecholamine-sensitive tissues to adrenergic agonists results in progressive attenuation of their ability to respond; mechanisms for these phenomena (termed "desensitization," "refractoriness," or "tachyphylaxis") are incompletely understood but multiple points of regulation appear to include receptors, G proteins, enzymes including adenylate cyclase, and cyclic nucleotide phosphodiesterase, with the pattern of refractoriness varying according to the extent that the different components are modified (Hardman, Limbird, et al., 1996). Acute "rebound" phenomena on discontinuation of a drug, which act in the reverse direction of the drug (due to development of downregulation in the signaling system(s)) are also widely known.   These include rebound hyperadrenergic effects following discontinuation of beta blockers or rebound insomnia following discontinuation of chronically or subacutely administered sleeping pills. (The consequences of cessation of nicotine administration in persons who stop smoking provides clear evidence of long-term consequences of cholinergic modification.)

For some substances, dramatic rebound effects occur early following withdrawal—such as the hypersomnolence following withdrawal of cocaine, the dramatic withdrawal syndrome following cessation of opiates, or even the withdrawal syndromes seen with cessation of selective serotonin reuptake inhibitors (Dominguez and Goodnick, 1995; Rosenstock, Keifer, et al., 1996; Haddad, 1997; Lejoyeux and Ades, 1997). These effects may contribute to the addiction process for some drugs. However, over the long term, somewhat more subtle but clinically important "rebound" effects may also ensue. Instances include the long-term effects following cessation of corticosteroids and opiates. For these drugs, withdrawal leads to far more long-standing, comparatively subtle changes that may be evident only in selected contexts. Physicians who care for former narcotics addicts are aware that such patients experience heightened sensitivity to pain (where pain constitutes the "challenge" to the opiate system), which may persist many years following cessation of opiates, perhaps even for life. Analogously, an inadequate corticosteroid response to major stress (such as the stress of surgery) is present for a highly variable duration (Wilson, Braunwald, et al., 1991)—from days up to a year, after as little as a week of pharmacological corticosteroid treatment; for this reason, physicians must remember to administer "stress doses" of corticosteroids if a major stressor is encountered during this time. Thus, different downregulatory effects occur, with different time-courses ranging from days to years. Indeed, several different time-courses may characterize different effects for the same drug.[1]

DOWNREGULATION IN THE ACh SYSTEM

Downregulation is also known to occur in the acetylcholinergic system and indeed has been cited as a factor that must be considered with respect to drug interactions in military personnel who have taken PB and who may require drugs as part of surgery for traumatic injury (Keeler, 1990). Regarding effects at the tissue level, there exists evidence from animal studies that changes in tissues result from excessive activity of ACh following administration of PB. In many cases these changes are "downregulatory," serving to counteract the excess acetylcholinergic activity while it occurs, leading to development of "tolerance" both to the therapeutic benefits (in myasthenia) and to the toxic effects, despite continued AChE inhibition. Downregulatory effects may include presynaptic effects, such as reduced production of ACh (fewer packets of ACh or less ACh in each packet); reduced release of ACh; or withdrawal of

---

[1]Nonpharmacological manipulations that produce a major surge or other alteration of signaling chemicals may also have lingering repercussions. Thus, rapid eye movement (REM) deprivation leads to REM rebound (the time-course has not been well characterized, but is believed to be on the order of several weeks). Neuroendocrine dysfunction produced by undernutrition or anorexia nervosa may persist despite complete recovery of body weight loss (Falk and Halmi, 1982). And serious psychological stressors, presumably at least in part through their neurochemical effects, may lead to lasting changes in neurochemical regulation in the condition termed Posttraumatic Stress Disorder (PTSD) (see section on "Stress").

cholinergic nerve terminals from their contacts. Postsynaptic effects may include reduced number or "density" of ACh receptors, reduced affinity of receptors for binding to ACh, or reduced sensitivity of receptors to the actions of ACh once bound. Moreover, increased breakdown of ACh (such as by production of increased AChE) may occur. These mechanisms may have different distributions—they may differ according to specific brain regions (or muscles); according to different "layers" of neurons, e.g., within the cortex, within a brain region; and according to the type of ACh receptor, contact cell, or AChE molecule. (In fact, effects may be in opposite directions for different brain regions, receptor types, etc.) Moreover, the varying changes may have different time-courses of appearance and of resolution. They may even lead to alterations in susceptibility to future ACh system exposures.

Data from the Neuromuscular Junction: Peripheral Nicotinic Receptors

Most of the basic-science evidence regarding downregulation derives from investigation of the neuromuscular junction and is reviewed in the chapter devoted to that issue (Chapter Twelve). (Additional discussion of certain elements of "downregulation" appears in the Chapter Fourteen, "Chronic Effects.") Changes that appear to take place at the neuromuscular junction following administrations of PB and other AChE inhibitors include presynaptic effects—such as withdrawal of nerve terminals, reduction in number of ACh quanta released following a nerve impulse, and reduction in ACh per quanta— and postsynaptic effects, such as reduction in receptor density and reduced receptor sensitivity. Just as excessive ACh action leads to downregulation, so abnormally depressed ACh action leads to upregulation; for instance, experimental denervation has been shown to increase receptor synthesis while stimulation suppresses it (Heinemann, Asouline, et al., 1987). Such changes serve to attenuate the effects of excessive ACh resulting from administration of PB or other AChE inhibitors while these agents continue to be given. Such changes would be expected to produce low acetylcholinergic activity once PB is withdrawn. Although the time-course of this altered regulation has not been characterized—that is, the speed with which it returns to normal following cessation of PB is not known—in studies in rats, at least some changes observed in the muscle or the neuromuscular junction have persisted even 60 days after *termination* of PB treatment, which is the farthest out such studies have been conducted (see Chapter Twelve, "Neuromuscular Junction"). Different effects appear to have different time-courses, even with the same drug—be it PB (see Chapter Twelve) or soman (Russell, Booth, et al., 1986). Functional manifestations of downregulatory effects, in the form of tolerance, are variable). However, these include a (mostly reversible) dose- and frequency-dependent reduction in the force of skeletal muscle contractions in response to nerve stimulation that occur with administration of PB (Adler, Maxwell, et al., 1984; Anderson, Chamberlain, et al., 1986).

As has been stated, most evidence regarding downregulation and tissue "subsensitivity" derives from the neuromuscular junction. This is in large part a consequence of the neuromuscular junction being the best studied and best understood of all synapses, "because of its accessibility to biochemical and electrophysiological techniques" (Heinemann, Asouline, et al., 1987); likewise, the muscle nicotinic ACh receptor is "the best characterized neuroreceptor to date" (Goldman, Evans, et al., 1987). Evidence is substantially less rich regarding nicotinic receptors present at other sites, or muscarinic receptors.

Data from Central (Brain) Muscarinic Receptors

Although downregulation is best documented at the neuromuscular junction, there exists some evidence to indicate that some such downregulatory changes may occur in the brain, and in the muscarinic system in particular (data from rodents) (Costa, Schwab, et al., 1982a; Schwab, Costa, et al., 1983; Stanton, Mundy, et al., 1994; Russell, Booth, et al., 1989), following administration of AChE inhibitors, including organophosphorus agents and carbamates (Costa, Schwab, et al., 1982a and 1982b). Administration of AChE inhibitors—e.g., soman—has been shown to lead to strongly reduced synthesis rate of ACh (Nordgren, Karlen, et al., 1992). Additional mechanisms of tolerance in the muscarinic system include receptor loss (Uchida, Takeyasu, 1979; Schiller, 1979; Schwab, Hand, et al., 1981; Schwab and Murphy, 1981; Ehlert, Kokka, et al., 1980a, 1980b; Costa, Schwab, et al., 1981; McPhillips, 1969; Brodeur and Duboi, 1964; Russell, Overstreet, et al., 1975; Schwab, Costa, et al., 1983); however, tolerance in some experiments has been detected prior to demonstration of reduced receptor number, indicating the presence of other mechanisms (Marks, Artman, et al., 1981; Schwab, Costa, et al., 1983). One apparent change is enhanced affinity of AChE for ACh (so that ACh is more likely to be broken down), which has been seen both peripherally and centrally following administration of an irreversible AChE inhibitor (Milatovic and Dettbarn, 1996). Some additional mechanisms have been proposed (El-Fakahany and Richelson, 1980, 1981), and many other remain unstudied (Schwab, Costa, et al., 1983). The relevance of these data to PGW veterans is limited by use of animal subjects (primarily rodents) and by the fact that the AChE inhibitors used were not PB. The effects differ from one tissue to another—and indeed, may be prominent in one tissue (e.g., ileum) and absent in another (e.g., heart) (Schwab, Costa, et al., 1983), a reminder that examination of one type of tissue may not be sufficient to ensure or exclude effects of this kind in other tissues. Regarding the issue of whether these changes might be prolonged, a single subcutaneous dose of chlorpyrifos led to long-lasting enhanced sensitivity to cholinergic antagonists (evidenced by exaggerated hyperactivity in response to scopolamine) in rats, which persisted for months although muscarinic receptor density and cholinesterase activity had returned to normal levels (Pope, Chakraborti, et al., 1992). Similarly, a single dose of fenthion led to apparently permanent alterations in intracellular communication of muscarinic receptors studied in rats (Tandon, Padilla, et al., 1994; Tandon, Willig, et al., 1994).

Data from Central (Brain) Nicotinic Receptors

Data regarding downregulation and central nicotinic function are complex. Nicotinic receptors are present not only in the neuromuscular junction but also in the CNS, as well as on autonomic ganglia and chromaffin cells in the adrenal medulla, where they participate in regulation of catecholamine release (Heinemann, Asouline, et al., 1987; Hardman, Limbird, et al., 1996). However, the brain receptors are not identical to those at the neuromuscular junction; for example, the receptors are not blocked by exactly the same complement of chemicals (Luetje, Patrick, et al., 1990). Indeed, many types of nicotinic receptors are in the CNS; the exact number is unknown, but it has been speculated that the CNS "might contain a large set of nicotinic receptors, each having different properties" (Heinemann, Asouline, et al., 1987). Certainly a number of pharmacologically different nicotinic receptors have been identified, with different distributions in the brain (Wada, Balivet, et al., 1987 ; Wada, Wada, et al., 1989; Wada, McKinnon, et al., 1990; Patrick, Sequela, et al., 1993; Luetje, Patrick, et al., 1990).[2] Not only are there different types of nicotinic receptors, but, further complicating the ability to extrapolate evidence with confidence from the neuromuscular junction, more than one type of nicotinic receptor can exist in one region (Alkondon and Albuquerque, 1993) or even on one cell type (Heinemann, Asouline, et al., 1987). There is some literature on the effects of stimulation of central nicotinic ACh receptors, much of which derives from efforts to understand nicotine addiction; but it appears that nicotine itself is a special case. It has been said that "there are many examples of receptor changes in the brain following repeated administration of drugs that increase or decrease receptor stimulation either directly or indirectly. These changes in

---

[2]The receptors are proteins composed of five subunits (Patrick, Sequela, et al., 1993). There are 11 known members of the gene family that encodes the subunits of the neuronal nicotinic ACh receptors): the genes and there products include alpha2–alpha9, beta2–beta4, so that many combinations are possible (Elgoyen, 1994; Patrick, Sequela, et al., 1993). Though not all possible combinations have been described, at least nine different receptors resulting from combinations of alphas with betas—or alpha alone—have been demonstrated (Duvoisin, Deneris, et al., 1989; Patrick, Sequela, et al., 1993). Those nicotinic receptors that occur at the neuromuscular junction are more homogeneous, containing two alphas, a beta, a gamma, and a delta; or the gamma may, depending on animal species and cell maturity, be substituted by an epsilon (Alkondon and Albuquerque, 1993).

receptors are usually reciprocal to the changes in stimulation, resulting in a pattern consistent with compensatory adaptation to the change in stimulation" (Schwartz and Kellar, 1983). This pattern (consistent with downregulation) is slightly modified in the case of nicotine, as we shall see, but the essential effect is apparently the same.

Factors in Downregulation. When agents that activate nicotinic receptors—other than nicotine—repeatedly stimulate nicotinic receptors, it leads to a reduction in receptor number—that is, receptor "downregulation." Administration of drugs—like AChE inhibitors—that cause "excessive" activation of muscarinic receptors leads to reduced numbers of muscarinic receptors, apparently as compensation, as noted above. A similar phenomenon is seen with activation of nicotinic receptors—except with nicotine itself. DFP (diisopropyl fluorophosphate) is an AChE inhibitor (as is PB), which—like other AChE inhibitors—produces a net increase in ACh action. In live mice, ten days of exposure to this agent (1 mg/kg tapered to 0.2 mg/kg daily under the skin) produces reduced nicotinic binding sites—that is, reduced density of nicotine receptors—consistent with the idea that *receptor* downregulation occurs after heightened nicotinic receptor activation (Schwartz and Kellar, 1983; Schwartz and Kellar, 1985). (For nicotine, it appears that depression of the nicotine system as a whole may occur following stimulation by nicotine, but receptor number may *increase*.) Thus, the effect on nicotinic receptors with DFP is more like the effect seen with muscarinic receptors—that is, reduced receptor number following activation.

Testing of carbamylcholine (also called "carbachol"), an "agonist" or stimulant of the ACh system, has been done in tumor cells from a clone of a type of tumor called a "pheochromocytoma"; these cells possess the type of nicotinic ACh receptors that are found on neurons (Robinson and McGee, 1985; Simasko, Soares, et al., 1986), and they serve as a "model" of neuronal-type nicotinic ACh receptors. (This is in contrast to the above studies, done in actual animals, looking at effects on their nicotinic receptors in vivo or in vitro). In addition to classically described desensitization of the receptors, a second process was found to occur that produced a nonrecoverable loss of neuronal ACh receptor activity. This process was termed inactivation (Simasko, Soares, et al., 1986). The onset was slower than for desensitization (15 minutes rather than three-fourths of a minute), depended on the concentration of carbachol, and was blocked by giving nicotinic antagonists (which prevented the carbachol from binding and having action on the nicotinic receptors). (Of note: Desensitization and receptor downregulation occur at a higher dose of carbachol than the one that produces maximum stimulation. The result is a biphasic response, with the response to carbachol increasing to a certain point, and then decreasing (Robinson and McGee, 1985). Thus, in some instances a monotonic "dose response" effect may not be seen.) Recovery was not seen in recovery buffer (over a two hour period). Inactivation did not seem to require desensitization (since strategies to reduce desensitization did not affect inactivation). It was suggested that inactivation might be a first step to receptor downregulation and could explain the rapid and prolonged tolerance to effects of nicotinic "agonists" (agents that bind and stimulate the nicotinic receptors) (Simasko, Soares, et al., 1986).

Factors in Upregulation. When nicotine binds to the nicotinic type of ACh receptor, there is an increase in the number of nicotinic ACh receptors—receptor upregulation. Nonetheless, the nicotinic ACh system as a whole appears to be depressed. Nicotine is an agent that binds readily to the "nicotinic" ACh receptors, activating them. Repeated or chronic exposure to nicotine, rather than reducing the number of ACh receptors, increases the number (Marks, Pauly, et al., 1992) (although there is no change in the affinity of receptors for nicotine—that is, in their inclination to bind to nicotine) (Marks and Collins, 1983). At least this is true for some types of receptors (Flores, Rogers, et al., 1992), in some parts of the brain (Pauly, Marks, et al., 1991). This seems to be in contrast to what occurs with activation of nicotinic receptors by other agents, and with activation of muscarinic receptors, in which receptor downregulation occurs. The special effect of nicotine may result from the ability of nicotine to desensitize or inactivate nicotinic receptors; the result is not fundamentally inconsistent with nicotinic *system* "downregulation" (in our use of the term). Once again, the effects that occur vary widely by area in the brain. Finally, the consequences have widely varying time-courses. Since effects differ by area of the brain and in time-course, there may be altered interactions among brain areas in consequence.

Following nicotine administration in animals—studies have mostly been done in mice and rats—the number of nicotinic receptors increases. Yet the nicotinic activity as a whole seems to be dampened rather than heightened following nicotine administration (nicotinic system "downregulation" in our terminology)—despite the increase in the number of nicotinic receptors. The most important evidence derives from the effects of later administration of nicotine. Treatment with nicotine for a time has been shown to abolish or reduce the response to nicotine given later, for a variety of responses, producing (in rodents) tolerance to effects of nicotine such as release of prolactin and of adrenocorticotropic hormone, depression of locomotion or "Y-maze activity" and rears, reduction in body temperature, change in heart rate, and effects on "rotarod" performance (Marks and Collins, 1983; Marks, Stitzel, et al., 1985; Collins and Marks, 1988; Hulihan-Giblin, Lumpkin, et al., 1990; Pauly, Marks, et al., 1991). (It has been observed that the "acute and chronic administration of nicotine might induce changes in central nicotinic cholinergic circuits that affect the adrenocorticotropic hormone and PRL responses to stress," suggesting a mechanism for a PB-stress interaction.)

How could there be an increase in receptors, and yet reduced response? This could occur if the increase in receptors were in turn partial compensation for reduced response occurring by some other mechanism. Nicotine appears to cause desensitization (or inactivation (Hulihan-Giblin, Lumpkin, et al., 1990; Pauly, Marks, et al., 1991)) of nicotinic ACh receptors. Indeed, one study—published in abstract form—has shown that prolonged incubation with low levels of nicotine, while causing little receptor activation, effectively blocks the nicotinic acetylcholinergic receptors, by stabilizing the desensitized state(s) of the receptor (Lester and Dani, 1994). This abstract alludes to the nicotinic receptor *up*regulation that also results—perhaps as a consequence of the desensitization. Tolerance may arise from such desensitization—and increased receptor number could result as a compensatory response to that effect. Indeed, chronic nicotine treatment results in an increase in nicotinic receptor number that parallels (and may be caused by) a decrease in sensitivity to nicotine (Schwartz and Kellar, 1985; Collins and Marks, 1988).

Tolerance (net "downregulation" of the system—though not of the receptors) results if the increase in receptor number is exceeded by the increase in number of receptors that are inactivated (Collins and Marks, 1988)—otherwise stated, if the increase in receptor binding by nicotine is more than offset by a loss in effect of binding. In fact, the number of binding sites may be inversely (rather than positively) related to effects produced by nicotine—the more receptors, the less the effect (Collins and Marks, 1988)—consistent with production of tolerance. Chronic treatment with nicotine leads to an increase in density of nicotine binding sites, in some but not all areas of rat brain (for instance, in the frontal cortex but not the striatum): If it is true that the increase in number of receptors accompanies—and may perhaps be secondary to—a reduction in measured aspects of function, then the same brain areas that show reduced function (such as nicotine evoked release of dopamine) should be those with increased receptor density, and indeed this appears to be true (e.g., again, frontal but not striatal), consistent with the possibility that the rise in receptor number is secondary to—and lesser in effect than—the reduction in receptor sensitivity (Wonnacott, Marshal, et al., 1994).

It has been suggested that strains (or individuals) that show more tolerance to nicotine may have receptors that resensitize slowly, whereas strains that develop tolerance less readily may have receptors that desensitize poorly or resensitize rapidly (Collins and Marks, 1988). (Actually, the story is undoubtedly more complex than this. For instance, increases in the number of receptors were seen before development of detectable tolerance to a challenge with nicotine; the attenuation by nicotine of stress-induced prolactin release appears to be independent of nicotine-induced desensitization to the stimulatory effect of subsequent injection of nicotine on prolactin secretion; and correlations between binding and acquisition and loss of tolerance to effects of nicotine vary according to which effect is being examined, indicating that other explanations for tolerance must be sought as well (Marks, Stitzel, et al., 1985; Sharp, Beyer, et al., 1987).)

In another way of characterizing similar information, some theorize that the time-averaged effect of nicotine is as an antagonist rather than an agonist (Hulihan-Giblin, Lumpkin, et al., 1990)—that is, it may do more, over time, to block activation of nicotinic receptors than to activate them. For instance, after a single injection of nicotine into rats, the prolactin response to a later injection is smaller; the investigators took this to mean that "nicotine is even more potent in stimulating desensitization of nicotinic cholinergic receptors than in stimulating prolactin release"; that after brief activation it causes protracted desensitization or inactivation of the receptors so that its "predominant" effect is that of an antagonist (Hulihan-Giblin, Lumpkin, et al., 1990). It has also been speculated that antagonist effects could occur perhaps through metabolites of nicotine, such as cotinine. Cotinine competes for ACh binding sites in the brain; and one or more metabolites of nicotine (possibly hydroxynicotine) confer protection against the lethal effects of nicotine in mice, which may support this idea (Schwartz and Kellar, 1983). Either way, it appears that increase in receptor number may be the consequence of reduced action of the nicotinic system, which in turn follows (and perhaps follows from) the increased activity initially provoked by nicotine.

Could some receptor types show a net increase in action resulting from nicotine? It remains possible, though the present literature review failed to uncover substantial support for this. Certainly, in instances in which ACh stimulation drives something else that is inhibitory, suppression of ACh could lead to stimulation of that other action.

Regional Brain Differences and Differences Between Types of Nicotinic Receptors. As mentioned, it has been shown that there are large differences in the effect (the increase in receptors—and perhaps the reduced sensitivity of receptors—in response to nicotine) in different parts of the brain. A study in mice found that in most brain areas, chronic nicotine infusion increased the number of nicotinic receptors (sites to which nicotine attached), but the extent of the increase and the dose response curve (how big of a dose is needed to provide how big of an increase) were "widely different among brain regions" (Pauly, Marks, et al., 1991) with some regions particularly "resistant" to change. Also, the type of nicotinic receptor may determine the degree of receptor change, and of functional tolerance. Binding by the agent alpha bungarotoxin (which binds to some nicotinic receptors but not to other types) was significantly increased in only 26 of 80 regions examined (Pauly, Marks et al. 1991), even at the highest dose, so that different receptor types behave differently, as well. Indeed, the point has been carefully made that these effects may well differ from one type of nicotinic receptor to another (Lester and Dani, 1994). Moreover, brain regions are not equivalent in nicotinic cholinergic regulation after stimulation with nicotine—for reasons due to and/or distinct from the types of nicotinic receptors in residence.

Individual Differences in Nicotinic Regulation. In animals, there are large differences from one strain to another in sensitivity to nicotine—and moreover in ability to develop tolerance to nicotine (Collins and Marks, 1988)—reinforcing the idea that there may be within-species individual differences in regulation of the ACh system. Strains that are high or low in nicotine binding (to one type of receptor) in certain brain regions are likely to be high or low in other regions— though binding to one type of receptors correlates poorly with binding to the other type (Collins and Marks, 1988).

The time-course of recovery from tolerance may be highly variable. Tolerance to the effects of nicotine has been shown to be lost at different rates for different tests in rodents. For instance, loss of tolerance (return to baseline or near baseline) occurred for Y-maze activity and rearings test in eight days; regaining control of body temperature required 12–16 days; and tolerance for a heart rate test persisted throughout a 20 day withdrawal period—although brain binding sites had returned to control levels by eight days after treatment, and alpha-bungarotoxin binding sites (representing a subset of nicotinic receptors) were normal at the first time tested (four days). This indicates that physiologic effects may persist after objective identified measures have returned to normal.[3]

Findings in humans appear consistent with findings in animals. It is not easy to study the brains of humans, at the cellular and subcellular level, while they are still alive, but studies have been done postmortem to compare nicotinic receptors (binding sites) in people who smoked with those in people who did not smoke. Consistent with findings in animal studies, smokers—presumably exposed chronically to nicotine—showed an increase in nicotine binding in an assortment of brain areas (like the hippocampus, cerebellum, and median raphe nuclei—involved in serotonin production)—but not in all areas (for

---

[3]Presumably these measured physiologic effects are consequences of neurobiological factors that should have objective measurable underpinnings, though it is not yet known what these objective correlates are and how to measure them. The fact that objective measures that correlate with the demonstrated physiologic effects have not been identified does not imply that mechanisms do not exist. This important point bears reflection when assessing symptoms in ill PGW veterans. A search for objective measures sensitive to the complaints of veterans must remain a priority, because absence of effect on existing tests can never be assumed to imply absence of organic mechanism.

instance the medulla oblongata) (Benwell, Balfour, et al., 1988). As in animals, the increase in binding appeared to result from an increase in number of receptors rather than an increase in affinity for receptors (Benwell, Balfour, et al., 1988). These findings corroborate that at least some of the findings from animals can be extended to people, including the variability of the effects from one part of the brain to another.

The Case of ACh Receptors in General. Clinically, there is indeed induction of "tolerance" with AChE inhibitors (Blick, Weathersby, et al., 1994; Russell, Over-street, et al., 1975; Rider, Ellenwood, et al., 1952; Sterri, Lyngas, et al., 1980; Schwab and Murphy, 1981; Bombinski and DuBois, 1958; Barnes and Denz, 1954; Smit, Ehlert, et al., 1980a, 1980b), including reduced clinical response to the same dose, such as reduced evidence of AChE inhibitor toxicity with later doses and with consistent inhibition of AChE, reduced response to subsequent higher doses following pretreatment with low doses, and reduced response to a later similar chemical (Schwab, Costa, et al., 1983). For example, the dose of the (AChE-inhibiting) nerve agent soman required to produce a performance decrement on a specific well-learned task in rhesus monkeys was two and a half times higher with continued use (e.g., more than five days) than initially; and required a substantially greater degree of AChE inhibition, reflecting develop-ment of tolerance to low levels of AChE activity (Blick, Weathersby, et al., 1994). Indeed, "tolerance" to the effects of PB is reported for patients with myasthenia gravis, who may require progressively increased doses (McEvoy, 1991); and is suggested by reports in PGW veterans, in some of whom side effects attributed to PB abated with continued use (Sharabi, Danson, et al., 1991).

Evidence of the effects of AChE inhibitor administration on later response to ACh *agonists* suggests reduced sensitivity. Evidence on the effects of AChE inhibitor administration on later response to ACh *antagonists* is less consistent. Some data relating to use of carbamates suggest that enhanced sensitivity to antagonists accompanies reduced sensitivity to agonists (Costa, Schwab, et al., 1982a and 1982b), amplifying the "downregulation" effect. Another study found no enhanced sensitivity to atropine (a muscarinic antagonist) after administration of PB and suggested this may reflect the relatively low doses of PB used in military prophylaxis (Matthew, Glenn, et al., 1993). Other evidence suggests that binding of antagonists, as well as agonists, may be reduced following AChE inhibitor, and affinity for binding may remain unchanged (Schwab, Costa, et al., 1983). Thus, the net effect of AChE inhibitor administration on response to ACh antagonists may differ according to which of a set of effects predominates, including reduced receptor number, unchanged or enhanced receptor affinity, and perhaps other consequences of AChE inhibitor administration. Supersensitivity, rather than downregulation, may occur with some receptor types in some conditions (Nilsson-Haransson, Lai, et al., 1990).

At the time this report was first circulated (including this chapter on dysregulation), ACh system dysregulation had not been previously proposed as a mechanism to consider in relation to illness in PGW veterans. Since then, additional evidence is emerging suggesting that such dysregulation may occur. More recent findings are included in an Addendum.

PREDICTIONS FROM THIS HYPOTHESIS

This hypothesis suggests that symptoms in ill PGW veterans should bear some relation to effects mediated by the ACh system.

General Comments. Both tissue and behavioral studies support the development of downregulation—or more generally dysregulation—of the acetylcholinergic system following administration of AChE inhibitors. Although existing evidence suggests that different ACh receptors, and therefore different functions of the ACh system, may alter their regulation in different ways and with different time-courses, existing evidence is insufficient to predict what functions should be influenced how. Overall, however, if symptoms result from cholinergic dysregulation, many or most should relate to functions under control of the ACh system. It remains to be asked, what might the expected consequences of such dysregulation be? Regulation of ACh turnover and concentration in synaptic junctions and neurons is believed to play an important role in conditions involving memory dysfunction (e.g., Alzheimer's disease), motor dyscontrol (e.g., tardive kinesia), and muscular fatigue (e.g., myasthenia gravis) (Lieske, Gepp, et al., 1993). The consequences of ACh dysregulation are at once potentially varied and dependent on the specifics of the dysregulation, with expected symptoms determined by the site and character of the cholinergic alteration.

Effects might be expected to occur in the periphery, due to presumably limited access of PB to the brain.[4] However, central consequences could ensue if PB

---

[4]If PB does not gain access to the brain, it is not inconceivable that some central effects could occur indirectly, through modulation of the peripheral nervous system, which interacts with and influences the CNS. Nicotinic receptors occur in the adrenal medulla and are involved in regulation of catecholamine release from chromaffin cells (although, in fact, catecholamine release by physostigmine appears to be a predominantly central process—as discussed elsewhere). Just as cholinergic function is subject to downregulation, so is the catecholamine system: exposure to catecholamines leads to reduced responsiveness of the catecholamine system, involving multiple points of regulation (Hardman, Limbird, et al., 1996). Enhanced exposure to catecholamines might occur through administration of PB, because PB would presumably increase ACh binding to nicotinic receptors in the adrenal medulla, producing increased catecholamine response and increased susceptibility to catecholamine downregulation. This effect would be heightened in circumstances of

does gain central access. This possibility is suggested by the high prevalence of apparently central symptoms that occurred in response to PB reported by Gulf War personnel (Sharabi, Danon, et al., 1991), as well as by some evidence from animals suggesting enhanced access of PB to the CNS in conditions of stress (Friedman, Kaufer, et al., 1996). In fact, because no troops in the same units were assigned to not receive PB, with whom PB recipients could be compared, it cannot be stated with certainty that the CNS symptoms were in response to PB. However, personnel interpreted these effects as occurring in response to PB, and effects were consistent with central effects of AChE inhibition, discussed in Chapter Three, and with side effects of PB reported by patients with myasthenia gravis, in whom some central effects of PB are reported (Hood, 1990).

Likely Impaired Functions. Functions known to be governed by the cholinergic system, in general, should be those most likely impaired by cholinergic downregulation or dysregulation. These include sleep, learning and memory, nociception (pain perception, in which ACh serves in a modulatory role) (Sitaram and Gillin, 1980), and neuromuscular action.

Indeed, prominent among symptoms reported by PGW veterans are problems with memory, sleep, pain, and musculoskeletal dysfunction. These are general terms, involving functions controlled by multiple mechanisms. A certain degree of greater specificity is desired; in the case of sleep, REM sleep in particular is governed by ACh and should be an object of scrutiny. (As noted later, sleep apnea may also have a cholinergic relation.) Where possible, more specific characteristics of the general functions that are under cholinergic control should be identified for investigation in PGW veterans.

Specific functions affected by cholinergic agents in normal people have been reported to include increased REM sleep (Sitaram and Gillin, 1980), and reduction of the P100 component of the visual EEG evoked response was reported. The "opposite" phenomena would be expected if downregulation has occurred and has produced effects uniformly opposite those of the specific cholinergic agonist used in those studies. These effects would be expected to include reduced REM, reduced arousal (perhaps having a clinical correlation in chronic fatigue or perhaps not), enhanced perception of pain, and reduced serial learning and memory (retrieval of clustered information).

---

stress, because the stress response itself would lead to enhanced release of catecholamines. Most symptoms reported by PGW veterans with PB administration appear more consistent with ACh system effects rather than peripheral catecholaminergic enhancement. Although it is conceivable that some delayed abnormalities in ill PGW veterans could involve dysregulation of the catecholamine system, neither the time-course of effects nor the nature of most reported effects seems closely consistent with this representing a major factor. (However, direct studies of autonomic function would be needed to preclude this possibility.)

Effects on mood would also be expected, though the direction of these effects is difficult to anticipate. The AChE inhibitor DFP may produce depression or lead to remission of mania, and its withdrawal may lead to precipitation of mania (Janowsky, El-Yousef, et al., 1974). Moreover, other evidence has suggested a "cholinergic supersensitivity" theory of affective disorder, suggesting that muscarinic upregulation and supersensitivity are associated with depression (O'Keane, O'Flynn, et al., 1992). (However, this may be a case of low baseline cholinergic action with concomitant heightened receptor expression.)

This might predict reduced incidence of depression in PGW veterans compared to controls with comparable health and environmental circumstances.[5] If positive mood effects occur, they might be counteracted by factors that depress mood, such as ill health and enhanced sensitivity to pain. Nonetheless, reduced depression might be predicted compared to a similarly symptomatic control group with unrelated illness. (This prediction is complicated by possible counteracting biochemical effects, if downregulation of serotonin function occurred following selective binding by carbamates to the serotonin-binding site on the ACh receptor; or if catecholamine downregulation occurred. These actions would be expected to act in the reverse direction and might attenuate or reverse positive mood effects resulting from changes in the cholinergic system, depending on which effects were most sensitive to chronic alteration.)

Some PGW veterans report eye and visual function problems. Increased tearing is among the acute effects of PB on the eyes. If cholinergic downregulation is in effect, ill PGW veterans might be expected to have reduced lacrimation, which can be assessed by a Schirmer test, rendering it one of the more cheaply and easily tested predictions.

Affected Brain Areas. Brain areas in which regional cerebral blood flow is most enhanced acutely by carbamates (physostigmine, which readily penetrates the brain) should be those brain areas in which regional cerebral blood flow reduction might be expected chronically, measured using quantitative SPECT (a technique that measures regional cerebral blood flow) or functional MRI. (More generally, with a dysregulation rather than a downregulation hypothesis, alterations in timing or degree of blood flow to these areas would be expected.)

Heightened regional cerebral blood flow with physostigmine acutely would be presumed to reflect heightened binding and activity of ACh. By hypothesis, this might coincide with regions in which chronic regional cerebral blood flow

---

[5]Alternatively, there could be increased mood lability and a heightened depressogenic effect of ACh acting agents if low ACh function were accompanied by compensatory muscarinic receptor upregulation; however, such receptor upregulation has primarily been reported for nicotinic receptors.

reductions are seen in ill PGW veterans, corresponding to reductions in ACh activity. Although there are reasons this might not be so (since areas acutely responsive to carbamates may not be those most subject to dysregulation), nonetheless the extent to which this is borne out (or not) adds (or subtracts) support from this hypothesis. These areas are discussed in greater detail in the next point, which looks at the functional correlates of this prediction.

Clinical symptoms in ill PGW veterans should correlate with functions governed by brain (and muscle) regions influenced by carbamates. Functions *governed* by brain areas most affected by carbamates (with physostigmine as an index) should be selectively affected in ill PGW veterans. (The prior prediction related to blood flow measures of activity across regions in the brain. This relates to functional and clinical correlates of activity in those regions.)

Regional cerebral glucose utilization in rats has been examined following administration of the related carbamate AChE-inhibiting compound physostigmine. Physostigmine, at doses of 0.2 and 0.5 mg/kg in rats, measurably increased local cerebral glucose utilization in 15 and 22 regions, respectively, out of 43 regions studied (Bassant, Jazat, and Lamour, 1993). Involved areas included the magnocellular preoptic nucleus (part of the hypothalamic pituitary axis, which is involved in neuroendocrine regulation), ventral thalamus (involved with the amygdala in conditioning), insular cortex (taste), cingulate cortex (concentration, attention), medial septal area (long-term memory), thalamus (gateway to the cortex), superior colliculus (eye movement control), interpositus nucleus (coordination of movement), and the septo-hippocampal system (episodic memory), but not the parietal cortex (sensory motor transformations) (Bassant, Jazat, and Lamour, 1993; and Sejnowski, 1997, for functions of brain regions). The regional topography of the changes in cerebral blood flow reportedly overlapped the distribution of the M2 muscarinic receptors and that of AChE activity, suggesting that the major effects of physostigmine on cerebral glucose utilization resulted from their anticholinesterase action (Bassant, Jazat, and Lamour, 1993).

Another study noted highly localized increased glucose utilization, in rats given physostigmine, in the superior colliculus (eye movements) and anteroventral thalamus (Dietrich, 1984). In humans, studies of cerebral glucose utilization show physostigmine was retained longest in areas rich in AChE, such as the striatum, compared to areas poor in AChE, such as the cerebral cortex (Pappata, Tavitian, et al., 1996). The cerebral distribution of radiolabeled physostigmine was putamen-caudate > cerebellum > brainstem > thalamus > cerebral cortex. Pending studies with finer levels of resolution, if ACh dysregulation is reflected in altered regional blood flow and if it contributes to illness in PGW veterans, then abnormal SPECT findings might be expected to follow this distribution (with the proviso noted above that areas with greatest acute effect might not be those most susceptible to dysregulation), predicting particular effect on the caudate-putamen.

If PB is postulated to be a cause of illness, with symptoms mediated by ACh dysregulation, such dysregulation might most likely occur in areas most affected by PB acutely. For predictive purposes, it is desirable to examine effects mediated by highly specific areas known to control specific functions. One such area is the superior colliculus, which featured in both the rat studies. Rat studies indicated that physostigmine concentrates in this region (Dietrich, 1984; Bassant, Jazat, and Lamour, 1993), and studies support similar involvement in humans, since physostigmine corrects errors in antisaccadic eye movements, in subjects with a condition termed "progressive supranuclear palsy" (Blin, Mazetti, et al., 1995). One prediction from the theory of cholinergic dysregulation is that superior colliculus function may be affected in some ill PGW veterans, producing abnormalities in eye movements, which are controlled by superior colliculus activity. This is one potential function for which sensitive tests should be devised. Some evidence suggests that objective measures of eye movement function are in fact significantly affected in some ill PGW veterans (Haley, Hom, et al., 1997), and efforts are ongoing to find more sensitive oculomotor measures.

In humans, positron emission tomography for AChE using radiolabeled 11C-physostigmine tracer (physostigmine again being closely related to PB) showed the following distribution of 11C-physostigmine, typical of AChE activity: putamen-caudate > cerebellum > brainstem > thalamus > cerebral cortex, with a striatal:cortex ratio of 2 (Barker, Loewenstein, et al., 1987). At times more than 20 minutes after the physostigmine injection, regional retention of 11C-physostigmine was consistent with the regional distribution of AChE activity and concentration in postmortem human brains. The average regional brain concentration of radioactivity at 25–35 minutes were as follows:

Putamen: 2.98±0.87

Cerebellum: 2.28±0.58

Brainstem: 1.94±0.49

Thalamus: 1.74±0.40

Amygdala: 1.83±0.52

Hippocampus: 1.70±0.40

Temporal cortex: BA 22, 21, 20, 38, 28): 1.63±0.50

Frontal associative cortex (BA 9,10): 1.47±0.40

Parietal associative cortex (VA 7,40): 1.49±0.37

White matter: 1.45±0.40.

This study did not report on fine resolution effects, so impact on the superior colliculus was not separately noted. Because of prominent effects in the putamen-caudate, PGW veterans should be monitored for possible early onset Parkinson's disease. Note that tremor has been reported following carbaryl exposure (Ray and Poddar, 1985), and early onset Parkinson's has been related to pesticide exposure, which also includes AChE-inhibiting agents, such as carbamates and OPs (Butterfield, Velanis, et al., 1993; Davis, Yesavage, et al., 1978).

Similarly, in PET studies in baboons, 11C-physostigmine uptake was higher in brain regions with high AChE activity and was prevented by preliminary perfusion by excess unlabeled physostigmine (Tavitian, Pappata, et al., 1993).

If symptoms in some ill PGW veterans result from cholinergic dysregulation, then administration of drugs that enhance or reduce ACh function should affect these symptoms.

Downregulation would be anticipated to produce low cholinergic action. If symptoms result from low ACh action, then ACh enhancing drugs should lead to benefit. This is empirically testable.

Similarly, symptoms known to be alleviated with cholinergic drugs might be expected to be present in ill PGW veterans, if ACh downregulation contributes to symptoms.

Symptoms of low cholinergic action may be helped by cholinergic drugs, and conversely symptoms helped by cholinergic drugs may (sometimes) result from low cholinergic action. (They need not always do so, however.) Some of these symptoms might occur in ill PGW veterans. (If one or two symptoms occur, this evidence by itself remains only suggestive, as ability of a nerve signaling chemical to assist in a function does not necessarily imply that reduced activity of that chemical contributed to the deficit. Presence of multiple such symptoms enhances the likelihood of a cholinergic relation to symptoms in ill PGW veterans. However, if altered regulation of ACh does not fit a simple descriptor of reduced or increased activity, all symptoms may not uniformly respond to agents that simply increase or reduce ACh action.)

Clinical Uses and Comparison to Symptoms

Examination of identified clinical uses of ACh-enhancing agents and comparison to symptoms in PGW veterans may thus be instructive.

- Learning and memory: AChE inhibitors physostigmine and tacrine have been shown to help reverse learning and memory deficits in some conditions involving memory disorders, which in some instances are believed to reflect cholinergic underactivity (Davis and Yamamura, 1978; Christie, Shering, et al., 1981; Murray and Fibiger, 1985) and to enhance memory in normal subjects (Davis, Mohs, et al., 1978). Specific functions enhanced include serial learning (Sitaram and Gillin, 1980), short-term consolidation of low-imagery words (Sitaram and Gillin, 1980), retrieval of clustered information (Sitaram and Gillin, 1980), and long-term memory (Davis, Mohs, et al., 1978). As noted earlier, subjective memory deficits are commonly reported in ill PGW veterans.

- Pyridostigmine has been used to assist in various conditions of fatigue and motor weakness, including myasthenia gravis, some HIV associated fatigue, "neurotic" fatigue (that is, for which no organic cause had been identified), and drop attacks in the elderly (See Chapter Three, "Characteristics of PB," section on medical uses).

- Nicotine has been used to treat sleep apnea; sleep apnea may occur at increased rates in ill PGW veterans. (See Chapter Fifteen, "Other Considerations").

- Nicotine has been used to treat diarrhea in ulcerative colitis; diarrhea has been reported at increased rates in ill PGW veterans (See Chapter Fifteen).

- Physostigmine has reduced eye movement errors in subjects with progressive supranuclear palsy, as above (Blin, Mazetti, et al., 1995). Some evidence suggests abnormalities in saccadic eye movements in ill PGW veterans, as noted earlier.

- Physostigmine has led to improvement on other neuropsychological tests in progressive supranuclear palsy, although not in that condition's motor deficits (Blin, Mazetti, et al., 1995). Some studies suggest that ill PGW veterans may have subtle deficits in neuropsychological tests; whether improvement in function would occur with ACh agents, or would occur more than in controls, is not known.

- Pain has been reduced with ACh agonists (Sitaram and Gillin, 1980) (see Chapter Fifteen for more detail). Pain is common in ill PGW veterans.

- Cortical arousal has been reportedly increased with ACh agonists (Sitaram and Gillin, 1980). Fatigue and reduced concentration and attention have been reported by ill PGW veterans.

LIMITATIONS OF THE HYPOTHESIS

"Downregulation" appears to be a common compensatory phenomenon in the face of pharmacologically heightened signaling, as a mechanism to counteract excessive nerve signaling. However, many concerns limit our ability to impute illnesses in PGW veterans to downregulatory phenomena. Most important, PB is normally excluded from central access, and would be poorly positioned to induce downregulation. (Chapters Six, Seven, and Eight discuss issues related to whether special circumstances may have been present that enhanced effect of PB, or central access of PB.) Second, data suggesting downregulation have been derived largely from animals, often using agents that more readily enter the CNS (particularly in studies looking at central effects), at doses that produce substantial AChE inhibition. Similar effects may or may not occur at lower doses and lesser levels of choline inhibition in humans, using PB in conditions of stress. Third, the time-course of different elements of the compensatory changes has not in all instances been assessed, but many of the changes are substantially reversed in a relatively short time. The time-course for different changes in regulation appears to differ (based on limited available evidence), which could be speculated to lead to loss of the normal coordination of signaling mechanisms. It is not known whether changes could persist or perhaps even evolve as a result of dyscoordination of regulation mechanisms leading to their own compensatory changes, following relatively low doses of PB (with or without other AChE inhibitor coexposures). Fourth, not all changes need be downregulatory—indeed, evidence suggests that opposite changes may occur in the muscarinic and nicotinic receptors, in rat brain, following the same exposure (Nilsson-Haransson, Lai, et al., 1990). On a related note, effects for cholinergic agonists and antagonists may occur differentially in different brain and body sites (Schwab, Costa, et al., 1983). While there is more evidence—clinically and at the tissue level—for downregulation than for other forms of aberrant regulation, the totality of alterations in regulation might most appropriately be termed "dysregulation."

Complicating the evaluation of this hypothesis, different effects of PB and other AChE inhibitors seem to obtain in different muscle groups and in different central sites in animals—perhaps reflecting such factors as different populations of ACh receptors, and different types of AChE (Kamal and al-Jafari, 1996). These differences are themselves a function of the particular AChE-inhibiting chemical (for reasons that are poorly characterized but presumably reflect differences in "specificity" of each agent). Moreover, regulatory changes in the acetylcholinergic system may differ substantially across species, even relatively close species, such as rats and mice. In mice, "denervation" leads to dramatic increases in ACh receptor–encoding genetic material, whereas muscle denervation has little effect in rats (Goldman, Evans, et al., 1987). Whether there also exist differences from one animal to another within a species has not been evaluated. Such individual differences—perhaps regional differences in susceptibility—might be more prominent in humans, since homogeneous groups of inbred animals reared in similar conditions are typically used to reduce individual variation in animal studies and since flexibility in brain development becomes more prominent as one "ascends" the phylogenetic spectrum.

In any case, the clinical consequences and time-course of cholinergic dysregulation, and the individual differences in ability to restore normal functioning, remain poorly defined. Evidence is insufficient to conclude that such differences do or do not contribute to illness in some PGW veterans.

OTHER NEUROTRANSMITTER SYSTEMS

As previously noted (Chapter Three), PB affects not only the acetylcholinergic system but also other neurotransmitter systems.

Glutamate

Glutamate is the major excitatory neurotransmitter in the brain. Moreover, ACh presynaptically modulates (enhances) release of glutamate. For this system, another form of "downregulation" or dampening of the transmitter system may obtain—in the form of "excitotoxicity." Excessive amounts of the intrinsic excitatory amino acid glutamate may excite brain neurons in a manner that results in death of these neurons. Moreover, excitotoxic neurodegeneration may occur with relatively low levels of excitotoxic substances (e.g., glutamate) when neuronal energy metabolism is impaired (Whetsell, 1996). A family of glutamate-sensitive receptors made up of subtypes that are selectively sensitive to a number of different glutamate analogs occur in the mammalian nervous system and respond differently to stimulation. Both "fast" and "slow" (also called "direct" and "indirect," "acute" and "chronic") excitotoxicity have been described (Whetsell, 1996).[6]

Whether excitotoxicity of the glutamate system has any reference to illnesses in PGW veterans is unknown. Additional work could seek to define the locations and characteristics of glutamate receptors that are potentially "sensitive" to carbamates—that is, for which increased ACh release (from AChE inhibition, from PB or similar agents) acts on presynaptic receptors of glutamate-releasing neurons to increase release of glutamate, leading to potential for excitotoxicity.

---

[6]Such excitotoxicity is thought by some to be involved in development of a motor-neuron condition termed amyotrophic lateral sclerosis. Both familial and sporadic cases occur, and GLU receptors, GLU metabolism, and/or GLU uptake mechanisms may all play a role (Whetsell, 1996). According to DoD sources, nine cases of amyotrophic lateral sclerosis have occurred among PGW veterans. The Oversight Report of the Subcommittee on Human Resources House Committee on Government Reform and Oversight appears to quote 1.4–1.7 cases as expected, but this is evidently the number expected in a single year, which would seem consistent with current reports of amyotrophic lateral sclerosis (Subcommittee on Human Resources, 1997 672).

Serotonin

Serotonin is believed to be the endogenous ligand (substance that binds), the special carbamate-binding site on nicotinic acetylcholinergic receptors to which physostigmine (and presumably pyridostigmine, if it enters the brain) binds. Physostigmine not only increases ACh by inhibiting AChE but also directly binds to this site, the "galanthamine"-binding site (named after another drug that also binds to this site), thus modulating ACh release. That is, such carbamates essentially mimic the action of serotonin (Albuquerque, Pereira, et al., 1997; Albuquerque, Alkondon, et al., 1997). The opiate codeine also binds to this site. Since the acetylcholinergic system is believed to be involved in pain regulation, as is the opiate system and the serotonergic system—in the case of fibromyalgia—it is justifiable to wonder whether this special binding site on the nicotinic receptor could reflect a common point of action. Further study may clarify whether excessive binding at this site leads to alterations that could contribute to enhanced pain of a character resembling "fibromyalgia," such as that reported by some PGW veterans.

Dopamine

Since the ACh system modulates dopamine release (see Chapter Three), there may be dysregulation of dopamine—upregulation, downregulation, or a combination—resulting from effects on the cholinergic system.

Catecholamines

The effect of ACh on release of catecholamines is discussed earlier in this chapter. ACh regulates catecholamine secretion from the adrenal medulla. Catecholamines are themselves subject to downregulatory influences (Hardman, Limbird, et al., 1996). Most but perhaps not all of these are of short time-course. It is not known whether low catecholamine function occurs as a result of catecholamine downregulation following delivery of PB. The combination of PB and stress would be expected to lead to a catecholamine surge, possibly producing at least temporary downregulation in the catecholamine system.

MORE COMPLICATIONS

As work continues to unravel potential effects of dysregulation or downregulation of ACh and perhaps of other neurotransmitter systems, the complexity of these systems must always be borne in mind. There exist a multiplicity of types of nicotinic and muscarinic receptors, which may behave differently. They are expressed differentially in different parts of the brain. A number of distinct choline types are also present, indicated by distinct isoenzyme bands (up to 20 bands have been described in the rat (Nagayama, Akahori, et al., 1996)). Impairments in a given system may be evident on challenge with one agonist but not another (Ghigo, Goffi, et al., 1992). There may be male/female differences in enzyme patterns; such differences have been demonstrated in other mammals (Nagayama, Akahori, et al., 1996). Many elements of regulation could be involved, each with possible individual differences and each potentially influenced by other specific properties of that individual's nervous system. Certainly native differences in regulation of different neurotransmitter systems have been identified, and such differences may play a role in individual susceptibility to dysregulation. (These differences have been related to functional differences in risk of addiction to selected substances, in harm avoidance, and in susceptibility to aggression, among other factors.)

CONCLUSION

Because the cholinergic system is known to be involved in many important functions, including memory, sleep, pain, and muscular activity, down-regulation or, more generally, dysregulation might be expected to produce abnormalities in these domains—domains reflected prominently in complaints of PGW veterans, for whom memory complaints, sleep disruption, and musculoskeletal complaints (including pain) have—along with rash—headed the list of complaints. (A possible role in the development of skin symptoms is discussed in Chapter Fifteen.) While complaints in these domains could arise from unrelated causes, there are reasons to seriously evaluate the possibility that PB may be a contributing factor. First, many ill PGW veterans were exposed to PB; second, changes resulting from administration of PB and lasting long after cessation of PB have been identified, though these results are primarily based on studies in neuromuscular junctions in animals; and third, changes of this type—if similar changes occurred centrally, arising from enhanced access of PB to the CNS in conditions of stress or chemical combinations, following doses of PB such as those given in PGW veterans—would be plausible causes or contributors to such symptoms as those described by ill veterans. (Musculoskeletal and even CNS problems might arise even without such central access by PB, through peripheral actions on the neuromuscular junction and on catecholamine release.) Nonetheless, the time-course and dosing characteristics of these changes have not been well characterized. It is unknown what magnitude of change in cholinergic function would be required to produce symptoms such as those described by PGW veterans (symptoms that, while important to veterans, do not produce readily detectable abnormalities on most neuropsychiatric batteries), and it is unknown whether the dose and time-course of the downregulatory effect—or of heightened sensitivity effects, if any—are compatible with such changes. It is possible that effects, which may differ for different brain areas and regulatory components, could interact to produce alterations that evolve over time, though this possibility is speculative.

At the time this report was first circulated (including this chapter on dysregulation), ACh system dysregulation had not been previously proposed as a mechanism to consider in relation to illness in PGW veterans. Since then, additional evidence is emerging that suggests that such dysregulation may occur. More recent findings are included in an Addendum.

SCIENTIFIC RECOMMENDATIONS

- Additional research is needed into the effects of AChE inhibition by agents—particularly carbamates—on central and peripheral nicotinic and muscarinic signaling. Such research should include investigation into effects on receptors (receptor density, binding affinity, sensitivity to action of ACh once bound), considering each identified receptor type separately; on nerve innervation (e.g., withdrawal of nerve terminals); production and release of ACh from signaling cells; and breakdown of ACh, including effects if any on AChE production and metabolism. Special attention should be paid to doses required for each effect, influence on each effect of the time-course of carbamate delivery, time-course of the effect (e.g., does it persist, increase, or reverse on discontinuation of the carbamate), regional brain differences in the effect (and their relation, or lack of relation, to specific receptor types that predominate in those brain areas), influence on these outcomes of individual differences in processing of PB and ACh (per Chapter Eight), and the influence of concomitant exposures with such agents as pesticides, nerve agents, cigarettes, and others (as per Chapter Nine). Both baseline "tone" of nicotinic and muscarinic systems, as well as reactivity to stimulation, should be assessed. (Evidence from several domains that low baseline function of a neurotransmitter system in some conditions is associated with high reactivity. This could occur, for instance, if there is reduced neurotransmitter release tonically but increased receptor density or binding affinity.)

- Similar tests should be performed to assess function of other neurotransmitter systems influenced by carbamates and by ACh, including the GABA-ergic, glutamatergic, serotonergic, and dopaminergic as well as catecholaminergic systems.

- Additional efforts should be made to assess, at as fine a scale as possible, baseline and task-specific regional blood flow with and without administration of physostigmine, using quantitative SPECT and functional MRI. (This makes the plausible assumption that, if PB crossed the blood-brain barrier, its regional effects would be similar.) Quantitative SPECT and functional MRI studies should be undertaken in ill PGW veterans and controls to examine regional cerebral blood flow. If abnormalities are seen in ill PGW veterans, the regions of altered distribution should be compared to regions altered with administration of physostigmine.

- Efforts should be made to identify objective tests of function related to brain areas in which physostigmine (a related carbamate that crosses into the brain) has been shown to alter regional glucose utilization. (These areas are discussed above.) Once again, it is reasonable to assume that if PB crosses into the brain, the areas affected will likely be similar to those affected with physostigmine, and areas in which effects of AChE inhibition with PB are greatest (indicated by alterations in glucose utilization) are a priori more likely to be areas in which altered regulation of function would ensue.

- Similar efforts should be made to identify sensitive tests for peripheral deficits that might relate to AChE dysfunction.

- Efforts could be made to institute consented, double-blind treatment trials employing agents that augment cholinergic function, such as nicotine, physostigmine, or antihistamines, which have AChE-inhibiting action and increase central ACh (Dringenberg, De Souza-Silva, et al., 1998; Laine-Cessac, Turcant, et al., 1993) or alternatively with agents that have anticholinergic effects. Such trials could test the hypothesis that symptoms in ill PGW veterans arise as a result of cholinergic dysregulation. Symptoms that might respond to cholinergic augmentation include sleep apnea—from which musuloskeletal pain, fatigue, and cognitive dysfunction might ensue—cognitive complaints, such as problems with memory or concentration; diarrhea; pain; and perhaps rash. (If the theory of cholinergic kindling for chemical sensitivities has merit, anticholinergic agents might be hypothesized to produce benefit for chemical sensitivities. However, most symptoms in ill PGW veterans appear primarily consistent with low cholinergic function.) Tests employing selective nicotinic, muscarinic, and antinicotinic or antimuscarinic agents might help to define whether or how dysregulation of the nicotinic and/or muscarinic systems contributes to symptoms in ill PGW veterans.

SUMMARY ANALYSIS

Exposure

Exposure to PB occurred in an estimated 250,000 to 300,000 veterans (Brake, 1997).

Compatible Symptoms

Symptoms of downregulation or dysregulation of the cholinergic system (which may include elements of depressed and heightened cholinergic responsiveness) would be expected to include problems with memory, learning, sleep, musculo-skeletal function, GI motility, and pain. Nicotine treatment has reportedly led to benefits for several of these conditions, including memory and cognitive dysfunction, diarrhea, and sleep apnea. Sleep apnea treatment in turn may lead to resolution of secondarily induced problems, including soft tissue pain (fibromyalgia), fatigue, and memory/cognitive dysfunction. These symptoms are prominent in ill PGW veterans. (Sleep and pain are discussed in greater detail in Chapter Fifteen.)

Link Between Exposure and Symptoms

No direct scientific evidence exists to either support or refute a link between cholinergic dysregulation and symptoms in ill PGW veterans.

Chapter Fourteen

CHRONIC EFFECTS

PB has been widely used in treatment of myasthenia gravis since it was licensed for this purpose by the FDA in the 1950s. No chronic adverse effects have been widely reported. However, there are two significant limitations to the evidence for safety in normal subjects: first, data from patients with myasthenia may not apply to normal subjects, or more specifically to PGW veterans; second, evidence of lack of chronic effects in patients with myasthenia is itself limited. Chronic adverse effects of time-limited administration of PB in large groups of normal individuals have not been studied, complicating the ability to comment on PB's safety for this group.

EXTRAPOLATION OF DATA FROM MYASTHENIA GRAVIS

Chapter Three included some discussion regarding potential limitations in extrapolation of data on use of PB from myasthenia to those without myasthenia. This chapter reprises and extends comments regarding why information regarding effects of PB use in myasthenia may not ensure safety in PGW veterans.

First, use of PB in myasthenia helps normalize nicotinic cholinergic activity, while use of PB in nonmyasthenics drives nicotinic cholinergic activity away from normal and might therefore have different effects.[1]

---

[1] There is precedent for such regulatory changes with drugs affecting many neurotransmitter systems, and the time-courses of the consequent effects are variable. Some are short lived, while others are long-lasting. Beta-blocker withdrawal leads to rebound hyperactivity—a short-lived but clinically important effect. Administration of hypnotic drugs to assist with sleep is problematic because tolerance develops quickly—within a couple of weeks—followed by rebound worsening of insomnia or withdrawal of the drug, an effect of ill-defined time-course. Narcotics, such as heroin, have well-known acute withdrawal effects in addicts, but many patients and physicians are familiar with additional long-term—perhaps lifelong—effects in the form of increased pain sensitivity (reduced pain threshold) experienced by prior addicts, presumably a consequence of down-regulation of the opiate neurotransmission system. Administration of exogenous corticosteroids for as little as a week is known by clinicians to lead to relatively prolonged (potentially one year) down-regulation in the form of suppression of the adrenal response to stress. (Such patients must then be

Second, patients with myasthenia continue to receive PB for life. If down-regulation of the cholinergic system occurs, initially in response to excessive cholinergic activity (see Chapter Thirteen, "Neurotransmitter Dysregulation"), the consequences might not be detected in persons continuing to receive cholinergic augmentation. In myasthenia, the body is responding to high levels of ACh (and high ACh activity at muscarinic receptors, though activity may be normal or low at skeletal muscle nicotinic receptors) by driving ACh response down. As long as PB administration continues—and doses must often be increased as "tolerance" to PB occurs in myasthenia, suggesting development of downregulation—effects of low ACh response will be masked by the presence of pharmacologically induced high ACh. If PB were discontinued, low ACh effects would be unopposed by augmented ACh, and symptoms could result; however, it is seldom possible to discontinue use of PB in patients with myasthenia.

Third, several critical PB interactions further complicate the extrapolation of "safety" (lack of identified long-term adverse effects) from myasthenia to PGW veterans. For instance, under ordinary circumstances, based on animal studies (and to some degree supported by reports of symptoms in people), little PB will cross the blood-brain barrier because of PB's charged quaternary ammonium structure. However, evidence (also from animal studies) suggests that more PB may cross the blood-brain barrier in the context of some forms of stress or severe chemical exposure (see Chapter Seven, "Blood-Brain Barrier"); stresses of this kind might more likely have been present for PGW veterans than for patients with myasthenia gravis (though whether stresses in the PGW were sufficient to induce similar effects is unknown). Thus, the de facto "exposure" from PB in PGW veterans may differ from the de facto exposure associated with PB use in myasthenics. Moreover, since PB may interact with other chemical exposures, for example by enhancing access of other chemicals to the CNS and by other chemical effects through competition for scavenging and metabolizing enzymes, chronic symptoms may result from the use of PB concomitantly with exposure to other chemicals, such as a low-level nerve agents, pesticides, or solvents. (See Chapter Nine, "Interactions Between PB and Other Exposures.") For these reasons, effects of PB in the PGW context might be presumed to differ from effects in patients with myasthenia gravis. Moreover, while a number of

---

given "stress doses" of corticosteroids when major stressors, such as surgery, are encountered.) Fenfluramine, a drug until recently given to enhance serotonergic function (until long-term side effects on heart valves were discovered) has been shown to be toxic to serotonergic neurons—an effect that is presumably long-lasting or permanent. Clearly, compensatory changes are made in regulation of many or most chemical-signaling systems in the body in response to pharmacological alteration of those signaling systems. The time-courses of these effects are highly variable. More-over, different compensatory changes in response to the same pharmacological challenge may have different time-courses. As mentioned in previous chapters, the time-course of such effects for the acetylcholinergic systems have not been well defined.

studies in small samples of military volunteers followed generally for short time periods provide confidence that acute effects of PB in these populations are modest (see the discussion of side effects and associated table in Chapter Three), these studies also would be expected to miss effects of PB in the context of stress or interactions. (Such studies have typically evaluated such physiological parameters as heart rate and temperature, side effects, and effects on performance. Although some such studies have been done in the context of "basic training" for the Israeli military, such basic training is "routine" and is undergone by the whole population, unlike in the United States. Persons in the Israeli military, queried during a fact-finding mission to the Middle East, did not regard basic training as particularly stressful, but likened it to "camp.") Indeed, evidence suggests that effects of PB in the context of war may indeed have differed from effects reported in military volunteers. In contrast to low rates of reported side effects in the latter group, a cross-sectional survey of Israeli soldiers who took PB during the PGW indicated quite high rate of symptom reporting (see Table 3.8) (Sharabi, Danon, et al., 1991).

Thus, differences in the circumstances of use between myasthenia patients and PGW veterans make it difficult to extrapolate evidence of long-term safety from myasthenic to nonmyasthenic subjects. Moreover, systematic evaluation of chronic effects of PB has seldom been performed for myasthenic PB users. The benefits of PB treatment in myasthenics (including maintenance of "activities of daily living" and prevention of death) so clearly outweigh the risks of use that subtle or even less-subtle adverse effects, if present, might fail to excite concern in patients or physicians, diminishing the ability to conclude that no long-term adverse effects are present. Furthermore, myasthenics have an identified neurological disorder, and evolving or chronic symptoms, if they occur, might be ascribed to the disease process or psychological response to this process, rather than to the treatment. The clear preponderance of benefit with PB treatment for myasthenics would render attempts to compare chronic consequences of active treatment to those of placebo in this group impractical and perhaps unethical. Nonetheless, if symptom-reporting serves as a guide, in fact more than 50 percent of myasthenia patients receiving PB report side effects they attribute to medication, including diarrhea and cognitive symptoms (Hood, 1990).   Of particular note, myasthenia patients have also reported that adverse effects of anticholinesterase medications were aggravated by stress and by extreme hot weather or sun exposure—both factors reported in animals to enhance permeability of the blood-brain barrier to PB in some conditions, by taking the medication on an empty stomach, by lack of adequate sleep, and by exercising immediately after a dose, among other factors that may have occurred in the PGW setting (Hood, 1990). Other factors to which PGW veterans may have been exposed that were also reported by patients with myasthenia gravis to aggravate symptoms included use of aspirin and other unspecified over-the-counter analgesics, use of Maalox and certain antibiotics, and consumption of dairy products, alcohol, and carbonated beverages (Hood, 1990).

Thus, many factors complicate the ability to compare chronic adverse effects in myasthenics and in normals. One class of chronic adverse effects from PB in myasthenics has been postulated. Specifically, research suggests that ultrastructural damage at the motor endplate resulting from use of PB is similar to ultrastructural damage at the motor endplate seen in myasthenics. It has been suggested that PB may contribute to these pathological changes, and thereby to the apparently reduced rate of cure seen in modern myasthenics. (The prevalence of myasthenia has risen significantly, despite no significant change in incidence or mortality (Phillips and Torner, 1996).) Evidence from animal studies clearly shows alterations in the motor endplates with use of PB— alterations that abate with continued use but may not disappear. Whether such alterations have clinical implications in humans is unknown.

In short, there exists "evidence" of the long-term safety of PB use by virtue of long-term use in myasthenics. But this "evidence" of safety consists primarily of absence of evidence of harm, in the context of absence of testing for harm, in persons in whom the evolution of some symptoms might be attributed to the underlying disease and in whom indefinitely continued use of PB might mask effects of cholinergic downregulation initially produced to help "normalize" function in the face of such use.[2] Tests for chronic adverse effects of PB would be difficult in myasthenics because of the problems associated with generating adequate controls. Moreover, little data exists on what becomes of myasthenics who have taken PB and then ceased to use it, because this is seldom possible.[3] Although controlled studies of the effects of PB in myasthenia are difficult for the reasons noted, observational studies do in fact suggest a high rate of side effect reporting in subjects with myasthenia gravis who receive PB (Hood, 1990). (However, they continue to receive it.) Meanwhile, chronic follow-up of large samples of military volunteers following short-term PB exposure, with neuropsychological tests designed to be sensitive for problems reported by ill PGW veterans or designed to sensitively test cholinergic function, have not been performed. Such factors render it difficult to exclude the possibility of chronic effects of short-term PB administration. Because PB may interact with other PGW exposures, for example enhancing access of other neurotoxic agents to the CNS, a contributory role for PB in long-term adverse effects due in part to

---

[2]Similarly, use of corticosteroids leads to a hypoadrenergic state—seen primarily in the face of adrenal challenge—that is unmasked only when the agent is discontinued.

[3]Anecdotally, many patients with myasthenia do experience central symptoms that are incorrectly attributed by their physicians to effects of the myasthenia (Haley, 1998).

other agents must also be considered when the issue of chronic effects is approached.

The aim in this chapter is to evaluate the plausibility of chronic effects by examining the evidence of long-term effects associated with PB and with other AChE inhibitors, where such evidence is available. This evidence is by its nature hypothesis-generating and is not intended to prove or disprove a relationship between PB and chronic effects. However, it can be used to direct further inquiry. It should be noted that interactions with many other exposures may play a role in determining susceptibility to chronic, as well as to acute, adverse effects; and individual differences in drug absorption, metabolism, elimination, cholinergic regulation, and levels of scavenging enzymes may condition which individuals (if any) experience long-term deleterious consequences when receiving PB alone or in combination with other exposures.

In an effort to evaluate the plausibility of chronic effects from administration of PB, this chapter will focus on the following potentially pertinent areas of investigation: Chronic EEG changes with AChE inhibitors, chronic changes in regional cerebral blood flow, other alterations seen in imaging studies following exposure to AChE inhibitors, chronic neuropsychiatric effects following exposure to AChE inhibitors and pesticides, chronic neurologic effects following exposure to AChE inhibitors, chronic neurochemical changes following exposure to AChE inhibitors, and the relation of acute exposure to chronic symptoms with AChE inhibitors. The implications of these findings for possible chronic effects of PB in PGW veterans will then be discussed.

EEG

Studies have evaluated effects of exposure to AChE inhibitors (predominantly OP pesticides and nerve agents) on the EEG. Acute and chronic EEG alterations have been reported in several but not all such studies.

Positive Findings

EEG changes were seen in primates with chronic low dose administration of pesticides (given for 18 months) without clinical signs (Santolucito and Morrison, 1971). Changes were seen for all four pesticides tested, including the carbamate pesticide carbaryl. (The other tested agents were the organochlorines DDT and dieldrin and the OP parathion.) Doses were "1,000 times" estimated consumption by humans based on market basket surveys (estimates of per capita use based on pesticide purchases); carbaryl was tested at 0.01 mg/kg/d, and 1.0 mg/kg/d. EEG changes included increased bilateral synchrony, reduction in high-amplitude slow waves, and reduction in low amplitude fast waves in pesticide-exposed monkeys (Santolucito and Morrison, 1971). This study evaluated the effect of chronic exposure but did not in fact evaluate for chronic effects following termination of the exposure.

Such an evaluation has been done for the cholinesterase-inhibiting nerve agent sarin. Rhesus monkeys were exposed to a single high dose of sarin (5 µg/kg) or to 10 low doses, which did not produce any "major" clinical symptoms (1 µg/kg at one week intervals) or to a placebo. EEGs were recorded before exposure and at 24 hours and one year after. Both large and small doses of sarin produced significant and persistent increases in the relative amount of high-frequency beta activity (13–50 Hz) in the EEG, changes that did not occur in control animals (Burchfiel and Duffy, 1982). These authors also conducted a retrospective study in 77 humans with past industrial exposure to sarin, occurring more than 1 year previously, comparing EEG findings to those in 38 unexposed controls from the same plant. Increased beta activity was again seen in the sarin-exposed population, as was increased REM sleep. In addition, increased slow activity (0–8 Hz, delta and theta) and reduced alpha (9–12 Hz) were reported. EEG findings were more pronounced in the "maximally exposed" group (n = 41), who had experienced at least three separate sarin exposures over the previous six years, than in the overall exposed group, suggesting a dose-response effect. Results appeared bimodal, with one mode corresponding to the mode of the control population, suggesting that differences in exposure or susceptibility may condition which individuals experience these changes (Burchfiel and Duffy, 1982). Of note: increased beta is also seen during drowsiness and sleep, aging, organic brain lesions, and with many drugs which produce beta as part of generalized desynchronization (Burchfiel and Duffy, 1982). (For more on possible long-term effects of nerve agents, see *A Review of the Scientific Literature As It Pertains to Gulf War Illnesses*, Vol. 5: *Chemical and Biological Warfare Agents* (Augerson, forthcoming).) Increased REM is a relatively uncommon pharmacological effect; many drugs, including alcohol, mood elevators, barbiturates, common tranquilizers, and amphetamine produce reductions in REM, but few produce increased REM. Indeed, REM sleep mechanisms are believed to be under cholinergic control, with pro-cholinergic drugs reducing latency to REM and increasing the duration of REM (Sitaram and Gillin, 1979).

In a study of 300 persons industrially exposed to pesticides requiring medical care and 300 controls, 15 percent of pesticide exposed versus 1 percent of controls showed (undefined) EEG abnormalities (Amr, Allam, et al., 1993). Abnormal EEGs have been reported by several other investigators, both following acute OP toxicity (Holmes, 1964; Metcalf and Holmes, 1969; Brown, 1971; Grob and Harvey, 1953; Korsak and Sato, 1977) and following chronic exposures to pesticides (Metcalf and Holmes, 1969; Korsak and Sato, 1977) or industrial exposure to sarin (Duffy, Burchfiel, et al., 1979).

Blinded assessment of EEGs in ill PGW veterans and controls, in sleep and awake, including assessment of beta-activity, is under way (Haley, 1998).

Negative Findings

No chronic EEG changes were reported in 100 OP-exposed cases compared to age, sex, SES, occupational level, and education-matched controls, despite pervasive differences in neuropsychological test results. However, this study does not discuss which EEG parameters were reviewed and compared (Savage, Keefe, et al., 1988). In one study of 20 ill PGW veterans, EEGs were performed as part of a battery of tests, and were stated not to demonstrate abnormalities. No control group was used, and there was no discussion of whether quantitative evaluation took place or of what EEG parameters were evaluated (Amato, McVey, et al., 1997).

Evidence supports the possibility that long-term changes in the EEG *may* occur following exposure to some AChE inhibitors, including the nerve agent sarin and the carbamate pesticides carbaryl. Some evidence involves relatively brief exposures or relatively low doses that do not produce overt chemical signs, although none involve long-term follow-up following a single low-dose exposure.

The EEG is a crude measure that is difficult to interpret. Chronic changes in this measure suggest widespread if subtle alterations in brain activity, but the relation to functional change is ill-defined. Moreover, the degree to which observed EEG abnormalities are agent-specific or represent the effect of exposure to AChE inhibition is unknown. Therefore, it cannot be stated that similar effects would be seen with PB exposure (although this is testable). PB exposure occurring together with pesticide or a low dose of a nerve agent might, by competing for scavenging and metabolizing enzymes, increase access of these other agents to the CNS and potentiate their ability to produce EEG effects, presumably resulting from alterations in underlying brain signaling.

EFFECTS ON CEREBRAL BLOOD FLOW

SPECT imaging has revealed abnormal regional cerebral blood flow in pesticide-exposed subjects. In one study, 40 cases (16 young, age 34±8, and 225 elderly, age 55±7) exposed to neurotoxic chemicals, including pesticides, glues, and solvents, and 30 controls (10 young and 20 elderly) underwent SPECT imaging. Results of Xenon regional cerebral blood flow showed diminished cerebral blood flow in cases compared to controls, which were worse in the right hemisphere, with random presentation of areas of hypoperfusion more prevalent in the dorsal frontal and parietal lobes (Heuser, Mena, et al., 1994). The findings were reported to be significantly different from those in patients with chronic fatigue and depression. The authors suggest a primary cortical effect (Heuser, Mena, et al., 1994).

It has been suggested that SPECT might be useful for identifying disease and tracking the response to treatment in neurotoxin-exposed subjects. In one case report, a woman exposed to an insecticide mixture (pyrethrin, phosphoro-thioate, piperonyl butoxide, and petroleum distillates), who had delayed chronic symptoms (including coarse tremor, hemiballistic movements of the right arm and leg, flaccid muscular tone, fasciculations of muscle groups, muscle cramps, and sensory disturbances) underwent SPECT imaging 34 months after exposure. SPECT revealed significantly reduced blood flow to the left temporal lobe and the right and left basal ganglia. A trial of medication (amantadine and selegiline) resulted in dramatic reduction in dysfunctional movements and ataxia, and posttherapy SPECT revealed significantly improved blood flow, suggesting that SPECT may both reveal abnormalities and their reversal with treatment (Callender, Morrow, et al., 1994). This study is severely limited in that it is a single case report with single SPECT scans before and after treatment. Larger trials examining response of SPECT to treatment are desirable, but depend on the existence of a treatment modality.

The role of SPECT (or alternatively, functional MRI, which allows a view of regional cerebral blood flow over time in the course of specific tasks and activities) in evaluation of toxin-exposed individuals remains to be defined. Alterations in regional cerebral blood flow are seen in many conditions (Schwartz, Komaroff, et al., 1994; Simon, Hickey, et al., 1994; Ito, Kawashima, et al., 1996; Krausz, Bonne, et al., 1996; Galynker, Weiss, et al., 1997; Iidaka, Nakajima, et al., 1997; Schmitz, Moriarty, et al., 1997). Distinctions in regional cerebral blood flow have been reported between conditions in some instances. For example, major depression produces a different profile than that seen in chronic fatigue and healthy controls (Fischler, D'Haenen, et al., 1996).) Additional work is needed to more clearly establish whether distinct patterns of deficit can be discriminated following neurotoxic exposures, and care will be needed to ensure blinded reading of SPECT images.

Recommendations

SPECT is a potentially important technique that may be sensitive to deficits produced with neurotoxins. This technique has been applied only to a very small group of ill veterans (see Chapter Eleven, "Multiple Chemical Sensitivity"). Evaluation of a larger sample of ill PGW veterans, who may be compared to healthy controls in blinded studies, may be desirable. If abnormalities are found, these can be compared to observed SPECT abnormalities in patients with depression, pesticide exposure, and chronic fatigue. There is no consensus regarding the source of illnesses in these veterans, and hypotheses include neurotoxic exposure and infection-related chronic fatigue, as well as psychiatric etiologies and "exaggeration" (Kotler-Cope, Milby, et al., 1996), among others. Therefore, SPECT should be evaluated for sensitivity and specificity regarding these diagnoses. (Absence of ability of SPECT, in isolation, to discriminate among these diagnoses does not necessarily preclude the utility of this test. Just as an elevated white blood count is compatible with several causes, which are distinguished by other tests, so supplementary testing may be needed to clarify the source of abnormal regional blood flow on SPECT imaging.) Moreover, ill PGW veterans should perhaps be compared to controls to establish whether objective findings, in the form of differences in regional cerebral blood flow compared to controls, characterize ill PGW veterans. If SPECT imaging is found to correlate with self-reported symptoms, it might offer an objective technique, as an adjunct to self-report, to track the stability, progression, or regression of CNS dysfunction in ill PGW veterans who report cognitive defects.

NEUROPSYCHIATRIC EFFECTS

The existing literature is mixed regarding whether chronic effects ensue following acute or low-dose chronic exposure to AChE inhibitors, including OP pesticides, nerve agents, and PB—although on balance the literature may be viewed as favoring such long-term effects (Jamal, 1995a; Jamal, 1995b). Short-term low-dose exposures, such as those likely to have been experienced during the PGW, may be less likely to lead to chronic sequelae, though little testing of this possibility has been performed.

Pesticides

Some studies have failed to find increased incidence of psychiatric disorders (Stoller, Krupinski, et al., 1965) or serious sequelae in humans (Tabershaw and Cooper, 1966), or abnormal behavior in animals (Clark, 1971) exposed to OP pesticides. For example, one study of 49 pesticide applicators and 40 comparison subjects (not well matched on education or language preference) found that after controlling for baseline performance, only one subtest showed worse adjusted postseason performance in cases than controls after one six-month season of pesticide application, in a group with "generally low, intermittent, and well-controlled OP exposure" (Daniell, Barnhart, et al., 1992). (In Chapter Eight, it was noted that in another study of pesticide applicators, all had the "resistant" PON phenotype, suggesting possible self-selection for the job; pesticide-sensitive individuals may selectively drop out and not undergo postseason testing. Something more akin to an "intention to treat" type of analysis, testing subjects before their first pesticide application and again later, would provide more persuasive evidence.)

In other studies, neuropsychiatric disturbances have been reported following acute (Rosenstock, Keifer, et al., 1991; Tabershaw and Cooper, 1966) or chronic low-dose (Richter, Chuwers, et al., 1992; Gershon and Shaw, 1961; Dille and Smith, 1964; Metcalf and Holmes, 1969; Rodnitzky, Levin, et al., 1975; Levin, Rodnitzky, et al., 1976; Maizlish, 1987; Korsak and Sato, 1977) OP exposure. For instance, EMG abnormalities have been reported in workers in OP production plants (Drenth, Ensberg, et al., 1972). In one study, of 300 persons industrially exposed to pesticides, only 30 percent were free of a set of neurological and behavioral symptoms compared to 80 percent of a group of 300 controls; and only 30 percent were free of a set of signs, versus 76 percent of controls (Amr, Allam, et al., 1993).

Chronic neuropsychiatric effects, including blurred vision, headache, weakness, and anorexia have been reported to persist in some workers months after exposure, when cholinesterase activity has returned to normal (Midtling, Barnett, et al., 1985). In one study, "poisoned" pesticide workers exhibited long-term deficits in memory, attention, visuomotor function, and motor skills (Rosenstock, Keifer, et al., 1991); in another, workers with chronic exposure to the OP pesticide fenthion showed significant changes in several neuropsychiatric tests (such as memory tests) suggestive of subclinical effects on cognitive function (Misra, Prasad, et al., 1994); exposed subjects performed worse on 15 of 17 tests, with equal scores on the remaining two. The differences were statistically significant in 7 of 17 tests.

Vibration sensitivity has been used as a model of sensory assessment in neurotoxicology (Maurissen, 1985). In one study, vibration thresholds in both hands (but not in feet) were significantly higher for 90 male pesticide "applicators" than for age-, sex-, and country-matched controls (Stokes, Stark, et al., 1995). Moreover, in pesticide applicators but not in controls, vibration thresholds increased dramatically with increasing age (Stokes, Stark, et al., 1995). Another study reports higher vibration thresholds, in hands and feet, in 36 OP-poisoned workers (McConnell, Keifer, et al., 1994).

Studies examining chronic effects following exposure to AChE inhibitors, particularly OP pesticides, have been criticized for not having one or more of the following: matched controls, complete documentation of acute exposures, sufficient quantitative neurologic and behavioral measures, and complete statistical analyses (Savage, Keefe, et al., 1988). A study that purports to correct these defects, by comparing results on a large neuropsychiatric battery in 100 OP-exposed cases and 100 controls matched to cases on age, sex, education, SES, occupational station, and other factors, found pervasive but subtle differences between cases and controls on many outcome measures (Savage, Keefe, et al., 1988). For instance, cases were significantly worse than controls on four of five neuropsychological summary measures, including the Halstead Impairment index, Average Impairment Rating, Wechsler Adult Intelligence Scale Verbal IQ ($p < .001$), and WAIS Full Scale IQ ($p < .001$) but not the WAIS Performance IQ ($p = .242$). Cases performed worse on 18 of 34 subtest scores for the Halstead Impairment Index. Twenty-four percent of cases versus 12 percent of controls performed in the range characteristic of documented cerebral damage or dysfunction. Subjects' subjective assessment of functioning were significantly worse in cases than in controls in 10 of 32 aspects of language and communication, memory, cognitive intellectual functioning, and perceptual function; while relatives' assessments of patient functioning were lower on four of 31 items as well as in four of 22 personality scale items (depression, irritability, confusion, and social withdrawal). No differences were found on basic neurological examination or EEG (Savage, Keefe, et al., 1988). This study is limited by a lack of data confirming baseline comparability on these measures in cases and controls prior to OP intoxication—that is, cases could have had test scores significantly different from controls in these many measures prior to OP exposure.

The findings of impaired functioning in OP-exposed cases, with diminished functioning as rated by patients and relatives despite technically "normal" performance on many tests, recalls the relatively subtle (as regards test outcomes, though not necessarily subtle to patients) deficits reported by PGW veterans across a variety of functions despite normal performance on tests. While loss of function within the "normal" range may seem unimportant to an observer, it may critically affect functioning of the individual, whose cognitive strategies evolved to capitalize on a set of strengths and skills that may have become impaired. On reflection, the potential for loss of function is obvious: most people test in the "normal" range on most tests, yet an extraordinary range of differences in skills and in ability to perform selected tasks is seen from one "normal" individual to another. Performance on tests that is reduced, even if still "normal," can clearly coincide with decrements in performance in daily tasks. (See Vol. 8: *Pesticides* (Geschwind and Golomb, forthcoming) for more detail on pesticide effects).

PB

One animal study, published in abstract form only, has evaluated persistent neurobehavioral effects of PB in rats. PB was given orally at a dose of 2 mg/kg (about 4.7 Gulf War doses) for seven days. Startle responses to noise were assessed using whole body and eyeblink EMG responses. These responses were unaffected 24 hours after the end of PB treatment, but enhanced startle responses emerged one to two weeks after treatment had ended (Natelson, Ottenweller, et al., 1996). These changes, though still present at 21 days, disappeared in 28 days (Ottenweller, 1998).[4]

Chronic Symptoms in Ill PGW Veterans

If AChE inhibitors are capable of producing chronic neuropsychological or other deficits, this is relevant to ill PGW veterans only if some of these veterans demonstrate these deficits. Several studies using selected groups of veterans have shown such deficits, though results are not uniform. This section will review some studies that have evaluated deficits in ill PGW veterans, including both neuropsychiatric deficits and, in some instances, other deficits, such as fatigue. Before reviewing the positive studies, it should be noted that some studies have failed to support neuropsychological or muscular deficits in ill PGW veterans—or have attributed those deficits to psychological factors (Goldstein, Beers, et al., 1996; Amato, McVey, et al., 1997; Sillanpaa, Agar, et al., 1997; Vasterling, Brailly, et al., 1998). Unfortunately, failure to show significant deficits does not necessarily signify absence of true deficits. Such negative evidence is persuasive only if factors that favor high variance or bias toward the null (factors that will produce false negative results) have been eliminated and only if a persuasive case can be made that the outcome measures employed constitute sufficiently sensitive measures of any potential deficits. (This a more difficult case to make persuasively in the presence of studies using other measures that show positive evidence of deficits.) Specifically, spurious null results may result from use of a poor case definition, leading to misclassification bias (producing bias to the null); inadequate power (from too small a sample for the amount of variance) to show a meaningful difference (virtually no such study performed power calculations); use of outcome measures that are insensitive to the deficits of ill PGW veterans; and design flaws, such as lack of actual statistical comparison to a control group or inferences not supported by the evidence. None of the negative studies is free of these factors. Although positive studies have had their own design imperfections, future research endeavoring to understand illness in PGW veterans must follow the trail defined by apparent positive findings, seeking to replicate and extend these findings or to refute them. Less attention is accorded negative studies because their failure to

---

[4]Although time-equivalents between animal species are function-specific, for many biological functions time periods in rats correspond to substantially longer periods in humans. However, neither the biological mechanisms for these particular changes, nor the correct time-correspondence in humans—presuming these findings are preserved at all—have been elucidated.

demonstrate deficits does not preclude existence of deficits defined by other measures or using other case definitions or in larger samples.

A study (published only as a several-sentence abstract) of 55 PGW veterans complaining of cognitive dysfunction found relative weaknesses in California Verbal Learning Test, Boston Naming Test, and Category Test performance in veterans compared to standard scores (Kotler-Cope, Milby, et al., 1996). Only two subjects had "a significant number" of scores more than two standard deviations below the standard score mean. However, the abstract does not state what constitutes "a significant number," in what group standard scores were derived, and whether the standard score group constitutes an appropriate comparison. The authors conclude that results are not consistent with a neuro-pathological process and suggest the influence of other factors, such as exaggeration, low premorbid functioning, and emotional distress. It is difficult to evaluate this study or these conclusions without more details regarding the study.

One survey of more than 1,000 (self-selected) PGW registry veterans is under way; preliminary evidence suggests a link between reported illnesses or symptoms and self-reported PB exposure. Moreover, a dose-response effect is suggested by greater reports of symptoms in those with reports of longer duration of PB exposure (Ottenweller, 1997). Although studies of this type are necessarily limited by self-selection and possible recall bias (at least some recollected doses are likely to be in error, since subjects have rarely reported taking PB tablets for as long as six months), self-report remains the best available measure for exposures in the PGW.

Several published peer-reviewed studies of selected PGW veterans find evidence of impaired neuropsychological function compared to controls, at least in the included subset. A pair of studies by Haley et al. found that report of side effects with PB use was associated with two of three primary factor-analysis derived syndromes in PGW veterans (Haley and Kurt, 1997), syndromes termed confusion-ataxia and arthro-myo-neuropathy (Haley, Kurt, and Hom, 1997). This study is limited by self-report of PB symptoms.

A third study from this group examines 23 veteran cases and 20 veteran controls (10 deployed and 10 not, from the same Naval Mobile Construction Battalion) in a nested case control study. The study found impairment in ill PGW veterans compared to controls on both of two global measures of brain dysfunction, the Halstead Impairment Index ($p < .01$), and the General Neuropsychological Deficit Scale ($p < .05$). Performance was worse on an assortment of other tests. Of 35 tests out of 165 on which cases and controls differed significantly or borderline significantly ($p < 0.1$ by Mann-Whitney U test), cases were more impaired than controls in 27 ($p < .001$ by binomial test). There were significant differences on 20 of 89 tests with endpoints that did not depend on volitional action by subjects (such as evoked potentials); cases were more impaired than controls on 18 of these. There were significant differences on 15 of the 76 tests with endpoints depending on volitional action; cases were more impaired on nine and controls on six (Haley, Hom, et al., 1997); findings were similar for those with each of the three factor-derived syndromes. Worse performance in ill PGW veterans was thus more rather then less evident in tests in which volition did not play a role, lending support to the substantive nature of the findings.

A fourth study from this group tested 26 cases and 20 controls (half deployed and half not, from the same battalion) on a different set of neuropsychological studies. The results were similar. A trend or effect toward greater impairment in cases than control was found in nine of nine measures of global brain function and 16 of 26 measures of specific brain function (in six there was no difference, in three a trend toward better performance, and in one significantly better performance). Of 71 total measures, PGW veterans performed worse on 59, significant by the binomial test at $p < 10^{-8}$ (Hom, Haley, et al., 1997). Of note: psychological profiles in ill veterans were found to be similar to those in general medical patients. The authors express the view that neuropsychological abnormalities seen in PGW veterans are likely to result from neurotoxic exposures in the PGW.

A study by a different set of investigators, with no control population, is potentially consistent with the construct of "confusion ataxia" syndrome described by Haley et al. (1997), in that, in a group of tested PGW veterans, motor incoordination ("ataxia") was significantly correlated with general cognitive functioning ($p < .01$) and executive functioning ($p < .01$) (Sillanpaa, Agar, et al., 1997). (There were few other correlations among assessed measures.) It is difficult to draw conclusions regarding either chronic symptoms or a relation to PB from this study: no control group was tested, and the measure of "exposure" was an *averaged* measure derived from self-report of exposure to each of the following: oil fire smoke, armored vehicles, shells, shell explosions, land mine explosions, battlefield sites, and burning enemy vehicles, sandfly bites, eating inadequately refrigerated food, and contact with reptiles, warm-blooded animals, prisoners, and corpses, as well as contact with unpurified water. (PB was not included as an exposure.) Obviously an averaged exposure measure of this type is inappropriate for assessing exposure-outcome links. However, such a measure may be useful for evaluating recall bias. The fact that this measure of exposure did *not* significantly predict neuropsychological variables and subjective complaints suggests against an important role for recall bias in exposure-outcome links for PGW veterans.

One study compared findings for 14 ill PGW veterans and 13 healthy civilian controls (matched on age, sex, physical activity, and handedness) on pre-defined outcome measures. The mean score for symptoms was substantially greater in the PGW veterans, and the mean score for clinical signs was also statistically significantly greater (p < .02). Of 22 individual tests performed, two were statistically significant after Bonferroni adjustment for multiple comparisons—namely, cold threshold and median nerve amplitude (Jamal, Hansen, et al., 1996).

Some studies have failed to demonstrate differences in neuropsychological function between ill veterans and controls. These differences in result may reflect subject selection and/or test sensitivity. Nonetheless, the existence of several studies finding objective evidence of impairment, albeit in selected subgroups of ill veterans, merits concern. Because there need be no single "Gulf War Syndrome," but rather there may exist several or many illnesses with distinct causes, it is appropriate to select those individuals with subjective neuropsychological complaints to undergo objective testing, just as would occur in the civilian population. Then it remains to be addressed whether frequency of these deficits is greater in ill PGW veterans than in nondeployed individuals, in those who received PB, or in those who responded adversely to PB.

Recently (since this report was initially sent for review), additional studies have found statistically significant alterations in neuropsychological function in defined sets of ill PGW veterans. These data are briefly reviewed here.

One study examined neuropsychological function in three cohorts of veterans including two followed since their return from the Gulf (abstract only) (White, Krengel, et al., 1998). These included the Fort Devens Reunion Survey sample, n~3000; a similar sample in New Orleans; and a cohort of National Guard members from Maine deployed to Germany rather than the Gulf. Deployment to the Gulf was reportedly associated with lower neuropsychological test scores on a number of tasks, which could not be explained on the basis of mood results or stress. The authors found relationships between self-reported exposures "to certain chemicals" and lower scores on specific neuropsychological tests, although the chemicals and tests are not named, and the results must in any event be viewed as exploratory and requiring subsequent confirmation.

Fatiguing symptoms have been considered a part of a Gulf War "syndrome" in ill PGW veterans by several investigators (Nicolson and Nicolson, 1995, 1997), and a case definition highlighting symptoms of fatigue, along with cognitive alterations, showed strikingly differential prevalence between deployed and nondeployed veterans (Fukuda, Nisenbaum, et al., 1998). In a study (abstract only) comparing performance on neuropsychological tests in registry veterans with fatigue as a major complaint who fulfilled clinical case definitions for chronic fatigue syndrome, idiopathic chronic fatigue, and/or multiple chemical sensitivity (n = 44) to performance of healthy PGW veteran controls (n = 23), group performance was found to differ on several tests, including the WAIS-R (Wechsler Adult Intelligence Scale) Digit Span Forward task, a simple Backwards subtest, the NES Complex Performance Test, and the PASAT (Paced Auditory Serial Addition Task) (Lange, Tiersky, et al., 1998a). Scores on a test of executive function, the Trail Making Test, were also significantly worse in fatigued than healthy PGW veterans. A strong trend toward significance was observed on all measures assessing visual-perceptual function. No verbal or visual learning or memory problems, or fine motor function problems (assessed by the Grooved Pegboard Test) were identified between the groups. There were no significant differences in alcohol consumption between the groups, with a trend toward lower consumption in fatigued veterans (Lange, Tiersky, et al., 1998a). Difficulties were believed similar to those in civilians with fatiguing illness.

Not unexpectedly, cognitive performance in another study was found to be worse in persons diagnosed with PTSD than in controls (Storzbach, Binder, et al., 1998). However, other studies have found that psychiatric disorders cannot explain symptoms in PGW veterans with fatiguing illness.

PSYCHIATRIC DISORDERS CANNOT EXPLAIN SYMPTOMS IN PGW VETERANS WITH FATIGUING ILLNESS

Registry veterans with fatigue as a major complaint who fulfilled case definitions for chronic fatigue syndrome, idiopathic chronic fatigue, and/or multiple chemical sensitivity (n = 53) were compared in DSMIII-R diagnoses to healthy PGW veterans (n = 42), who did not report health problems since the war. Forty-nine percent of fatigued PGW veterans had psychiatric diagnoses similarly distributed to those in healthy veterans, while the profile was significantly different in the remaining 51 percent (abstract) (Lange, Tiersky, et al., 1998b). Thus, psychiatric problems were present in some ill PGW veterans, but were not required for development of fatiguing illness.

Moreover, although PGW veterans who had psychiatric illness (in addition to fatigue, n = 29) were, as might be expected, the most impaired on measures of *psychological* well-being, they did not demonstrate reduced *physical* functioning compared to other fatigued veterans (n = 19), in whom reduced function and well-being were observed relative to healthy PGW veterans (abstract) (Tiersky, Tiersky, et al., 1998b). Thus, psychiatric disturbance did not appear to be responsible for functional decline in fatigued PGW veterans.

Consonant with these results, another study in a stratified subset of PGW veterans (n = 198) reporting high or low rates of health symptoms related to their

Gulf War deployment found that although PTSD and major depression were each significantly linked to report of health problems, nearly two-thirds of those reporting moderate health problems and one-third with severe health problems had no psychiatric diagnosis (Wolfe, Proctor, et al., 1998c). Moreover, comparison to personnel deployed to Germany rather than the Gulf showed that health symptom rates for PGW veterans were higher regardless of psychiatric status. This study also reported that lifetime PTSD and major depression (7 percent and 23 percent respectively) were "comparable to those provided by recent national comorbidity studies, suggesting no appreciable elevation of psychiatric disorders" (Wolfe, Proctor, et al., 1998c). In fact, however, unless age adjustment was made, an increase may have been present. It is crucial to reinforce that psychiatric symptoms can be sequelae of physical exposures and illness that may be part of or distinct from the causal pathway for other symptoms and that coexistence of psychiatric conditions must be considered as a possible concomitant and not exclusively as a possible cause.

NEUROLOGIC EFFECTS: OP-INDUCED DELAYED POLYNEUROPATHY AND INTERMEDIATE SYNDROME

Intermediate Syndrome and OPIDN represent examples of delayed and long-lasting or permanent clinical conditions that arise following exposure to selected OP AChE inhibitors. (For details, see Vol. 8: *Pesticides* (Geschwind and Golomb, forthcoming).) A brief discussion of these conditions is included to show instances of identified conditions in which delayed neurological illness follows neurotoxic exposure.

OPIDN

Some investigators perceive symptoms in PGW veterans to be consistent with OPIDN (Hom, Haley, et al., 1997). OPIDN illustrates that delayed and long-lasting clinically significant effects of AChE-inhibiting agents may occur. Classic OPIDN is not classically associated with PB or other carbamates in isolation (though the view has been put forward that all agents capable of inhibiting the enzyme "neurotoxic esterase" may have the potential to do so (Moretto, Bertolazzi, et al., 1992)). Indeed, carbamates given before some OPIDN-producing OPs may confer protection against OPIDN; however, carbamates given after OPs may enhance the severity of OPIDN or even induce OPIDN that would otherwise not have occurred (Lotti, 1991; Lotti, Caroldi, et al., 1991; Lotti and Moretto, 1993; Moretto, Bertolazzi, et al., 1994). Moreover, carbamates may induce OPIDN when potentiated by other agents (Moretto, Bertolazzi, et al., 1992). Symptoms of classic OPIDN are not consistent with symptoms reported by most PGW veterans.   Similar or unrelated mechanisms of delayed neurotoxicity could conceivably play a role in these conditions.

Briefly, OPIDN is a condition in which chronic combined central and peripheral axonopathy with secondary myelinopathy, leading to combined sensory and motor deficits, occurs one to several weeks following exposure to certain OPs and lasts for months or sometimes permanently.   Clinical symptoms of OPIDN are divided into a progressive phase (primarily a peripheral neuropathy) lasting three to six months after symptom onset, first involving pain, burning, tingling, or tightness in the lower extremities followed later by hypoesthesia in a "stocking and glove" (or "stocking" only) distribution; weakness of legs possibly spreading to the hands; foot drop, with steppage gait, positive Romberg, and in severe cases bilateral flaccid paralysis (paraplegia or quadriplegia) (Abou-Donia and Lapadula, 1990).   This is followed by a stationary phase, lasting from three to 12 months after symptom onset, in which sensory symptoms disappear but paraplegia or quadriplegia persists, and an improvement phase, from six to 24 months after onset of neurological deficits, with improvement occurring in reverse order to symptom onset.   In mild cases, recovery is complete.   In severe cases, hands show great improvement but paralysis remains below the knees. Later stages of neurologic deficits involve central, not peripheral lesions, in the spinal cord.   These persisting lesions are unmasked as peripheral neuropathy is diminished, and are characterized by spasticity (excessive muscle tone) and exaggerated knee jerk (Abou-Donia and Lapadula, 1990).

OPIDN also occurs preferentially in some species (e.g., rats are relatively refractory; cats, primates, and hens develop OPIDN more readily).   It is thought that induction of OPIDN requires at least 70 percent inhibition of the enzyme neurotoxic esterase (NTE, also called neuropathy target esterase), a membrane-bound carboxylesterase.   Not all agents that inhibit NTE equally produce OPIDN, and, like carbamates, those that do not typically produce it protect against it if administered before a neurotoxic OP (Pope, Tanaka, et al., 1993; Pope and Padilla, 1990).   Of note, inhaled sarin (5 mg per cubic meter for 20 minutes a day for 10 days) produced OPIDN (first symptoms occurring on day 14) in female mice.   The report does not cite the presence of clinical symptoms prior to development of delayed neurotoxicity (Husain, Vijayaraghavan, et al., 1993).   "Nonneuropathic" OPs, as described above for carbamates, may actually potentiate OPIDN if administered after the neuropathic OP (Pope, Tanaka, et al., 1993; Pope and Padilla, 1990); or may even produce it in animals who would not have been susceptible from the neuropathic OP exposure alone (Pope, Tanaka, et al., 1993).   The mechanism of potentiation is unknown but has been proposed to be independent of NTE (Moretto and Lotti, 1993).

Intermediate Syndrome

While we naturally perceive the state of science and medicine to be advanced (perhaps because the only comparison we have is the past, in which science was, almost by definition, less advanced), many medical conditions and biochemical factors, even critical ones, continue to be defined. Thus, *Helicobacter pylori* was recently discovered as the major cause of peptic ulcers;[5] leptin was recently identified as a hormone;[6] and human pheromones were only just shown to exist (Stern and McClintock, 1998). Likewise, neurotoxic effects, like other medical conditions, are continuing to be defined.

Intermediate syndrome is an instance of a condition of delayed neurotoxicity that was described relatively recently. Like OPIDN, it is a condition in which delayed symptoms occur following AChE inhibitor exposure. Although the symptoms and time-course are not consistent with illnesses commonly described in PGW veterans, intermediate syndrome will be reviewed as additional example of (mildly) delayed clinical effects that may occur with AChE-inhibiting compounds.

Intermediate syndrome (also called type II paralysis) results from an OP exposure and causes an associated muscle-weakening condition which occurs 24 to 96 hours after exposure, occurring subsequent to an acute OP cholinergic crisis (which typically happens within the first 24 hours) but before the development of OPIDN (two to three weeks later). It is characterized by acute onset of muscle weakness or paralysis affecting neck flexors, motor cranial nerves, proximal muscles of the limbs, and respiratory muscles (Leon-S, Pradilla, and Vezga, 1996; Mani, Thomas, et al., 1992). Deep tendon reflexes are commonly absent. It is often associated with respiratory insufficiency, and artificial ventilation may be required. It may occur with many OPs including fenthion, methyl-parathion, parathion, dimethoate; though it may occur more commonly with certain compounds (perhaps those with high lipid solubility), it is not confined to a few distinct compounds (De Bleecker, 1993). Prognosis for recovery is good, and occurs within four to 18 days (Leon-S, Pradilla, et al., 1996b; Mani, Thomas, et al., 1992). The necrotizing myopathy seen with AChE inhibitors (including PB) had been suggested as a cause (Senanayake and Karielledde, 1987), but some data suggest against this hypothesis, and some have suggested persistent AChE inhibition as the mechanism (De Bleecker, 1993), possibly due to toxicokinetic properties of the OP ester involved (e.g., fat solubility),

---

[5]There were four citations in the MED85 MEDLINE database (extending from 1985–1990), compared to 985 in the MED90 database (from 1990–1993) with the key words "helicobacter" and "peptic."

[6]As of August 1, 1998, there were 878 citations in the latest MEDLINE database with the keyword "leptin"; there are 0 in the MED90 database, which extends from 1990 to 1993.

individual variation in the safety factor of neuromuscular transmission, and delayed metabolism and clearance (De Bleecker, 1993). Of note: One study found that biochemical, electromyographic, and morphological data were unable to discriminate between patients with and without a symptom-free episode (De Bleecker, 1993).

NEUROCHEMICAL EFFECTS

Little work has been done to determine whether chronic neurochemical effects ensue following cholinergic manipulation with carbamates, and particularly with PB, though work is currently in progress (Albuquerque, 1997). As seen below, examination of such effects will be complicated by the potential for regional and measure-specific differences in effect and by differences in the time-course of an effect. In this section, evidence regarding the existence of delayed and chronic neurochemical changes with AChE inhibitors (usually AChE inhibitors distinct from PB, because little literature exists on chronic effects of PB) will be examined. Emphasis will be given to the emerging complexity of our understanding of the cholinergic system, with regional differences, differences in time-course of different effects, and differences in receptor characteristics complicating the process of extrapolating evidence on ACh and AChE function to new settings.

Delayed Effects

Effects associated with the delivery of AChE-inhibiting drugs may occur with differing temporal characteristics. In particular, not all drug effects of cholinesterase inhibitors quantitatively or even qualitatively parallel AChE inhibition in their time-courses. The existence of OPIDN and Intermediate Syndrome, among other effects, supports this point. For example, muscarinic receptor numbers fall in rats (receptor downregulation) following exposure to AChE inhibitors, an effect that does not show up at three days postexposure, but will by six days in rat pups exposed to chlorpyrifos at age 21 days (Stanton, Mundy, et al., 1994).

Even within a selected area of the brain, the time-course of effect of an AChE-inhibiting agent may differ depending on which measure of effect is evaluated. In OP-exposed rats, a shift was seen from greater AChE inhibition early, to greater BChE inhibition later, as tolerance to the behavioral effects emerged. (From this finding it was surmised that pseudocholinesterases may be involved in the development of tolerance and the reduction of toxicity (Swamy, Ravikumar, et al., 1992). The time-course, therefore, differed for AChE and for BChE inhibition. This finding reflects the general principle that distinct effects of the same drug may have distinct time-courses. Thus, demonstrations that one or several effects of a drug are constrained to a specific temporal framework is not necessarily an assurance that other effects will be similarly circumscribed in time.

Moreover, changes in neurochemistry with cholinesterase inhibition occur differentially in different brain regions, a finding determined primarily from studies in rodents. For example, while cholinesterase inhibition occurred in both the cortex and hippocampus in one study, only the cortex showed muscarinic receptor downregulation (Stanton, Mundy, et al., 1994). In rat studies using OPs, the cerebral cortex was affected more initially, but striatum was affected more during later dosings (Swamy, Ravikumar, et al., 1992). This study performed measurement while OP administration continued. Such regional differences in effect complicate efforts to extrapolate effects, or the lack of effects, determined from one area of the brain to other areas. Even within an area, different effects may follow a different time-course.

Differences may also occur based on receptor type. Some studies have shown evidence of muscarinic receptor downregulation (Russell, Booth, et al., 1989). However, central nicotinic receptors may behave differently, demonstrating increased receptor number in some areas of the brain following AChE inhibition, possibly as secondary compensation to reduced receptor affinity (see Chapter Thirteen, "Neurotransmitter Dysregulation"). Further complicating the picture, there exist different structural and perhaps functional forms of nicotinic receptors. These may have distinct regulatory properties, perhaps accounting for some regional differences in nicotinic receptor response.

Evidence of Long-Standing Alteration in Neurochemistry After Brief Chemical Exposure. The question remains whether all effects of cholinergic dysregulation are relatively transitory and fully reversible, or if there exist long-term changes that coincide with the time-course of illnesses in PGW veterans. For most phenomena examined thus far, substantial reversibility occurs early, though in some instances full reversibility has not been demonstrated even with prolonged follow-up. There exist additional reports indicating that the neurochemistry of animals may be permanently altered after a single exposure to AChE inhibitors. A single subcutaneous dose of chlorpyrifos led to long-lasting enhanced sensitivity to cholinergic antagonists (evidenced by exaggerated hyperactivity in response to scopolamine) in rats, which persisted for months although muscarinic receptor density and cholinesterase activity had returned to normal levels (Pope, Chakraborti, et al., 1992). (See Chapter Thirteen.) Similarly, a single dose of fenthion led to apparently permanent alterations in intracellular communication of muscarinic receptors studied in rats (Tandon, Padilla, et al., 1994; Tandon, Willig, et al., 1994).

The existence of long-term neurochemical and behavioral consequences to temporally defined exposures is well known in other systems and is manifested in such other widely recognized phenomena as addiction, sensitization, and habituation. The above studies suggest that long-term changes in neurochemical properties may occur with AChE inhibitors. It is not known whether these or other changes occur with subacute administration of low doses of PB in humans. Neither is it known whether such changes, if they occur, provide the substrate for cognitive and behavioral changes reported following exposure to AChE inhibitors.

RELATIONS OF SYMPTOMS TO DRUG LEVEL OR MEASURE OF "DRUG EFFECT"

It is often assumed that symptoms resulting from AChE inhibitors require concurrent AChE inhibition to be manifest. Indeed, it is commonly assumed that drug levels determine drug effects. Yet there are many examples of drugs in which a time lag exists between the plasma or biophase drug concentrations and the time-course of pharmacodynamic response (Jusko and Ko, 1994). One example is corticosteroids, for which adrenal suppression may persist long after cessation of the drug.

As noted elsewhere, symptoms have been shown to persist beyond the time of AChE inhibition when AChE-inhibiting drugs are administered. Effects of carbamate insecticides (using screening tests recommended by the U.S. EPA, including a Functional Observational Battery and motor activity) were shown to last for days after cholinesterase inhibition returned to normal (Padilla, 1995; Moser, 1994). Adverse effects of both OP and carbamate insecticides have been reported weeks after an initial dose in rats (Ehrich, Shell, et al., 1993) and longer-term clinical and behavioral effects have been reported to differ from short-term effects (Padilla, 1995). (Clinical aspects are reviewed in the section on "Chronic Neuropsychiatric Effects" findings.)

RELATION OF ACUTE TO CHRONIC SYMPTOMS

It is widely thought that chronic symptoms following AChE inhibitor exposure require the presence of antecedent acute symptoms. However, this assumption may not be valid.

One study examined 77 16–65-year-old male British sheep-dippers. This study failed to find a relation between acute symptoms of OP toxicity, determined by a change from baseline to 24 hours after sheep-dipping exposure, and chronic neuropsychiatric symptoms, ascertained a minimum of two months following exposure (Stephens, Spurgeon, et al., 1996). The OP (AChE-inhibiting) drugs to which the sheep-dippers were exposed included Diazinon, a mixture of Diazinon and chlorfenvinphos, or propetamphos. This study is limited by investigation of acute symptoms on only one sheep-dipping occasion, which may miss more marked effects from prior sheep-dipping events; lack of baseline data on the chronic symptom profile; lack of usable comparison data on cases and controls; and a control group (quarry workers) of uncertain "baseline" comparability on the chronic effect profile. The study concludes that "the chronic effects found in this group ... appear to occur independently of symptoms that might immediately follow acute OP exposure," though this conclusion is not necessarily justified by the data.

To the contrary, another study found that 45 California pesticide workers who had been temporarily pulled from carbamate and OP pesticide application work because of red blood cell cholinesterase values under 70 percent of normal, or plasma cholinesterase values under 60 percent of normal but who had no evidence of toxicity, did no worse on a battery of neuropsychological tests than 90 non-age-matched controls (friends brought in by pesticide workers), using regression analysis. Limitations of this study include aborting of subtoxic exposure, which may reduce chronic toxicity compared to more subchronic or chronic AChE inhibition exposure; strong differences in age between cases and controls (with younger controls), which may produce collinearity of pesticide exposure with age in the regression analysis, leading to the spurious appearance of no association following age adjustment; and a small sample, in which toxicity to a subset, or subtle effects to all, could be missed. The authors conclude that this study gives some support to the notion that protection from acute effects also confers protection against chronic neuropsychological sequelae. Of note: The Haley and Kurt study (1997) found that self-reported experience of acute effects with PB (reported retrospectively) was associated with subsequent illnesses in PGW veterans, a finding that, if accepted, may be consistent with this report.

Interactions

In a slightly different vein, chronic neurochemical and behavioral effects have been seen in rodents in the absence of acute symptoms of toxicity, when pyrethroid insecticide exposure (bioallethrin) as adults occurred following organochlorine exposure (DDT) as neonates (Johansson, Fredriksson, et al., 1995). (Pyrethroid insecticides have some esterase-inhibiting activity.) Those exposed to DDT alone as neonates had an apparently permanent decrease in muscarinic receptor density, with increased low- compared to high-affinity muscarinic binding sites. Those exposed to DDT also had an (apparently permanent) increase in susceptibility to bioallethrin-induced increase in muscarinic receptor density, also accompanied by increased low- to high-affinity binding sites. (No changes in nicotinic receptors were observed in these groups.) Animals receiving bioallethrin showed difficulty learning a skill, the swim maze of the Morris water maze type. While some behavioral effects occurred in animals not receiving prior DDT, these abated with time, whereas permanent changes in muscarinic receptor density and behavioral variables were seen in the animals with prior DDT exposure. No studies have been identified that assess whether similar findings ensue with pyrethroid use following adult exposure to organochlorines or whether similar findings occur when the first exposure is to an AChE inhibitor, such as an OP (or carbamate). This study makes the point that complex interactions between exposures may occur despite separation in time between such exposures, prior exposures may serve to influence individual differences in susceptibility or response to drugs, and permanent alterations in neurochemical and behavioral susceptibility or permanent neurochemical and behavioral effects can occur following time-limited exposure to drugs. This may occur specifically within the muscarinic cholinergic system, at least in animal studies. No data were identified to assess whether analogous phenomena may occur with adult exposures in animals, in humans, or with exposures to AChE inhibitors, such as those experienced during the PGW.

OTHER CHRONIC EFFECTS

Porphyria. Porphyria refers to a set of genetic and acquired disorders in the synthesis of heme, an iron complex critical to many body functions that serves as a prosthetic group to proteins, including hemoglobin and mitochondrial proteins essential to life (Wilson, Braunwald, et al., 1991). Carbamates have been found to cause experimental porphyria in liver cell cultures (Matters, 1967). More relevant is the finding that carbamate poisoning precipitated clinical porphyria in a 17-year-old Caucasian woman who accidentally drank a glass of carbaryl liquid. Symptoms included abdominal cramping, nausea, and vomiting (commencing two days after ingestion); limb weakness (commencing four days after ingestion and progressing to quadriparesis with hypoactive tendon reflexes); and behavioral changes (beginning 21 days after ingestion). Porphyria was confirmed by elevated levels of uroporphyrin and coproporphyrin (Sargin, Cirak, et al., 1992). The high carbamate exposure greatly exceeded that experienced by PGW veterans, and the symptomatology is not strongly reminiscent of symptom reports by most ill PGW veterans. However, the finding of behavioral changes that commenced 21 days after exposure reinforces the observation that delayed neuropsychiatric changes in response to drugs including carbamates may occur through a variety of identified and unidentified mechanisms. Though one ill veteran has testified that porphyria was among the new diagnoses he received following the PGW (Zeller, 1997), it is difficult to draw conclusions regarding causality from a single case. Some researchers state that abnormalities in porphyrin metabolism are present in many ill PGW veterans, with measured values outside of normal ranges although the findings do not meet clinical criteria for porphyria (Donnay, 1999). It would be reasonable for these findings (presently unpublished) to undergo replication or refutation. As noted elsewhere (Chapter Fifteen, "Other Considerations"), identification of specific objective findings in ill PGW veterans constitutes an important priority, as candidate etiologies—including PB and others—can then be tested in animal studies to assess for production of corollary findings, thus abetting the process of understanding the possible causes and contributors of illnesses in PGW veterans, which may in turn assist with identification of potential treatments and prevention of similar problems in the future.

Conditioned Taste Aversion. PB as well as other carbamates and anticholinesterase nerve agents have been found to produce conditioned taste aversion in rats (McPhail, 1981; Romano and Landauer, 1986; Romano, King, et al., 1985; Romano and King, 1987), in doses that did not affect response rates in a rat operant paradigm (Modrow and McDonough, 1985). An animal may develop an enduring aversion to a "conditioned stimulus" (such as a taste, when it has been paired with an unconditioned stimulus such as PB) following a single association of the two—another instance in which a brief exposure may produce lasting effects.

Whether such enduring aversions relate to new chemical sensitivities, such as those reportedly experienced by some PGW veterans, is open to speculation.[7]

SUMMARY AND CONCLUSION

Although PB has been given to myasthenics for many years with few concerns regarding long-term adverse effects, the circumstances of use are quite different for patients with myasthenia and for PGW veterans. Despite use of a lower dose of PB in PGW veterans than in myasthenics, the possibility that PB could produce chronic effects in some PGW veterans cannot be excluded: PGW veterans differ from myasthenics in their cholinergic state, in short-term rather than lifelong PB use, and in the presence of concomitant stress and a diverse assortment of potential chemical and environmental exposures that have been demonstrated in animal studies to interact with PB.

---

[7]Perhaps surprisingly, not only do PB and physostigmine produce conditioned taste aversion, but so also does the anticholinergic agent atropine (Romano and King, 1987). Thus, dysregulation of the cholinergic system—perhaps in either direction—may produce lasting aversion to coadministered chemicals.

Few studies examine chronic effects of PB, perhaps in part because under normal unstressed conditions little PB enters the CNS. (Under conditions of stress and chemical coexposure, however, PB does penetrate the blood-brain barrier and produce central cholinesterase inhibition in animal studies.) Though few studies look at the chronic effects of PB, many studies examine other AChE inhibitors, and these were briefly reviewed. Additional information on effects of pesticides and nerve agents can be found in Vol. 5: *Chemical and Biological Warfare*, and Vol. 8: *Pesticides* (Augerson, forthcoming; Geschwind and Golomb, forthcoming).

The neurochemical effects of AChE inhibitors, including PB, on the cholinergic system are complex. The precise nature of these changes—and regional differences in their character or time-course—remain to be fully elucidated. At present, we can neither confirm nor exclude the theory that PB (assuming circumstances that allow it to cross the blood-brain barrier) precipitates longstanding or permanent changes in CNS neurochemistry or that PB in combination with other exposure facilitates the ability of these coexposures to do so. Nonetheless, some evidence indicates that long-term or permanent changes may occur in the cholinergic system and in other neurotransmitter systems, following time-limited exposures to agents. Lasting alterations in muscarinic receptor number and affinity are seen with exposure to AChE inhibitors, and interactions between early and later exposures have been demonstrated—one exposure may evidently prime an animal to experience a marked effect with a much later exposure. Regional brain and temporal differences arising from different effects of the same AChE inhibitor have been demonstrated. A single exposure to AChE inhibitors can produce a lasting aversion to coadministered chemicals in rats, perhaps suggesting a mechanism for chemical sensitivities such as have been reported by some veterans. The possibility of chronic effects on the motor endplate are discussed in a separate chapter (see Chapter Twelve, "Neuromuscular Junction Effects"). In the absence of entry into the CNS, there remain mechanisms by which changes in some elements of neuropsychiatric function could take place, involving dysregulation of release of catecholamines from the adrenal medulla, a process regulated by ACh.

In humans, AChE-inhibiting drugs have been shown to produce delayed and chronic effects. Chronic EEG abnormalities have been demonstrated with pesticides and nerve agents; chronic changes have been isolated in SPECT brain scans in subjects exposed to pesticides; and neuropsychiatric tests have demonstrated variable deficits in such subjects. Many of these findings are preliminary and require replication. Moreover, whether PB may have contributed to similar chronic effects in PGW veterans, alone or through potentiation of actions of pesticides or other exposures, is uncertain. Subjects exposed to pesticides, and relatives of these subjects, report development of functionally significant chronic changes that may occur despite relatively subtle deficits on neuropsychological testing. This appears to parallel the experience of PGW veterans and suggests that more targeted tests sensitive to the deficits perceived by veterans need to be identified. It is critical to note that reductions in function that occur within the "normal" range may still produce marked functional impairment in real-world tasks. For instance, two individuals may both score "normal"—although one excels in a challenging job (or school) and another struggles at a substantially less challenging enterprise. Development of tests sensitive to deficits experienced by individuals with pesticide exposures may prove useful in evaluating the characteristics and possible etiology of illnesses in ill PGW veterans.

Some studies in PGW veterans indeed report (modest) neuropsychiatric abnormalities that appear to be widespread rather than confined to one or two specific functions, potentially consistent with the pervasive influence of ACh in the brain and body. (Nonetheless, efforts should be made to develop neuro-psychiatric tests sensitive to functions likely to be potently regulated by ACh, as discussed in Chapter Thirteen.)

These findings, taken together, suggest that chronic effects from PB cannot be excluded. Such effects could occur from PB exposure alone (in the context of stress) or perhaps more likely in combination with other chemical exposures. Chronic biological and clinical effects have been demonstrated with related agents that share the capacity to inhibit AChE. Some, but not all, of these effects have been shown to be restricted to a subset of AChE-inhibiting agents. Preliminary neuropsychiatric studies offer support, in some cases, for chronic neuropsychiatric effects in subsets of ill PGW veterans, and additional studies continue.

In short, it remains undetermined whether PB produces chronic effects that in turn contribute to illnesses in PGW veterans. However, findings from PB and related agents suggest that chronic neurochemical and neuropsychological effects are possible following exposure to AChE inhibitors under certain conditions.

SCIENTIFIC RECOMMENDATIONS

- Efforts to evaluate the connection between PB exposure or adverse response to PB and subsequent chronic neuropsychiatric symptoms should continue.

- Sensitive testing techniques, able to capture the deficits reported by PGW veterans, are imperative to adequate evaluation of their chronic cognitive and neuropsychiatric complaints. Continued efforts should be made to find neuropsychiatric tests sensitive to the functional level and to the possibly "mild" cognitive deficits reported by some ill PGW veterans (which may nonetheless produce marked changes in functional ability for those in more-demanding occupations). A test of executive decisionmaking has been shown to correlate with job success with a correlation coefficient of 0.6, compared to 0.3 for IQ tests, and has been shown to identify functional impairment in patients with mild head injury when other tests fail to do so (Streufert, Satish, et al., 1997). This test is quite costly and time-intensive, but consideration should be given to devising similar tests to supplement current testing in a trial of ill PGW veterans and controls.

- Prior to future deployments in which PB may be given, at least some personnel and some controls who will not be deployed should receive baseline neuropsychological testing using sensitive instruments (preferably instruments that preliminary data suggests may differ between ill PGW veterans and controls), to allow comparison of pre- and postresults if PB exposure occurs as part of deployment. Although delicate ethical issues are associated with conducting research on military personnel, the greater ethical breach is to fail to perform such testing of an intervention and then administer it to hundreds of thousands of individuals.

- Consistent with recommendations in Chapter Thirteen, a trial of (blinded) SPECT imaging might be appropriate in PGW veterans with chronic cognitive complaints, particularly those who report neurotoxic exposures. SPECT has been reported to identify abnormalities in individuals exposed to pesticides that are distinct from those of individuals suffering from depression and chronic fatigue. Thus, objective differences on quantitative SPECT, if present, might distinguish among several possible etiologies of illnesses in PGW veterans. Challenge studies in which pro- and anti-cholinergic agents are given and regional blood flow evaluated by SPECT may help to clarify short-term and chronic effects. Moreover, SPECT might provide an objective marker of cerebral dysfunction in subjectively impaired individuals and may conceivably offer a marker for treatment effect.

- Basic research in cholinergic function in the CNS should continue (see recommendations from Chapter Thirteen), with emphasis on the character and time-course of effects, and particularly on identifying and assessing chronic effects.

Chapter Fifteen

OTHER CONSIDERATIONS

OVERVIEW

This chapter briefly presents evidence related to several topics explored in lesser detail. These topics include fertility, hormonal and stress effects, sleep, mood, dermatologic effects, birth defects, and violent death.

While the cholinergic system is involved in reproduction, and thus alterations in fertility might be theoretically possible, there is presently no evidence of reduced fertility in PGW veterans.

PB is known to affect certain hormones, including growth hormone. No evidence has been identified to suggest that growth hormone abnormalities are associated with illnesses in PGW veterans, though there is no evidence to exclude this possibility.

PB affects the cholinergic system, which in turn affects sleep, and many PGW veterans complain of sleep abnormalities. Increased incidence of sleep apnea may occur in ill PGW veterans, and studies suggest that nicotinic cholinergic stimulation may ameliorate symptoms of sleep apnea. Nonetheless no *direct* evidence supports or excludes the possibility that PB use alone or in conjunction with exposures to other AChE inhibitors is associated with current sleep complaints among veterans. Sleep abnormalities merit further evaluation because of the possible link to the one identified source of excess mortality in deployed PGW veterans, namely death by unintentional injury.

Many ill veterans report rashes, hair loss, or other symptoms related to the dermatologic system. One prior report characterizes a woman who repeatedly experienced hair loss on institution of PB for myasthenia. Literature suggests some mechanisms by which skin effects could occur. Although it is not possible to attribute skin symptoms or hair loss in ill veterans to use of PB, neither is it possible to exclude PB as a contributor to reported skin symptoms and hair loss.

No literature suggests severe birth defects with PB use in pregnant myasthenics. PB use in myasthenia may be linked to the development of neonatal myasthenia; however, this effect occurs with high-dose PB delivered for long periods. Moreover, epidemiologic evidence does not suggest increased rate of severe birth defects in children of PGW veterans. Risk of birth defects was increased (borderline significance: RR 1.12, 95 percent CI 1.00–1.25) in children of deployed women, although the increase was no longer significant after adjustment for race/ethnicity, marital status, and branch of service (Cowan, De Fraites, et al., 1997). PB has been shown to demonstrate some teratogenic of developmental effects in rats and chickens. Gross structural effects were seen in chickens exposed to high doses of PB. More subtle behavioral effects and regional brain function changes were seen in rats exposed to low doses of PB in their neonatal period, doses more comparable to exposures occurring in PGW veterans.

PGW veterans have experienced increased death by unintentional injury. While many factors could contribute to this increase, subjective complaints of difficulties with sleep and concentration by ill veterans—complaints that may or may not relate to abnormal ACh function and prior PB use—merit scrutiny as contributing factors.

FERTILITY

Data identifying the presence of ACh and AChE in sperm, ovaries, and other reproductive tissues suggest a role for the cholinergic system in reproduction, leading to the question whether alterations of cholinergic activity could produce changes in fertility. Ongoing fertility problems would likely (but not necessarily) require the presence of long-standing changes in cholinergic function following exposure to PB (and other AChE-inhibiting coexposures, such as a nerve agent or pesticides). It is unknown whether such long-standing changes occur.

A role for cholinergic function in reproduction is suggested by the presence of cholinesterases in ovarian follicles, cholinergic villi, and human oocytes, and cholinergic signaling has been implicated in chorionic villi, which express the BChE gene, and in sperm motility, as suggested by presence of ACh, AChE, and choline acetyltransferase, as well as BChE in mammalian sperm. One µM of an agent that inhibits ACh production depressed sperm motility by 95 percent; while ACh itself may either augment or depress sperm motility (Schwarz, Glick, et al., 1995).

An effect of PB on fertility has not been demonstrated. Following return from the Gulf, PGW veterans experienced a higher birth rate then nondeployed controls. While it is conceivable that this increased birth rate was less than the increase in procreation behavior would warrant, there is no evidence to allow assessment of this possibility. If concerns regarding fertility remain, birth rates farther out from the time of deployment should be evaluated.

HORMONE AND STRESS EFFECTS

Differences in the influence of PB on growth hormone or other pituitary-adrenal axis hormones could themselves be postulated to play a role in individual differences leading to illnesses in some PGW veterans and not in others. PB is used in the evaluation of growth hormone status and acts to cause a surge of growth hormone presumably by inhibiting release of somatostatin, a growth hormone suppressant, from a region of the brain termed the hypothalamus (Wehrenberg, Wiviot, et al., 1992). Marked differences in growth hormone response to PB have been documented; these may interact with other factors that influence hypothalamic regulation of growth hormone secretion, as noted above. Moreover, PB interacts with other factors that regulate functional growth hormone release. For instance, PB administration significantly augments the exercise-induced increase in growth hormone release (Cappa, Grossi, et al., 1993) and the delayed growth hormone response to glucose administration (Valcavi, Zini, et al., 1992); it also partially reverses the inhibition of growth hormone response to the growth hormone–releasing hormone found in corticosteroids (Trainer, Kirk, et al., 1991).

In turn, differences in growth hormone may influence other systems in the body. For instance, growth hormone is involved in regulation of blood glucose, muscle mass response to exercise, and has been shown to enhance cardiac function (Valcavi, Gaddi, et al., 1995).

More generally, acetylcholinergic stimulation (e.g., with physostigmine) appears capable of producing a stress response in which cortisol, prolactin, and growth hormone are all elevated (Davis and Davis, 1979). (Corticosteroids, such as cortisol, are considered the quintessential stress hormones, although in acute stress, catecholamines are released as well. AChE inhibitors also promote release of catecholamines—see below.) In vitro studies suggest stimulation of corticotropin-releasing factor from the hypothalamus in rats (Bradbury, Burden, et al., 1974). The effect is believed to be largely nicotinic, since nicotinic blockade reduces the effect while a muscarinic agent (bethanecol) had no effect (Hillhouse, Burden, et al., 1975). (Although a number of studies suggest that the stress-induced secretion of cortisol has a muscarinic acetylcholinergic basis, there are reasons to doubt this. For instance, infusion of the muscarinic antagonist atropine into the fluid-filled ventricles of the brain (or implanting of atropine pellets into the hypothalamus of the brain) inhibits the stress response. however, this does not occur when doses of atropine are used that are specific for blockade of muscarinic receptors (0.4 mg/kg) (Davis and Davis, 1979).) More data on stress and the cholinergic system are provided in a foot-note.[1]

PB may influence other hormones as well, perhaps including calcitonin and TRH (the hormone from the hypothalamus that incites release of thyroid-stimulating hormone from the pituitary). PB (120 mg orally, or four Gulf War doses) has been shown to increase plasma levels of calcitonin gene-related peptide in normal humans ($p < .01$) (Trasforini, Margutti, et al., 1994). If cholinergic "downregulation" (see Chapter Three, "Characteristics of PB") occurs following PB withdrawal, the effect on calcitonin may be viewed with interest in PGW veterans who report pain, in light of increasing evidence for, and increasing specialist use of, calcitonin as a pain-reducing agent. (Of more direct relevance is evidence that nicotinic ACh function is perhaps more directly involved in pain control—discussed in greater detail in the section on pain, below.) PB suppresses hypothalamic somatostatin; and somatostatin suppresses thyroid-stimulating hormone from the pituitary. Tests indicate that PB (at a dose of 180 mg; six Gulf War doses, or two "daily" doses) can augment the thyroid-stimulating hormone response to TRH in a normal man (Yang, Woo, et al., 1995). Others find effects on the thyroid-stimulating hormone response to TRH only in patients with Cushing's disease (Giustina, Bossoni, et al., 1992). No data have evaluated whether subtle long-term effects may characterize thyroid hormone function or response following subchronic use of PB.

----

[1]Administering the ACh-mimicking drug "arecoline" (at 4 mg/kg) to rats increased elevation of serum corticosterone particularly in rats bred to be sensitive to ACh (Overstreet, Janowsky, et al., 1986). (It also produced greater suppression of behavioral activity in ACh-sensitive rats (Overstreet, Janowsky, et al., 1986), which show more immobility in the face of stress to begin with (Overstreet, Janowsky, et al., 1986).)

Of note: rats chronically treated with and subsequently withdrawn from the muscarinic blocking drug scopolamine (2 mg/kg once daily) or the antidepressant drug amitriptyline (10 mg/kg once daily), which has muscarinic actions, were also significantly more immobile (Overstreet, Janowsky, et al., 1986; Overstreet, Russell, et al., 1988), consistent with the idea that depressing the cholinergic system with drugs may render it more sensitive on withdrawal.

Rats bred for sensitivity to cholinergic agonists, the Flinders Sensitive Line (FSL) rats, exhibited on autopsy lower concentrations of the Corticotropin Releasing Factor receptors in the median eminence, locus ceruleus, and prefrontal cortex but not in 13 other brain regions (Owens, Overstreet, et al., 1991). (The Corticotropin Releasing Factor is released by the hypothalamus and stimulates the pituitary to release the adrenocorticotrophic hormone, which in turn stimulates the adrenal glands to release corticosteroids.) They had significantly lower plasma adrenocorticotrophic hormone concentration, but no difference in corticosterone in comparison to Flinders Resistant Line rats (Owens, Overstreet, et al., 1991). The density of Corticotropin Releasing Factor receptors in the anterior pituitary was elevated. This was taken to suggest that cholinergically "supersensitive" Flinders Sensitive Line rats may have diminished hypothalamic-pituitary-adrenal activity (Owens, Overstreet, et al., 1991).

A variety of hormonal effects have been noted following exposure to other AChE inhibitors, specifically to the nerve agent soman, including increases in serum corticosterone, thyroxine, and triiodothyronine concentrations; reduction in adrenocorticotrophic hormone levels; and reduction in testosterone (Clement, 1985). Whether long-standing hormonal effects occur with AChE inhibitors has not been evaluated. Specifically, studies have not been identified that evaluate chronic effects on hormones from PB alone or in combination with other AChE inhibitors.

One of the more widely touted hypotheses with regard to illnesses in PGW veterans has been the stress hypothesis. Some postulate that stress predisposes people to illness by influencing "stress hormones," such as adrenal hormones, as well as catecholamines. These neuroendocrine actions, when produced by stress, are postulated to result in sequelae. Although it is clear that stress results in defined syndromes (such as PTSD) and enhances risk to other established medical conditions (such as myocardial infarction)—perhaps mediated through changes in intermediate factors (such as hemoconcentration and hypertension that are promoted with adrenergic arousal, or in the instance of PGW veterans, perhaps through enhancement of permeability of the blood-brain barrier, as discussed in Chapter Seven)—it is less well established (that is, not at all established) that stress might result in symptoms conforming to the frequency distribution seen in ill PGW veterans. However, if stress is postulated as an etiology for these symptoms, acting through acute neuroendocrine changes, then acute neuroendocrine actions precipitated by other etiologies, such as PB, would also need to be considered as possible sources of illness in veterans. PB exposure is estimated to have occurred in 250,000 to 300,000 PGW veterans (Brake, 1997). However, the effect of PB on hormones, including stress hormones, and the relation of these hormonal effects to chronic illness remain to be better elucidated.

CATECHOLAMINE EFFECTS

Catecholamines, such as epinephrine (adrenaline) and norepinephrine (noradrenaline), are part of the "fight or flight" response and part of the stress response. Central (brain) ACh stimulation appears to produce release of epinephrine. For example, physostigmine (a "carbamate," like PB, that differs from PB by more readily crossing the blood-brain barrier and by being shorter acting) has been shown to produce marked increases in epinephrine levels and to a much lesser degree, norepinephrine levels—with profound increases in pulse rates and blood pressure (Janowsky, Risch, et al., 1985; Janowsky, Risch, et al., 1986). This effect occurs not through peripheral action of ACh on the adrenal medulla, where epinephrine is produced but through central (brain) effects. For example, if physostigmine is given together with agents that block action of ACh in the body (the periphery), the effect still occurs: pronounced release of epinephrine along with increased pulse and blood pressure (with a dose of 0.022 mg/kg of physostigmine) (Kennedy, Janowsky, et al., 1984). As further evidence that the effect is central, neostigmine, a carbamate that like PB does not act centrally but only increases peripheral ACh levels, does not lead to similar increases in pulse and blood pressure in humans (Janowsky, Risch, et al., 1985). Nonetheless the effect is relevant to PB because in times of stress, PB may cross the blood brain barrier (see Chapter Seven, "Blood-Brain Barrier"), and PB may induce central effects, including those enhancing function of such "catecholamines" as epinephrine. (Importantly, since stress is associated with catecholamine release, PB may in turn augment the effects of stress.)

PAIN

Activating ACh receptors of the muscarinic type (for example, by administering the drug physostigmine, which is related to PB), stimulates release of the "endogenous opiate" or pain reducing substance termed ß-endorphin (Risch, Janowsky, et al., 1981; Risch, Janowsky, et al., 1982a; Risch, Janowsky, et al., 1982b; Risch, Kalin, et al., 1983). Thus, downregulation of the muscarinic system would be expected to produce reduced release of ß-endorphin, presumably associated with reduced analgesia—or heightened pain sensitivity. Thus, muscarinic downregulation could contribute to symptoms of pain in ill PGW veterans.

Perhaps more important, neuronal nicotinic downregulation could enhance symptoms of pain. Interest in the role of neuronal nicotinic ACh receptors in pain-processing has been rekindled by the discovery of epibatidine, a naturally occurring neuronal nicotinic ACh receptor agonist that has antipain activity more than 200 times greater than that of morphine (Donnelly-Roberts, Puttfarcken, et al., 1998). Work is ongoing to understand the role of these receptors in pain-signaling, and to develop agents selective for the neuronal nicotinic ACh receptors without binding to ganglionic and neuromuscular ACh receptors, to provide specific agents capable of pain relief (Barlocco, Cignarella, et al., 1998; Holladay, Wasicak, et al., 1998; Puttfarcken, Manelli, et al., 1997; Khan, Yaksh, et al., 1997; Damaj and Martin, 1996; Rao, Correa, et al., 1996; Bannon, Gunther, et al., 1995; Rupniak, Patel, et al., 1994; Damaj, Creasy, et al., 1994; Donnelly-Roberts, Puttfarcken, et al., 1998). Of note, development of tolerance to the antipain effects of epibatidine (downregulatory effects) has been found to show a different profile and characteristics compared to nicotine (Damaj and Martin, 1996). A nicotinic agent is currently being marketed for pain (by Abbott Laboratories).

Additional possible mechanisms of pain, mediated through effects on sleep and serotonin, are discussed below.

Of incidental note, Flinders Sensitive Line rats, bred to have cholinergic "hyperresponsiveness," have higher pain thresholds than Flinders Resistant Line rats, bred to have low cholinergic responsiveness, when tested by the "jump-flinch" method (Pucilowski, Eichelman, et al., 1990). Depressives (who are generally more vulnerable to pain) show muscarinic supersensitivity to beta endorphin release (as well as to pituitary adrenocorticotrophic hormone release) (Risch, Janowsky, et al., 1981); heightened sensitivity may accompany low baseline activity.

MOOD AND BEHAVIOR

Mood

A body of literature has linked ACh to mood, and both cholinergic and cholinergic-adrenergic models of mood disorders have been put forth (as have more complicated models which also incorporate other neurotransmitters) (Janowsky, El-Yousef, et al., 1974; Risch, Kalin, et al., 1981; Janowsky and Risch, 1984; Janowsky and Risch, 1986; Janowsky and Risch, 1987; Janowsky, Risch et al., 1988; Janowsky and Overstreet 1990; Janowsky, Overstreet, et al., 1994; Janowsky and Overstreet, 1995). Cholinergic agents have acute effects on mood, including induction of depression, anergia, and behavioral inhibition and suppression of manic symptoms when given alone or combined with other agents (El-Yousef, Janowsky, et al., 1973; Janowsky, El-Yousef, et al., 1973; Janowsky, Risch, et al., 1983). Cholinergic system "downregulation" would, then, not be expected to be prodepressive and could conceivably have an anti-depressive effect. Counterbalancing this in ill PGW veterans is the effect of chronic illness itself, which may be expected to favor the genesis of depression.

Evidence suggests that depressed individuals may have a sensitive muscarinic system, with increased vulnerability to cholinergic stimulation (possibly leading to increased vulnerability to affective and neuroendocrine disturbance), per-haps, it has been suggested, with muscarinic receptor "upregulation" (Janowsky, Risch, et al., 1980; Risch, Kalin, et al., 1981; Overstreet, Janowsky, et al., 1989; Gillin, Sutton, et al., 1991; Janowsky, Overstreet, et al., 1994). Thus, muscarinic stimulation (for instance with the drug arecoline, a muscarinic receptor agonist, or drug that mimics the effect of ACh on muscarinic receptors) produces greater effect on some tests (such as induction of REM sleep) in depressed subjects than in controls. However, other central cholinergic effects, such as the profound increase in serum epinephrine levels that normally occurs with such cholinergic-acting drugs as physostigmine, are relatively blunted rather than exaggerated in depressed individuals (Janowsky, Risch, et al., 1986).

The relation of these factors to illnesses in Gulf War veterans remains unclear. Many ill veterans have some depressive symptoms, but these may not occur more than would be expected in patients with a comparable degree of chronic illnesses. Ill veterans have been shown to have psychological profiles similar to those found in medical patients (Hom, Haley, et al., 1997). Mortality data indicate that, at least in the period 1991–1993, the suicide rate did not increase in PGW veterans; the adjusted mortality rate ratio from suicide was 0.94 for PGW veterans (n = 695,516) compared to other veterans (n = 746,291) (95 percent CI 0.79–1.12) (Kang and Bullman, 1996), suggesting that severe depression associated with suicide does not occur with increased frequency in PGW veterans, despite the significant pain and illness reported by many. Information on suicide rates for ill PGW veterans compared to (matched) medical patients has not been published. Thus, it is not known whether counter-depressive effects from ACh downregulation serve to partially offset factors disposing to depression and suicide, or whether rates of suicide are comparable to those with other medical illness.

Behavioral Effects

Limited behavioral information related to ACh is available from studies in animals. Rats selectively bred for increased cholinergic sensitivity (Flinders Sensitive Line), which seem to have low baseline ACh action but increased ACh responsiveness, are marked by reduced action in the face of stress. For instance, they performed poorly in a tone-cued two-way active avoidance task in comparison with the control Flinders Resistant Line of rat (Overstreet, Rezvani, et al., 1990). Such rats also exhibit a high degree of immobility in a forced swim test (Overstreet, Rezvani, et al., 1992). But Flinders Sensitive Line rats have increased cholinergic *and* serotonergic sensitivity, and the immobility in the swim test (assessed by the amount of time spent immobile in a five minute swim test) appears to segregate with the serotonergic rather than the cholinergic sensitivity. (These were assessed by looking at the "hypothermic" response (reduction in body temperature) to a serotonin activating drug (a chemical termed "8-OH-DPAT" or "8-hydroxy-2-(di-N-propylamino)tetralin," which stimulates the serotonin 1A receptors); and to an ACh-activating drug (the anticholinesterase "oxotremorine" (0.2 mg/kg)) (Overstreet, Janowsky, et al., 1994).

MEMORY AND COGNITIVE EFFECTS

There is widespread evidence of effects of ACh on learning, memory, and attention (Levey, 1996; Barkai and Hasselmo, 1997; Levin, Torry, et al., 1997; Sarter and Bruno, 1997; Segal and Auerbach, 1997). Cholinergic underactivity is believed to underlie some human memory disorders, including Alzheimer's disease (Davis and Davis, 1978). Nicotinic and muscarinic ACh receptors are important for maintaining optimal memory performance (Levey, 1996; Felix and Levin, 1997; Ohno, Kobayashi, et al., 1997; Vannucchi, Scali, et al., 1997). Nicotinic and muscarinic antagonists have been shown to impair performance in learning and memory tasks (Kohler, Riters, et al., 1996; Felix and Levin, 1997; Harder, Baker, et al., 1998; Vannucchi, Scali, et al., 1997). Physostigmine can relieve the mental confusion produced by scopolamine (Ketchum, Sidell, et al., 1973; Granacher and Baldessarini, 1975; Mohs, Davis, et al., 1979), and can reverse the memory deficit produced by anticholinergics like scopolamine (Drachman, 1977; Ghoneim and Mewaldt, 1977). Acetylcholinergic drugs like physostigmine and arecoline enhance learning and memory in animal studies (Robbins, McAlonan, et al., 1997), as well as in normal humans (Davis, Mohs, et al., 1978) and in subjects with memory disorders, including Alzheimer's (Peters and Levin, 1977; Agnoli, Martucci, et al., 1983; Christie, Shering, et al., 1981). (Physostigmine, at the correct dose, may improve memory in those with certain memory problems but may be ineffective or perhaps harmful at too high or too low a dose (Peters and Levin, 1977; Mohs, Davis, et al., 1979).) The effects of ACh on cognitive function are diverse (Safer and Allen, 1971; Drachman and Leavitt, 1974; Ghoneim and Mewaldt, 1975; Drachman, 1977; Ghoneim and Mewaldt, 1977; Peterson, 1977; Mohs, Davis, et al., 1979; Beatty, Butters, et al., 1986) and difficult to summarize (Deutsch and Rogers 1979; Sarter and Bruno, 1997) (though difficulties with some tasks involving visual attention, sensory integration, intermediate and long term memory, and spatial memory have been described) and generalizations from animal studies to human behavior have been described as not straightforward (Mohs, Davis, et al., 1979).

In short, ACh is vital for learning and memory, and disruption of ACh function—particularly low function but perhaps also too high of function impairs learning and retrieval of learned memories. Cognitive and memory impairment, which has been reported in some studies of ill PGW veterans (see Chapter Fourteen), might be an expected consequence if ACh dysregulation occurred following use of PB.

DERMATOLOGIC FINDINGS: SKIN SYMPTOMS AND HAIR LOSS

Skin symptoms (particularly rashes) have figured prominently in assessments of symptoms reported by ill PGW veterans. For example, rash represented the second most common complaint in an analysis of complaints of 17,248 ill or concerned veterans in the Veterans Affairs Persian Gulf Health Registry (as of June 1994), cited by 17 percent of such veterans (Persian Gulf Veterans Coordinating Board 1995); and rash was reported by 35 percent of 125 reservists of the 123rd Army Reserve Command (De Fraites, Wanat, et al., 1992), and rash or dermatitis by 38 percent of 18,075 participants in DoD's Comprehensive Clinical Evaluation Program (CCEP) (DoD, 1996). There are many causes of rashes, including drugs, systemic infection, skin infection or disease, endocrine disease, autoimmune disease, and cancer. No reports have been uncovered in which PB was clearly linked to subsequent development of rashes. However, "central"-type nicotinic receptors have been identified in skin cells termed keratinocytes that may be involved in cell migration and adhesion (Grando, Horton, et al., 1995; Conti-Fine, Horton, et al., 1994). It is possible that if dysregulation of this system occurred, increased susceptibility to skin abnormalities presenting as rashes and other skin complaints would result. Some veterans have reported increased susceptibility to injury with "challenge," such as shaving or abrasion. This suggests that a test could be devised to measure skin susceptibility to injury with such challenge.

Many reports have surfaced that PGW veterans report dental problems, such as loose teeth, bleeding gums, or rapid dental decay (De Fraites, Wanat, et al., 1992; DoD, 1996; Gordon 1997). For instance, 47 percent of a group of 79 reservists from the 123rd ARCOM reported dental complaints; dental complaints were prominent in a list of symptoms by 33 ill British PGW veterans; and bleeding gums were reported by 8 percent of 18,075 CCEP participants (DoD, 1996). Whether problems with cell migration and adhesion resulting from AChE inhibition could contribute to bleeding gums or loose teeth remains a matter for future investigation.

Hair loss (alopecia) has also been reported among symptoms in ill PGW veterans from the United States (De Fraites, Wanat et al., 1992; DoD, 1996) and from the United Kingdom (Beale, 1994). For instance, hair loss was reported by 12 percent of 18,075 participants in the DoD's CCEP (April 1996 report) (DoD, 1996). Hair loss may be caused by many conditions, ranging from endocrine disorders (such as hypothyroidism) to autoimmune diseases (such as lupus), drugs, infections (including leishmaniasis), and dermatological disorders. ("Telogen effluvium," in which the normally asynchronous growth/death phase of follicles becomes synchronous, causing much of the hair to fall out at once, may occur with stress, pregnancy, and severe systemic illness (Adler, Lam, et al., 1994).) PB is among the drugs that have been reported to possibly cause alopecia. One report describes a 69-year-old woman who received 360 mg/day of PB (four times the PGW PB daily dose, in a patient with myasthenia gravis) in whom extensive generalized hair loss occurred several months after initiation of PB. PB was reinstituted one year later, and striking hair loss reoccurred after five weeks of use, with hair regrowth three months thereafter (Field, 1980).

Because many causes of rash and of hair loss are known, PB cannot be presumed to cause these symptoms in ill PGW veterans. However, because PB has been previously implicated in hair loss (albeit in one published case) and because ACh may influence skin cell behavior, a role for PB in skin symptoms and reported hair loss cannot be excluded.

DIARRHEA

Diarrhea is commonly reported by ill PGW veterans. For instance, 20 percent of 18,075 participants in the DoD's CCEP reported diarrhea, and for 2 percent it was the chief complaint. Diarrhea was reported as an acute symptom in patients who received PB. Indeed, muscarinic ACh symptoms, discussed in Chapter Three, include enhanced GI peristalsis. In addition, however, there is evidence of a connection to diarrhea for both high and low nicotinic ACh function.

Diarrhea, particularly in ulcerative colitis, has been treated successfully with nicotine (Griffel and Das, 1994; Guslandi and Tittobello, 1994; Pullan, Rhodes, et al., 1994; Silverstein, Lashner, et al., 1994; Nilsson, 1995; Rhodes and Thomas, 1995; Thomas, Rhodes, et al., 1995; Watson and Lewis, 1995; Birtwistle, 1996; Forbes, 1996; Guslandi and Tittobello, 1996; Pullan, 1996; Thomas, Rhodes, et al., 1996; Bonapace and Mays, 1997; Green, Thomas, et al., 1997; Sandborn, Tremaine, et al., 1997; Thomas, Rhodes, et al., 1998). Cigarette smoking is associated with protection against ulcerative colitis (with a risk ratio of 0.13 in one case control study, 95 percent confidence interval 0.05–0.38) (Silverstein, Lashner, et al., 1994), and cessation of nicotine has in some instances been linked to onset or exacerbation of this diarrheal condition (Birtwistle, 1995; Birtwistle, 1996), with those who smoked most heavily perhaps showing the greatest increase in risk (Birtwistle, 1996). Several factors reduce the impact of this finding—that nicotinic stimulation may ameliorate diarrhea, and nicotinic (ACh) withdrawal may produce diarrhea—as an explanation for diarrhea in ill PGW veterans. First, diarrhea in most ill PGW veterans has not been associated with inflammatory bowel disease. Although it is possible that low nicotinic function is responsible for diarrhea in ill veterans, and/or that nicotine will ameliorate symptoms of diarrhea, this has not been tested. Moreover nicotine may exacerbate rather than ameliorate symptoms in another inflammatory bowel disease termed Crohn's disease (Bonapace and Mays, 1997; Thomas, Rhodes, et al., 1998).

SLEEP

This section briefly discusses the presence of sleep disorders in PGW veterans; the possible relationship between sleep abnormalities and neurochemical changes, specifically related to ACh and to serotonin; and the possible relationship between sleep disorder and other adverse outcomes in PGW veterans, including pain and death by unintentional injury.

Sleep Disorders in PGW Veterans

Sleep difficulties figure prominently in complaints of ill PGW veterans. In one early report, sleep abnormalities constituted one of the two most common complaints, along with headache (Newmark and Clayton, 1995); they were also the second most common (after fatigue) among a group of 79 reservists of 123rd ARCOM, endorsed by 57 percent of reservists (De Fraites, Wanat, et al., 1992) and the second most common specific diagnostic subcategory, after malaise and fatigue, among 6,517 CCEP participants with primary or secondary diagnoses of "Symptoms, Signs, and Ill-defined Conditions," in whom sleep disturbances constituted a primary or secondary diagnosis of approximately 32 percent (Joseph, 1997). A more modest 5 percent of 17,248 ill or concerned veterans in the VA Persian Gulf Health registry (June 1994) reported sleep disturbances (Persian Gulf Veterans Coordinating Board, 1995). Ill PGW veterans from the United Kingdom also report sleep abnormalities (Beale, 1994).

Sleep apnea appears to be emerging as a prominent contributor to sleep abnormalities in ill PGW veterans. An evaluation of sleep disorders in 14 PGW veterans revealed that six had abnormal sleep studies, including three with obstructive sleep apnea, two with narcolepsy with abnormal multiple sleep latency test, and one with periodic movements of sleep with abnormal polysomnogram. (Narcolepsy is associated with decreased REM latency, consistent with abnormal ACh action—in this case, heightened ACh effect.) The most common diagnosis in this series, however, was "unspecified sleep disorder" (Newmark and Clayton, 1995). Another study has found a high prevalence of sleep apnea in self-referred PGW veterans with symptoms believed consistent with sleep disorder who were evaluated for sleep apnea; 15 of 46 evaluated, and 15 of 192 presenting met criteria for sleep apnea (Peacock, Morris, et al., 1997), suggesting that somewhere between 8 percent and 33 percent of these ill veterans had the disorder (since some who were not tested for the disorder might have tested positive). A study of consecutive CCEP participants found that sleep apnea was the primary diagnosis in 7.4 percent, and any diagnosis in an additional 5 percent of those PGW veterans who were registered (Roy, Koslowe, et al., 1998). (An additional 11.7 percent had any sleep problem as the primary diagnosis, and 19 percent as any diagnosis (Roy, Koslowe, et al., 1998).) Efforts are ongoing to characterize sleep disorders in a controlled, blinded fashion at the University of Texas Southwestern Medical Center at Dallas (Haley, 1998, citing work with R. Armitage and R. Hoffman).

ACh and Sleep Apnea. As noted, sleep apnea is the most common identified sleep abnormality in tested ill PGW veterans with sleep complaints (Peacock and Marris, 1997). A possible relation of sleep apnea to the ACh system (and ACh downregulation) is suggested by (mixed) evidence that nicotine may be useful in treating sleep apnea (Davila, Hurt, et al., 1994; Hein, Kirsten, et al.,

1995; Wali and Kryger, 1995; Wirth, 1995; Obermeyer and Benca, 1996; Schrand, 1996). Although this is consistent with the hypothesis in Chapter Thirteen that ACh downregulation as a possible sequela of PB administration may contribute to symptoms in ill PGW veterans, it does not constitute persuasive evidence for this hypothesis.

ACh and Sleep: Other Information. The acute effect of PB on the acetyl-cholinergic system is increased cholinergic activity. Long-term effects of PB (such as changes in the neuromuscular junction) have been demonstrated in animals. However, whether similar or unrelated long-term changes also occur in central muscarinic or nicotinic cholinergic synapses in humans is presently unknown, though animal data suggest that some similar effects may occur at central muscarinic sites. Elsewhere it is postulated that long term ACh dysreg-ulation—and perhaps downregulation—may occur (see Chapter Twelve, "Neurotransmitter Dysregulation"). Sleep quality is believed to be affected by low brain ACh activity, and indeed the anticholinergic effects of antiparkinson drugs are believed to contribute to sleep quality disturbance in Parkinsonism.

ACh is known to be involved in regulation of REM sleep in particular. ACh (and agents that stimulate its action) increases REM sleep (Sitaram and Gillin, 1979; Kok, 1993). Effects of ACh on sleep have been shown by administering pilo-carpine, a muscarinic "direct agonist" (agent that acts on muscarinic receptors directly to mimic the effects of ACh acting on those receptors). ACh-like mus-carinic action in a double-blind study of 13 healthy males produced shortened REM sleep latency (time taken to first enter REM sleep, the phase of sleep in which dreaming occurs) and increased total REM time, REM percent (percent of time asleep that is spent in REM), and duration of the first REM period, and it reduced stage IV sleep and Delta sleep (Berkowitz, Sutton, et al., 1990). In this small, short study, subjective sleep experience was not affected. In another study, arecoline (another agent that stimulates the muscarinic type of ACh receptors) was shown to induce REM sleep in both depressed subjects and controls, in a dose-dependent fashion, when compared to placebo infusions; depressed patients entered REM more rapidly than control patients with a higher dose of arecoline, suggesting that depressed individuals might have a more sensitive muscarinic system (perhaps due to muscarinic receptor up-regulation) (Gillin, Sutton, et al., 1991).

Of note regarding possible long term effects of AChE inhibition: one study reports *enhancement* of REM more than one year after nerve agent exposure in the industrial setting (Bushfield and Duffy, 1982). (This appears to suggest ACh upregulation or activation for the REM system, rather than downregulation or depression with these agents.) Since the long-term effects of PB on the cholin-ergic system remain to be elucidated, whether such REM alterations occur long-term following PB (alone or with co-exposures, in selected individuals) remains unknown. Short-term mild sleep deprivation, which ordinarily means selective REM deprivation because REM is more prevalent later in the course of sleep, produces mood elevation. Indeed, some antidepressants are thought to exert part of their action by shortening the duration of REM. Alteration of sleep architecture in the form of increased REM might be expected to lead to relative dysphoria.

The finding of prolonged increased duration of REM observed following exposure to soman suggests that, at least with that OP nerve agent in primates, long-lasting enhanced rather than reduced cholinergic function occurs in REM regulation, more consistent with the concept of cholinergic *dys*regulation, rather than exclusively downregulation. It is not known whether similar effects, no effects, or opposite effects (consistent with downregulation) would occur following exposure to PB—alone or in combination with other exposures—if it gains access to the brain. Cholinergic *down*regulation would be expected to result in increased REM latency and perhaps reduced REM duration. Ongoing sleep studies are evaluating sleep, including REM, in ill PGW veterans and controls, and results of these studies will allow these possibilities to be narrowed down (Haley, 1998b, 1998c). (The complexities of such evaluations are reinforced by the findings noted previously: effects on ACh function from AChE inhibitors may differ from one brain area to another, perhaps reflecting different properties of the resident ACh receptors; thus it is conceivable that lasting effects of AChE inhibitors on sleep regulation (if any) need not parallel effects of AChE inhibitors on other functions regulated by different brain areas or involving different classes of ACh receptors.)

Serotonin and Sleep. Sleep and serotonin may each influence the other. Serotonin may influence sleep because serotonin is the precursor of melatonin (Hardman, Limbird, et al., 1996), which is involved in regulation of sleep. Sleep may in turn influence serotonin because serotonin is preferentially produced during stage IV sleep (Duna and Wilke, 1993).

PB may affect sleep, as noted previously, perhaps through enhancement of REM. If total sleep time is preserved, REM enhancement may lead to absolute or relative reduction in stage IV sleep, which could influence serotonin production. However, it remains unsupported that long-term changes in REM or stage IV sleep occur following short-term administration of PB.

As noted previously, PB appears to bind to the serotonin binding site on the ACh receptor, offering a possible avenue for disruption of serotonergic mechanisms from PB not mediated through sleep (see Chapter Three). (For example, if altered regulation of ACh receptors—increase or decrease—takes place, then a commensurate increase or decrease in serotonin binding capability results, which may, though feedback mechanisms, lead to further changes in regulation of the serotonin system.) Whether such disruption occurs with PB, or in Gulf War veterans, has not been established.

In war-related PTSD, elevated awakening thresholds in sleep stages III and IV have been demonstrated, although overall sleep data were within normal limits (Dagan, Lavie, et al., 1991), and no evidence of change was found in the proportion of slow wave sleep. This finding may serve as a caution that sleep that appears "normal" by crude sleep measures may in fact differ in more subtle characteristics, perhaps with neurochemical correlates (as a cause or effect).

Possible Sequelae of Sleep Alteration in PGW Veterans

Sleep, Pain, and Fibromyalgia. Fibromyalgia is a condition of chronic pain entailing widespread pain; and pain with finger pressure over at least 11 of 18 designated "tender point" sites. Fibromyalgia occurs predominantly in females in the civilian population (Bennett, 1995), but fibromyalgia and similar pain syndromes are common in ill PGW veterans (about 93 percent of PGW veterans are male). For example, muscle and/or joint pain was the fourth most common symptom among 7,248 ill or concerned veterans in the VA Persian Gulf Health Registry, June 1994, represented in 14 percent of registrants (Persian Gulf Veterans Coordinating Board, 1995). Diseases of the musculoskeletal system and connective tissue constituted the most common primary diagnosis among a group of 20,000 CCEP Gulf War participants, occurring as a primary diagnosis in 19 percent and as a secondary diagnosis in 30 percent (Joseph, 1997). "Joint pains" were reported by 54 percent of reservists of the 123rd ARCOM (n = 79) (De Fraites, Wanat, et al., 1992)—tied for the third most common complaint. In a series of consecutive PGW veterans referred to a CCEP, rheumatological consultation was the most common elective subspecialty referral (56 percent); among those referred, 59 percent had soft tissue syndromes, in which fibromyalgia was prominent (17 percent) (Grady, Carpenter, et al., 1998).

In light of the high prevalence of soft tissue pain in ill veterans and the high prevalence of sleep disorders, the known relation between sleep disorder and fibromyalgia merits discussion.

Non-REM stage IV sleep is disrupted in fibromyalgia (Saskin, Moldofsy, et al., 1986; Bennett, 1995). If stage IV sleep is disrupted intentionally in normal controls, fibrositic symptoms develop (symptoms akin to those in patients with fibromyalgia) (Duna and Wilke, 1993). Although periodic leg movements are the most common sleep disorder diagnosis associated with fibromyalgia, sleep apnea is a relatively common finding in men with fibromyalgia (Bennett, 1995).

Serotonin is preferentially produced in stage IV sleep, and these patients are reported to have reduced levels of serum serotonin and CSF 5-HIAA, a metabolite of serotonin (Duna and Wilke, 1993). Moreover, if tricyclic anti-depressants are given, which raise serotonin levels and enhance stage IV sleep, symptoms abate (Duna and Wilke, 1993). It is thought that reduced serotonin from stage IV sleep deprivation may lead to lowered pain thresholds and "activation" of latent tender points by one of two possible mechanisms: atten-uating the pain-modulating effects of endogenous opiates called "endorphins" (Duna and Wilke, 1993; Vaerøy, Helle, et al., 1988a); or altering the function of a neurotransmitter involved in signaling pain, called "substance P," so that sen-sory stimuli are more likely to be interpreted as pain (Duna and Wilke, 1993; Murphy and Zelman, 1987). Serotonin deficiency may explain the elevated CSF levels of substance P found in patients with fibromyalgia (Vaerøy, Helle, et al., 1988b; Duna and Wilke, 1993). (In turn, substance P may enhance cholinergic receptor desensitization, and is viewed by some as an inhibitory modulator at nicotinic cholinergic sites (O'Neill, 1981; Stallcup and Patrick, 1980) (see chap-ters on neuromuscular junction and neurotransmitter dysregulation)); thus stage IV sleep deprivation, if present, could theoretically potentiate any effects of cholinergic downregulation.

Sleep and Accidents. Sleep disruption has been a prominent symptom in PGW veterans in some reports (noted previously). Increased deaths from motor vehicle accidents have also been reported in ill PGW veterans (Kang and Bull-man, 1996).

Motor vehicle accidents are strongly associated with sleep deprivation, cir-cadian disruption, and sleep disorders (Gold, Rogacz, et al., 1992; Maycock, 1996; Findley, Weiss, et al., 1991). The risk has been particularly well studied for sleep apnea, which as noted above may be increased in ill PGW veterans. Studies report from a twofold to a more than sevenfold increased risk in all or (particularly) single car accidents, or in those for which subjects were at fault (Haraldsson, Carenfeldt, et al., 1995; Findley, Unverzagt, et al., 1988; Stoohs, Guilleminault, et al., 1994); one reports a twelvefold higher risk of single-car accidents adjusted for miles driven (Haraldsson, Carenfeldt, et al., 1990). The risk may rise with increasing severity of sleep apnea (Findley, Fabrizio, et al., 1989). Moreover, treatments (such as nasal continuous positive airway pres-sure, or uvulopalatopharyngoplasty) that reduce symptoms and signs of obstructive form of sleep apnea also have been reported to significantly reduce the rate of accidents in obstructive sleep apnea sufferers (Flemons and Tsai, 1997; Cassel, Ploch, et al., 1996; Haraldsson, Carenfeldt, et al., 1995). (Such treatment also benefits mood and cognitive effects associated with sleep apnea (Flemons and Tsai, 1997).) Special driving simulation tests may predict which patients with sleep disorders are at increased risk for automotive accidents (Findley, Unverzagt, et al., 1995), and such tests could be considered for use in ill PGW veterans with identified sleep abnormalities.

Increased injury deaths have been reported in PGW veterans (see "Violent Death" section in this chapter). While other mechanisms may be postulated for this increase in violent death, the presence of widespread reports of sleep abnormalities requires that sleep disruption be investigated as a contributing factor.

Summary. Whether sleep disruption reported by PGW veterans relates to use of PB (alone or with anticholinesterase coexposures) remains unknown. If long-term cholinergic or serotonergic changes are produced by PB, a matter that remains unresolved, then alterations in REM sleep or stage IV sleep, respectively, may be produced. Sleep apnea, which has been the most prominent specific sleep disorder in ill PGW veterans, has been associated with fibromyalgia and could contribute to symptoms of pain reported by PGW veterans. Whether or not sleep abnormalities relate to prior use of PB, both subjective and objective sleep abnormalities, including particularly sleep apnea, have been documented in a substantial fraction of tested PGW veterans reporting sleep problems. Because sleep disorders (particularly sleep apnea) and sleepiness have been strongly linked to increased risk of automotive accidents in several studies, reported and identified sleep disorders in ill PGW veterans are a possible or even likely contributor to the increased rate of accidental death observed in PGW veterans (see section on "Violent Death").

Because sleep disruption is widely reported in ill PGW veterans and can have serious sequelae including pain and death from injury, additional effort should be made to characterize the sleep abnormalities of ill PGW veterans, to determine the nature of the abnormalities and if possible devise effective treatments. Consideration *could* be given to a trial of nicotinic agonists for ill PGW veterans with sleep apnea.

TERATOGENICITY AND DEVELOPMENTAL EFFECTS

Birth Defects in Children of PGW Veterans

Epidemiological studies indicate that children of PGW veterans are no more likely than controls to exhibit serious birth defects (Cowan 1997). However, risk of birth defects was increased in children of deployed women (borderline significance: RR 1.12, 95 percent CI 1.00–1.25), although the increase was no longer significant after adjustment for race/ethnicity, marital status, and branch of service (Cowan, De Fraites, et al., 1997). This study has been criticized on the grounds that by confining evaluation to births of active-duty personnel in military hospitals, those with illness (who would have been preferentially separated from the military) would have been preferentially excluded (Haley, 1998b, 1998c). If exposures of some kind associated with Gulf

War service are responsible for illness, and also for birth defects, then the very population at risk for birth defects would have been excluded from evaluation.

One study reported that children of 52 National Guardsmen from two Mississippi National Guard units deployed to the Persian Gulf had a frequency of minor and major birth defects, premature births, low birth weight, and other health effects (based on examination of medical records of 54 of 55 children born to those veterans) supposedly similar to that in the U.S. general population (Penman, Tarver, et al., 1996). However, this conclusion was rendered from this small sample in the absence of statistical analysis.

One study examined the presence of Goldenhar's syndrome (or "oculoauricular vertebral dysplasia"), one of the birth defects that had been described in the popular press) among 34,069 infants of Gulf War veterans and 41,345 infants of non–PGW deployed personnel conceived after return from the Gulf (or after December 31, 1990, for non–PGW deployed) born in military hospitals before October 1, 1993, from parents still on active duty (Araneta, Moore, et al., 1997). Goldenhar's syndrome is characterized by abnormal facies (facial appearance), including ear abnormalities (microtia, anotia, or preauricular tags), asymmetry or hypoplasia of the face or mandible, unilateral cysts on the eyeballs (epibulbar dermoids), defects ("colobomas") of the upper lids, and lateral facial clefts, as well as vertebral anomalies. Medical records, subsequent hospital admissions, and genetic evaluations of all infants diagnosed with anomalies of the face or skull, or those with defects associated with Goldenhar's syndrome, were examined by two pediatricians blinded to Gulf War status. A threefold excess risk of Goldenhar's syndrome was derived from small numbers of affected infants and was not statistically significant (RR 3.03, 95 percent CI 0.63–20.57). Again, by confining evaluation to offspring of active-duty personnel born in military hospitals, it is possible that those at greatest risk for birth defects may have been preferentially excluded from analysis, although it cannot be presumed that inclusion of those individuals would not necessarily buttress the case for increased incidence of Goldenhar's syndrome.

An ongoing VA Cooperative Study of PGW veterans and their families plans to look at severe birth defects only (Murphy, Kang, et al., 1998). Confinement to severe birth defects necessarily restricts the number of endpoints evaluated, possibly reducing the power to detect an effect; moreover, since prior study suggested the possibility of increase in all birth defects but not severe birth defects in offspring of female veterans (Cowan, De Fraites, et al., 1997), this plan precludes analysis of those defects that existing evidence suggests may be increased.

A study is under way evaluating birth defects among children of British Gulf War veterans (Doyle, Roman, et al., 1997).

PB: Fetal and Developmental Effects

As noted in Chapter Three ("Characteristics of PB"), PB may cross the placenta. Controlled trials cannot be done in humans to evaluate the effect of PB on fetal development. Controlled studies can be done in animals, and observational studies are possible in humans.

PB use during pregnancy in myasthenics has been postulated as a contributor to neonatal myasthenia (Blackhall, Buckley, et al., 1969), a condition involving transient weakness of the infant seldom persisting beyond six weeks after birth; however, the condition may primarily arise from maternal antibodies to the ACh receptor circulating in the fetus. Reports have not been identified indicating teratogenicity from PB administration in myasthenics, despite the fact that substantially higher doses of PB (e.g., 600 mg/d; or 6.7 times the PGW dose) are given in this population, and treatment occurs for a more prolonged period. This situation provides additional reassurance that gross fetal abnormalities are not common with PB administration during pregnancy.

Animal studies evaluating "teratogenic" or developmental effects of PB have been done in rats and chickens. In rats, developmental concerns of PB occur for adult male offspring of females exposed while pregnant, although some of these data derive from studies employing neonatal rather than in utero PB delivery: Neonatal delivery of PB (2 µg/day for four days, then 10 µg/day for 10 days) was found to permanently increase male sexual behavior in those rats that exhibited even slight hypoplasia of seminal vesicles in neonatal life, reinforcing the notion that changes of neurotransmitter concentrations and/or turnover rates induced by psychotropic drugs can affect sex-specific brain differentiation (Dorner and Hinz, 1978). Moreover, adult male rats treated neonatally with PB (2µg/day for four days—or 0.03 GWE—then 10 µg/day for 10 days in 20–25 g rats—or 0.31 Gulf War daily doses) showed a slight decrease in the noradrenaline concentration in the hypothalamus. It was concluded that PB (and other psychotropic substances) may exert "teratogenetic" effects, which are mediated, at least in part, by unphysiologic concentrations and/or turnover rates of neurotransmitters during brain differentiation (Dorner, Hecht, et al., 1976; Dorner, Staudt, et al., 1977).

Studies in chicken embryos with cholinomimetic agents, including neostigmine (in doses from 0.1 to 0.6 mg), PB (in doses of 10 mg/egg or more), physostigmine, carbachol, decamethonium, and others found that all these compounds led to abnormalities of the cervical vertebrae, or the whole vertebral column (Landauer, 1975). Hypoplasia of leg muscles occurred with lower incidence. A high degree of synergism was seen when two cholinomimetic compounds were used in combination (Landauer, 1975). PB results were not reported in detail, but PB showed among the stronger effects, exceeding those of neostigmine, and accounting for short crooked necks and muscular hypoplasia of the legs. Physostigmine produced additional abnormalities including syndactylism (webbed digits), micromelia (shortened limbs), and abnormalities of the "visceral skeleton" and of the eyelids (Landauer, 1975).

Other studies looking at gross survival and morphological findings in rodents do not provide strong support for teratogenic concerns. When female rats were given 50–60 times the human dose of PB (on a mg/kg basis) in their drinking water on days 6–16 of pregnancy, there was reportedly no adverse effect on pregnancy, litter size, resorption rate, malformation rate, or fetal development (Wetherell, 1992). Although amount of PB actually consumed was not reported, the highest dose reportedly led to marked signs of toxicity and initial weight loss. Of course, this does not preclude effects of PB during developmental periods outside days 6–16 of pregnancy. When female rats were given PB from 15 days before mating to day 20 of gestation, no adverse effects were identified on mating, fertility, resorption rate, litter size, gestation length, malformation rate, or skeletal development. There was a slight reduction in postnatal pup weight gain but no effect on pup survival or time of developmental landmarks or visual or auditory function. When male rats were given PB in their drinking water for 18 weeks, mating performance and fertility were reportedly not affected. When female rabbits were given 93 times the human dose (on a mg/kg basis) of PB in their drinking water (no data were given showing how much was actually consumed), PB was stated to produce no "treatment related effect" on pregnancy, resorption rate, or malformation rate (Wetherell, 1992). It was concluded that these agents were safe for use in men and in women of childbearing age.

Clearly, teratogenic effects may be species- and dose-dependent. The data presented here suggest that monitoring for effects is appropriate, particularly for the small number of female veterans who received PB while pregnant. Moreover, while identification of gross abnormalities may occur by inspection, identification of delayed behavioral effects may not be readily apparent at birth or even in later life, without suspicion and careful investigation. Of note: alteration in the ratio of male to female births (a relative reduction in males—presumed to be opposite to the effect that might be expected from gender-selective abortion) has been reported in several industrial countries and is proposed as a possible "sentinel health indicator" (Davis, 1998). If this is correct, this ratio most likely relates to exposures distinct from AChE inhibition. Nonetheless, consideration could be given to comparing the sex ratio of children born to PGW veterans to the ratio in controls, or in the general population (considering female veterans and controls separately).

PREGNANCY AND PGW

Pregnant women were not knowingly deployed to the PGW, though some women were later determined to have been pregnant at or during the time of deployment. Pregnancy was cited as a reason for women personnel to consult medical personnel prior to taking PB (see Chapter Four, "PB Use in the Persian Gulf War"). Children of these women would seem to be those at greatest risk of manifesting effects, if any, resulting from maternal PB exposure. The number of children possibly affected by this exposure would be small, and these children should be easily identified.

If changes in brain development do result from in utero exposures, resulting behavioral alterations might not be identified until years after birth, and then perhaps only with careful study and may not be attributed to PB. An analogous experience can be cited from women in the 1950s who were given progestins to prevent miscarriage—daughters of these women reportedly exhibit characteristic differences in sex-typical behavior that begin to be evident in childhood. In addition, some but not all experienced minor birth defects, such as clitoromegaly. It is unclear whether testing for behavioral differences would have been performed, and behavioral differences identified, in the absence of identified physical changes at birth in a subset.

Consideration could be given to performing case control studies of behavior and cognition in children of female myasthenics who took PB while pregnant. While children of female PGW veterans who took PB while pregnant could also be evaluated, the sample would be quite small. These studies would have limited impact on future military use, because pregnant women are not knowingly deployed.

VIOLENT DEATH (DEATH FROM UNINTENTIONAL INJURY)

While illness mortality has not been elevated in PGW veterans (adjusted mortality rate ratio for "disease related causes" of death in PGW veterans compared to other veterans was 0.88, with a 95 percent confidence interval (CI) of 0.77–1.02, adjusted for age, race, sex, branch of service, and type of unit), mortality from unintentional injury was increased in deployed compared to nondeployed veterans (Kang and Bullman, 1996). Mortality rate ratios for all external causes were 1.17 (95 percent CI 1.08–1.27); for all accidents 1.25 (1.13–1.39); and for motor vehicle accidents 1.31 (1.14–1.49) (Kang and Bullman, 1996). This increase in accidental death was sufficient to produce increased overall mortality in PGW veterans compared to veteran controls. Despite no increase in illness mortality, and indeed a trend toward reduction, the adjusted overall mortality rate ratio showed a 9 percent increase, and this increase was statistically significant (95 percent confidence interval 1.01–1.16) (Kang and Bullman, 1996).

In the year from August 1, 1990 through July 31, 1991, more than half of all non-battle deaths in PGW era active duty personnel were from unintentional injury; and more than half of these from motor vehicle accidents (Committee to Review the Health Consequences of Service During the Persian Gulf War; IOM, 1996). The relative risk, or risk in deployed veterans divided by risk in non-deployed veterans, was 1.54, indicating a 50 percent increase in Gulf War deployed personnel; the 95 percent confidence interval was 1.32–1.77, signifying that, with 95 percent confidence, the smallest true increase supported by the statistics was 32 percent (Committee to Review the Health Consequences of Service During the Persian Gulf War; IOM, 1996). As noted above, mortality follow-up of PGW veterans supports a continued increase in the rate of injury death in the postwar period (Kang and Bullman, 1995; Kang and Bullman, 1996).

There are many possible causes of accidental death in PGW veterans, including some that may relate to PB. Several possible PB-related alternatives include cholinergic overactivity; sleep abnormalities, dependent on or independent of cholinergic changes; and possibly changes in serotonergic activity. Substance abuse relates strongly to violent and accidental death. However, Department of Veterans Affairs studies shortly after demobilization indicated a relatively low prevalence of substance abuse of 1.7 percent (Committee to Review the Health Consequences of Service During the Persian Gulf War; IOM, 1996); no comparison numbers were provided.

Cholinergic Activation

Many men were said to report enhanced aggression after taking nerve agent pretreatment sets with PB (Currie, 1995). Consistent with an AChE-inhibiting mechanism for this effect, aggressive behaviors have also been reported following exposure to other cholinesterase inhibitors including OPs and carbamates (Devinsky, Kernan, et al., 1992). Aggression by a person is related to nonillness mortality (death from injury or violence) in that person. Violent deaths, including homicide, suicide, and accident are interrelated and tracked together as nonillness mortality in international studies (Holinger and Klemen, 1982). Death by these three modes are linked etiologically through low serotonin (see below), through alcohol, through substance abuse, and through psychiatric disease (in which an apparent "accidental death" may in some instances represent a covert suicide or occur as a consequence of grossly impaired judgment). However, in PGW veterans, these causes of violent death are dissociated. Rates of death from suicide and homicide do not appear to have increased commensurately with accidental death in the PGW veteran population (see below). Other mechanisms may more selectively affect accidental death.

Sleep Deprivation

Sleep deprivation and sleep disorders are known to be strongly associated with death by motor vehicle accident. Many veterans report sleep abnormalities; therefore this etiology should be strongly considered (see section on "Sleep," above).

Reduced Serotonin

Natively low or experimentally lowered serotonin has been strongly associated with impulsive violent behaviors, risk-taking behaviors, and violent outcomes in many studies in humans and animals (Grant, Coscina, et al., 1973; Kulkarni, 1968; Kantak, Hegestrand, et al., 1980; Miczek and Donat, 1989; Miczek, Mos, et al., 1989; Olivier, Mos, et al., 1989 ; Kostowski and Valzelli, 1974; Åsberg, 1994; Eichelman, 1979; Coccaro, 1989; Coccaro, Siever, et al., 1989; Brown, Goodwin, et al., 1982; Brown, Ebert, et al., 1982; Brown, Goodwin, et al., 1979; Brown and Goodwin, 1986a; Brown and Goodwin, 1986b). However in humans, reduced serotonin is strongly associated with suicide in particular, an effect that cuts across psychiatric diagnoses (whether persons have unipolar depression, personality disorder, or schizophrenia, it is the low serotonin subgroup that is at greatest risk for suicide attempts (Grant, Coscina, et al., 1973; Kulkarni, 1968; Kantak, Hegestrand, et al., 1980; Miczek and Donat, 1989; Miczek, Mos, et al., 1989; Olivier, Mos, et al., 1989; Kostowski and Valzelli, 1974; Åsberg, 1994; Eichelman, 1979). While suicide was a significant cause of death in personnel who were on active duty in the PGW and elsewhere (with 216 deaths from suicide among the 1,622 total nonbattle deaths from August 1, 1990, to July 31, 1991), the relative risk for suicide among PGW-deployed compared to non-PGW deployed veterans was 0.34 during this period (95 percent CI 0.16–0.63) (Writer, De Fraites, et al., 1996), signifying a markedly *reduced* rate of death from suicide during the war. Data from after the war, derived from a comprehensive study of mortality among all 695,516 personnel who served in the Persian Gulf from August 1990 to April 1991, compared to 746,291 personnel who served elsewhere during the same time, found the postwar suicide rate in men to be comparable in PGW veterans to that in controls; women showed a nonsignificant trend toward increased suicide and homicide (Kang and Bullman, 1995; Kang and Bullman, 1996). The mortality rates for PGW veterans versus controls in 1991–1993, based on death certificate information, adjusted for age, race, sex, branch of service, and type of unit were as follows: for suicide 0.94 (0.79–1.12) and for homicide 0.85 (0.67–1.08). Suicide and homicide were not increased, while all accidents and motor vehicle accidents were. These data do not support either a low serotonin state or substance abuse as major contributors to death from injury in PGW veterans and add credence to an alternative mechanism involving impaired neurocognitive function, such as impaired concentration or decisionmaking, whether due to sleep disruption, altered neurochemistry from PGW exposures (perhaps including PB), or other sources.[2]

Increased accidental deaths have been reported following other conflicts, including World War II prisoners of war (Eberly and Engdahl, 1991); and Vietnam veterans (Watanabe and Kang, 1995). In Vietnam veterans, the relative risk of death from "external causes" was 1.21 (95 percent CI 1.0–1.47) (Watanabe and Kang, 1995). Greatly elevated rates of PTSD were noted particularly among prisoners of war. Associated sleep and concentration disruption from PTSD and perhaps substance abuse may have been etiologic following these conflicts.

Both similar and different exposures occurred in the different conflicts, and similar and different etiologies for violent death may be at play. In contradistinction to the PGW, increased incidence of suicide has been reported for Vietnam veterans (Watanabe and Kang, 1995); this adds support to etiologies of violent death that include accident and suicide (as many do), rather than etiologies more specific for accidents. Thus, PTSD, alcohol and substance abuse, and serotonin dysregulation may play a more significant role in the increased violent deaths observed in Vietnam veterans, while these etiologies are less strongly supported for ill PGW veterans.

DEFINING CASES AND CONTROLS FOR RESEARCH ON ILLNESSES IN PGW VETERANS

Because there was no particular location in previous chapters for discussion of how Gulf War veteran cohorts should be defined for the purpose of clinical studies (which may be different from definitions for other purposes), such a discussion is included here. Subjects selected as representing ill PGW veterans for case-control studies should ideally be those with more characteristic and perhaps more severe symptoms: use of all PGW veterans, all who chose to enter registries, or all who report any illness will dilute the sample and complicate the ability to detect true associations. Moreover, use as healthy controls of all veterans who do not enter registries is particularly problematic, because preliminary work suggests that many who have not elected to participate in registries may experience similar symptoms. Some groups are beginning to generate case definitions of illness in PGW veterans for the purpose of studies they are conducting. One group uses degree of compatibility with factor-analysis defined syndromes in ill PGW veterans (Haley, Kurt, et al., 1997) for this purpose (Haley,

---

[2]Comment: Data emerging after this writing suggest an increase in suicide may be present, with a risk ratio of 1.53; homicides, however, were not increased (RR 0.85).

1998); this permits assessment of how "typical" symptoms are, at least according to the factor-analytic standard.

The soundness of the factor-analytic strategy would be strongly enhanced if the results were replicated using cross validation, or if other techniques, such as unsupervised neural networks, were shown to categorize subjects similarly. However, while this standard can be questioned, case assignment error resulting from use of this strategy would likely produce bias toward the null and would *not* be expected to engender spurious positive findings.

"Healthy" controls should be selected to have none of the characteristic symptoms—no unusual fatigue, headache, joint and muscle pains, or sleep disturbance and no new onset of diarrhea, rash, mood alteration, headache, chemical sensitivities, or difficulty concentrating. A separate group of "unhealthy" controls could be defined in whom symptoms are present but quite distinct from those of persons with "characteristic" illness. The goal is to separate groups at extremes of symptomatology, just as studies of cardiovascular risk factors may compare those in the highest quintile on some factor—either exposure or outcome—to those in the lowest quintile, to increase potential for assessment of the link between exposure and illness. The criteria employed for the purpose of study are expressly intended to identify the more typical cases (thus, those most likely to be part of a coherent syndrome in which risk factors may be identified), and while they may not be selected as cases, it should not be presumed that others with atypical or lesser symptoms are necessarily "free" of illness.

SCIENTIFIC RECOMMENDATIONS

- Sleep studies should be considered in PGW veterans who complain of fatigue; evaluation for sleep apnea should be included.

- Sleep studies in PGW veterans who complain of sleep difficulties or fatigue should specifically examine sleep parameters known to be related to cholinergic dysfunction, such as REM sleep latency and duration.

- Sleep studies in PGW veterans who complain of sleep difficulties should specifically evaluate stage IV sleep patterns, including duration, timing (including latency), proportion of total sleep, and awakening.

- Consideration should be given to evaluating other indices of serotonergic function, including peripheral and central measures.

- Investigation of circadian functioning (e.g., of neurotransmitter and hormone levels and responsivity, and such autonomic indices as temperature and blood pressure) should be done in ill PGW veterans and controls.

- Consideration should be given to evaluating automobile accident risk in PGW veterans with fatigue and/or identified sleep disorders, using driving simulation tests that have been shown to correlate with accident risk in sleep-disordered drivers.

- Additional work should be done to evaluate contributors to death by unintentional injury. Persons with hospitalization for unintentional injury may be compared to controls on measures that may relate to injury risk. Candidate measures include subjective fatigue; subjective and objective sleep measures; sensitive neuropsychiatric measures, such as those involving attention, psychomotor speed, or visual function; and perhaps measures of cholinergic and possibly serotonergic function and substance abuse.

- Strong emphasis should be placed on research performed to identify specific objective abnormalities that may characterize subsets of ill PGW veterans. This may include clinical tests of vestibular function, eye movement, neuropsychiatric function, autonomic function, such laboratory tests as tests of cytokine function or porphyrin metabolism, and such imaging tests as tests of regional blood flow. Identification of such abnormalities in ill veterans will be essential to pursuing tests of etiology in animal models. Specifically, different candidate exposures can be tested for production of similar objective findings, thus abetting the process of identifying causative or contributory exposures. This recommendation is applicable to study of etiologies and contributory factors discussed in all chapters.

- Clinical case-control studies should endeavor to define cases and controls in a manner that would permit assessment of a link to risk factors, if such a link is present. Thus, cases should consist of those with more "characteristic" clusters of symptoms; healthy non-PGW (and perhaps PGW) controls should consist of those who lack both characteristic and equivocal or less typical symptoms, and unhealthy non-PGW (and perhaps PGW) controls can be defined as those in whom health symptoms are present, but do not include characteristic symptoms, or equivocal or less typical symptoms, of ill PGW veterans. As scientific advances are made, objective correlates of illnesses in PGW veterans may be identified. Subsequent case definitions may then be modified to incorporate those findings. There is ample evidence that ill PGW veterans are ill from more than one cause. (A small number, for example, have been found to have viscerotropic leishmaniasis, but this is unlikely to account for illness in most ill veterans.) Strategies for clustering data should be considered for defining symptom clusters, in an effort not to confute findings by mixing different illnesses in one "case" definition. (Note: since this report was originally sent for review, additional efforts toward such case definitions have been generated, notably that by the CDC (Fukuda, Nisenbaum, et al., 1998).)

SUMMARY ANALYSIS

This chapter discusses an assortment of etiologies and hypotheses relating PB to physiological function or outcomes. These hypotheses are evaluated in lesser detail than in other sections, and summary analyses for each area presented in this chapter are not provided.

Chapter Sixteen

CONCLUSIONS

This report endeavors to identify theories which may relate use of PB to development of chronic illnesses in PGW veterans and to review the evidence regarding these theories. The theories on safety are sorted into two categories: those that discuss mechanisms for heightened susceptibility to effects of PB or increased effective exposure to PB and those that suggest mechanisms by which PB exposure—perhaps enabled by such heightened susceptibility—could produce chronic illnesses. Theories relating to mechanisms of increased susceptibility to PB include the following:

- Conditions of stress in the PGW may have produced breaches of the blood-brain barrier, allowing PB to enter the brain, producing effects of PB that would not normally occur, or would occur only at far higher doses.

- Different individuals have physiological variations that result in marked individual differences in processing of, and susceptibility to, PB.

- Interactions between PB and other chemicals to which veterans may have been exposed may result in toxic effects occurring at far lower doses than if exposures had occurred separately.

Theories suggesting mechanisms by which PB exposure could produce subsequent chronic symptoms—in the face of these factors that enhance susceptibility—include the following:

- Ingestion of bromide in PB may (according to the theory) produce bromism, which can cause multiple neuropsychiatric symptoms.

- PGW veterans may have developed a (not universally accepted) condition termed "multiple chemical sensitivity," which is associated with many of the symptoms seen in ill PGW veterans.

- PB may lead to disruption of the neuromuscular junction.

- PB, which abnormally elevates ACh, may cause changes in regulation in the ACh and perhaps other neurotransmitter systems.

Some other considerations are discussed in less detail, relating PB to changes in hormones, sleep, serotonin, violence, and other factors, although these can be viewed as consequences of the mechanisms mentioned here.

THEORIES OF HEIGHTENED SUSCEPTIBILITY

We now describe the theories regarding heightened susceptibility in slightly more detail.

The first postulate suggests that permeability of the blood-brain barrier in PGW veterans may have been enhanced due to stress and other conditions of war, permitting increased access of PB to the brain and that, moreover, PB itself may increase access of other agents to the brain. (The "blood-brain barrier" refers to special ability of certain cells to exclude access to the brain of chemicals and organisms that circulate in the blood—including PB.) Data demonstrating breach of the blood-brain barrier, allowing increased access of PB to the brain in conditions of stress, derive from rodents. (Some evidence suggests that heat may potentiate permeability effects.) However, human data suggest a possible increase in central side effects of PB during the war compared to peacetime, which could reflect increased access of PB to the brain in circumstances of stress in humans. The degree to which the blood-brain barrier may have been infringed, thus allowing entry of PB into the brain, determines the possible contribution of several other of the theories that have been discussed. For example, "downregulation" of the cholinergic system, at least central down-regulation (described in more detail below), is not likely to result from administration of PB unless PB gains access to the brain. Therefore, if central cholinergic downregulation is to be proposed as a contributing mechanism for memory, learning, and sleep deficits in ill PGW veterans, then PB must have entered the brain—or other AChE inhibitors must have done so, perhaps facilitated by PB. Another animal study reports that PB itself may enhance permeability of the blood-brain barrier.

The next postulated factor that may contribute to a connection between PB and chronic illnesses concerns individual differences in processing of PB, leading to individual differences in susceptibility. How is it, if PB is a contributor to chronic illnesses in PGW veterans, that some PGW veterans who received PB became ill, while others who received a similar amount did not? Evidence was found for individual differences in PB processing at many levels. Differences occurred in the dose of PB actually taken by troops and the duration of treatment. Moreover, individual differences in "absorption" of PB pills from the gut to the blood contribute to different blood levels for the same administered dose. Different rates of clearance of PB from the blood also contribute to different blood levels of PB. These different rates of clearance occur because of enzyme "polymorphisms" and individual differences in enzyme quantities. (Different individuals have different DNA coding for the enzymes, producing enzymes that are different in structure and function. Moreover, the same enzyme may be present in widely differing amounts.) Differences in AChE enzyme inhibition may occur, even if the same blood level of PB is obtained. Finally, differences in toxic effects may occur, even for the same degree of AChE inhibition—perhaps resulting from underlying differences in the ACh system—and in cholinergic "responsiveness"—which have been shown to occur in people.

These widespread differences in intake and processing of PB could contribute to important differences in the effect of administered PB from one individual to another. Indeed, from a clinical standpoint, individual differences in *acute* susceptibility to PB obviously occur, as reflected in differences in side effects experienced in response to PB. (Individual differences in "tolerance" to PB given therapeutically are also seen in patients with myasthenia gravis, a medical condition in which there is low action of ACh at the muscle, leading to weakness.) The same differences in susceptibility that lead to acute differences in response—or perhaps other differences in susceptibility, unrelated to those producing acute differences in response—may be postulated to condition development of long-term effects, if any, in response to PB. There is weak evidence that the acute susceptibility differences may arise from mechanisms relevant to differences in chronic symptoms in PGW veterans, since one study finds a relation between certain chronic illness "syndromes" (derived from factor analysis) in ill PGW veterans and self-reported adverse acute response to administration of PB. If PB is a contributor to chronic illnesses in some PGW veterans (perhaps for reasons discussed below), then individual differences in susceptibility almost certainly (and almost tautologically) play a role in determining which individuals are affected.

Another postulated factor that may play a role in the connection between PB and illnesses in PGW veterans involves possible toxic interactions between PB and other exposures. Studies performed in animals indicate that toxicity of PB is enhanced—indeed, in a synergistic fashion—with concomitant exposure to other chemicals, such as pesticides, to which some troops may have been exposed. (Synergistic toxicity means the toxic effects from a group of chemicals is more than the sum of the toxic effects from the individual chemicals.) These other exposures may include pesticides and insect repellents, as well as caffeine, perhaps nerve agents, and stress (which also figures in the relation of PB to illness in the blood-brain barrier theory—and which could be considered to have a role in the individual differences theory, since responses to stress may differ from one individual to another based on individual differences in neuro-chemistry and experience). The degree to which these interactions between PB and other factors may play a role in PGW veterans is unclear, for several reasons. First, we do not have good data regarding who received which exposures, which complicates performance of epidemiological studies looking for the effect of these interactions. (Epidemiological studies using self-report data could, however, look to see whether incorporating an "interaction term" between PB and other self-reported exposures increases the explanatory power of the statistical model.) Second, the data from animal studies are difficult to extrapolate to PGW veterans because extremely high doses of drugs—both of PB and of the interactants—were used in these animal studies, doses many times higher than those experienced by PGW veterans. To address the question of whether important synergistic effects would occur with lower doses—more comparable to those administered to PGW veterans—is not simple. Even supposing administration of those low doses in animals produced effects comparable to those reported by ill veterans, there is no good way to assess the presence of those effects. (We have enough trouble assessing them in humans, who can tell us what they feel; in humans we have not, or not yet, found good "objective" tests to coincide with reports of symptoms.) In existing animal studies, relatively crude measures, such as gross incoordination in walking or death, are often employed. If lower doses of drugs are studied, more sensitive measures will need to be found to gauge the possibility of synergistic effects between PB and other exposures. Because evidence of synergistic toxicity exists—albeit in animals, using high doses and different routes of administration from those experienced by PGW veterans—interactions between PB and other agents or exposures remain a possible avenue by which increased effect or toxicity of PB may have occurred in some veterans.

THEORIES CONCERNING POSSIBLE CONTRIBUTION BY PB TO CHRONIC SYMPTOMS

The relation of such increased effect to long-term illnesses requires introduction of other theories, discussed below.

The first seeks to link PB exposure to development of chronic illnesses and suggests that illness results from excessive accumulation of bromide following PB administration. However, bromism emerges as an unlikely cause of chronic illness, because the cumulative doses of bromide given and the time-course of illnesses in PGW veterans are incompatible with available knowledge regarding bromism. Although it is possible that bromism could have contributed to illness in a small number of veterans with specialized circumstances, bromism appears unlikely to be a significant contributor to chronic illness in most ill veterans.

The second proposes that symptoms in ill PGW veterans have much in common with those of patients with a putative—but not universally accepted—condition termed "multiple chemical sensitivity" (MCS). MCS is a symptom complex involving multiple self-reported "sensitivities" or adverse subjective responses to a host of apparently unrelated foods and chemicals. Many ill veterans are said to have new chemical sensitivities (though peer-reviewed data on frequency of these reports are not available); MCS patients have other symptoms in addition to chemical sensitivities, symptoms said to parallel those of ill PGW veterans (again, not peer-reviewed data); and many or most ill PGW veterans and MCS patients report prior exposure to AChE-inhibiting agents—PB and perhaps nerve agent and pesticides in Gulf War veterans and pesticides and organic solvents in MCS patients. Moreover, the genesis of MCS has been proposed to relate to exposure to excessive ACh activity, or reduced AChE activity, which may presumably have been experienced by PGW veterans exposed to PB. However MCS is poorly positioned to serve as an explanation for illness in PGW veterans, because MCS itself is not well understood (or even universally accepted as a syndrome by scientists or clinicians). Like illness in PGW veterans, there is no widely accepted case definition (though several have been proposed); and there is as yet no identified objective marker that distinguishes those who report symptoms from those who do not. At present, MCS cannot serve as an explanation for illnesses in any PGW veterans. However, it can be hoped, whether or not MCS and illnesses in PGW veterans are found to converge in any way, that ongoing research for each condition into possible cholinergic mechanisms will assist in pursuit of understanding for the other.

A third theory relating PB to development of chronic illnesses in PGW veterans involves effects of PB on regulation of ACh.

- The first component of this discussion relates to the effects of AChE inhibitors at the neuromuscular junction.

Nerves signal to skeletal muscles using ACh, at receptors termed "nicotinic" receptors. Binding of ACh to these nicotinic receptors at the neuromuscular junction causes the muscle to contract. Administration of AChE-inhibiting drugs, including PB (leading to excessive signaling by ACh at the neuromuscular junction), has been shown in animals to produce destructive changes to the muscle tissue and to produce "presynaptic" and "postsynaptic" changes in the neuromuscular junction. These changes begin after a single dose of PB. Though some effects of destruction (effects visible with light or electron microscope) begin to recede even if use of PB is continued, partially restoring the appearance of the muscle and of the neuromuscular junction, such restoration has not in all cases been complete even long after administration of PB has been stopped—indeed, as long out as anyone has looked. Findings at the neuromuscular junction are potentially important for two reasons: first, because some of the symptoms reported by PGW veterans include musculo-skeletal problems and fatigue—to which effects of PB at the neuromuscular junction could conceivably contribute—and second, because this junction is the most accessible cholinergic synapse and therefore is the best studied. It is partly presumed, partly hoped, that effects evident at the neuromuscular junction will accurately reflect effects at central acetylcholinergic synapses, at least the nicotinic ones, and may help to explain central effects from AChE inhibitors. (Evidence to date supports both similarities and differences between the skeletal muscle nicotinic receptor and central nicotinic receptors.)

Data from the neuromuscular junction support development of "dysregulation" of the nicotinic and muscarinic acetylcholinergic systems—particularly but not exclusively for "downregulation" (that is, attenuation or suppression of those systems)—following use of AChE-inhibiting drugs, such as PB. That is, effects occur that tend to counteract the abnormally high activity of ACh induced by delivery of PB (or other AChE inhibitors) by suppressing ACh production, release, and response. Such changes include "presynaptic" changes—changes associated with the nerve cell sending the signal—including withdrawal of nerve terminals from the muscle; reduced production of ACh; reduced release of ACh, including reduced number of packets or "vesicles" (also called "quanta") of ACh released with a nerve signal; and reduced number of ACh molecules in each such packet. Such changes also include "postsynaptic" changes—changes at the cell (in this case, muscle cell, but in the brain, another nerve cell) that receives the signal—such as reduced number of ACh receptors (the receptor is a five-subunit protein to which ACh binds; this binding leads to fluxes of ions that produce a chemical signal to the muscle cell, signaling it to contract) and reduced affinity by, and sensitivity of, ACh receptors to ACh.

- The second component of this theory relates to effects on ACh regulation produced by AChE inhibitors "centrally," in the brain.

Although changes consistent with dysregulation have been best demonstrated in the neuromuscular junction, evidence from the brains of rodents suggests that dysregulation changes (again, especially but not necessarily exclusively downregulation) may also occur centrally (that is, in the brain and perhaps spinal cord) for both the nicotinic and muscarinic systems. These central changes have been demonstrated in animals, using AChE inhibitors that gain central access and typically at doses that achieve higher levels of AChE inhibition than those to which veterans were exposed. Clinical effects of down-regulation may be referred to as "tolerance" to a drug when they are reflected in reduced response to that drug or "rebound" when effects opposite to those produced by the drug occur when the drug is discontinued. Tolerance to PB has been described, in the form of reduced therapeutic effect of PB, and reduced production of side effects by PB with continued use has been described. It is not known whether symptoms described by PGW veterans could in some instances be manifestations of a prolonged form of rebound effect.[1] If PB gains central access, therefore, discontinuation of PB might be associated with effects of abnormally reduced activity of the nicotinic and muscarinic systems in the brain.

Though evidence for this possibility is substantially less extensive, there may be—alternatively, or more likely in addition—ACh upregulation producing increased activity for some receptor types, in some brain areas.

Evidence indicates that different effects have different time-courses. Some are short-lived and may dissipate even while PB continues to be given. These cannot of themselves plausibly contribute to chronic illnesses in PGW veterans. However, other effects appear to be long-lasting and may continue long after discontinuation of PB. The normal coordinated functions of the brain could be disrupted by differentially altered elements, and the resulting interactions could, hypothetically, produce their own consequences and result in evolution of effects over time. Even if upregulation is not a significant factor (other than upregulation of nicotinic receptors, which may occur in some brain regions after acetylcholinergic stimulation), existing evidence that different degrees of downregulation occur in different brain (and peripheral) areas and with different receptor subtypes suggests that "dysregulation" rather than "downregulation" may more accurately characterize the full spectrum of alterations in regulation that might occur following exposure to AChE-inhibiting agents in susceptible individuals. Neurotransmitter "dysregulation" constitutes the fourth "theory" relating PB to illness (though actually it is really an extension of the findings at the neuromuscular junction—or, otherwise viewed, the findings at the neuromuscular junction are a lead-in to this theory).

The actual contribution of dysregulation to symptoms in humans is not known, because evidence for dysregulation derives primarily from animal studies and basic science research. However, it is known that the cholinergic system is vitally involved in regulation of muscle action, sleep, pain, and learning and memory. Thus, a downregulated "hypocholinergic" (or dysregulated "dyscholinergic") state might be expected to lead to problems with muscle action (or fatigue), memory, learning, and sleep, and increased sensitivity to pain—problems that figure prominently in complaints of ill PGW veterans.

---

[1]PB may affect many systems that interact, including not only the ACh neurotransmitter system but the GABA system, the glutamate system, the catecholamine systems, and the 5-hydroxytryptamine (5-HT or serotonin) system; because these systems have complex interactions and are characterized by an assortment of different time-courses of regulation, effects distinct from simple rebound, here given the general term "dysregulation," may occur.

Indeed, treatment with ACh-activating drugs has been used in other populations to treat most of the symptoms most commonly reported by ill PGW veterans. Pyridostigmine itself has been used to treat fatigue from various causes. Moreover, nicotine, which stimulates the nicotinic subtype of ACh receptors, along with other cholinergic drugs, has been reported clinically to reduce diarrhea (in patients with ulcerative colitis), to enhance cognitive function (in animals (Abdulla, Bradbury, et al., 1996; Zarrindast, Sadegh, and Shafaghi, 1996; Arendash, Sanberg, and Sengstock, 1995; Socci, Sanberg, and Arendash, 1995); in patients with Parkinson's disease and Alzheimer's disease (Christie, Shering, et al., 1981; Fagerstrom, Pomerleau, et al., 1994; Lena and Changeux, 1997), in normal subjects (Davis, Mohs, et al., 1978; Baldinger and Schroeder, 1995; Foulds, Stapleton, et al., 1996), and especially in former smokers (Foulds, Stapleton, et al., 1996), and to improve attention (in smokers (Ghatan, 1998) and in patients with attention deficit disorder (Benowitz, 1996; Levin, Conners, et al., 1996; Lena and Changeux, 1997). Moreover, nicotine has been used in treatment of sleep apnea, which appears to be the most common sleep disorder identified in ill PGW veterans. (Sleep apnea has in turn been linked to fibromyalgia, particularly fibromyalgia in males, and to fatigue and to mood and cognitive dysfunction.) And recently it has been shown that nicotinic stimulation has powerful pain-relieving effects, stronger than those of morphine. Since nicotinic stimulation may lead to improvement in memory, attention, diarrhea, sleep, and pain—areas that figure prominently in complaints of ill PGW veterans—central nicotinic dysfunction or depression might reasonably be postulated to explain many symptoms in ill PGW veterans.

Little is known about the time-course of ACh dysregulation (centrally or peripherally), following pharmacologically heightened ACh activity, and more needs to be understood about the doses of drug and the durations of use that might produce such dysregulation. At present, the idea of cholinergic downregulation (or neurotransmitter dysregulation) as an explanation for illness in PGW veterans is speculative. Although existing literature supports the possibility of a link between ACh dysregulation and each of the symptoms commonly reported by ill PGW veterans and some evidence suggests that such dysregulation may occur with PB in animals, this does not mean that ACh dysregulation necessarily occurred in PGW veterans or is in fact the cause of any of these symptoms. (The consistency across many symptoms is suggestive, however.) Additional research is needed to clarify what role, if any, such dysregulation might have in development of chronic symptoms.

Issues relating to whether chronic symptoms might plausibly arise from acute administration of PB are discussed in a separate chapter. Evidence suggesting the possibility of chronic effects by AChE inhibitors, including but not confined to PB, is reviewed. Data regarding chronic effects, particularly from low-dose exposures not producing acute symptoms, are meager, and studies are frequently of poor quality. Bearing this in mind, some evidence suggests the possibility of chronic effects, at least for some AChE inhibitors, perhaps even at dosage levels that do not produce obvious symptoms acutely. Some such studies have suggested the possibility of chronic changes in nerve and muscle function, EEGs, regional cerebral blood flow, or neuropsychological tests, typically with exposure to AChE-inhibiting pesticides or to nerve agents. Other studies fail to show such findings. Of course, if chronic effects, and particularly neuropsychological effects (which, along with musculoskeletal effects might be the effects most plausibly related to PB, stemming from PB's prominent action on acetylcholinergic function), are not present in PGW veterans, then neither PB nor any other exposure will need to be invoked as an explanation. Therefore, we have reviewed some evidence regarding chronic neuropsychological findings in ill PGW veterans.

Several studies suggest that selected ill veterans have statistically lower scores on neuropsychological batteries than do well controls. Often, although they do less well than controls, their scores remained in the "normal" range. Although it appears that *some* ill veterans do have diminished neurocognitive function compared to healthy controls when sensitive tests are selected, we would expect that some *non*veterans reporting similar complaints of memory and attention problems would also have lower scores. The extent to which an excess number of veterans do so remains to be clarified. The reductions in function that have been observed do not appear to relate to one or a small number of neurocognitive abilities. However, since the acetylcholinergic system plays a prominent role in many functions of the brain, if effects were mediated through dysregulation of the ACh system, the effects might be expected to span many functions.[2] The additional important issue is whether such impairment is related to use of—or adverse response to—PB. One small study (mentioned above) suggested a connection between adverse acute response to PB and current neuropsychological syndromes. Moreover, a recent

---

[2]Moreover, there are large differences from one skill to another in where one person "ranks" compared to other people. For instance, in school one person may have been good in spatial reasoning but bad in algebra; excellent in computation but average in mathematical abstraction; a person may have an adequate short-term memory but abysmal visual tracking ability. Therefore even if the drug's effects were in some sense "uniform" across the functions affected (presumably primarily the many functions influenced by the acetylcholinergic system; perhaps to a lesser degree by serotonergic, glutaminergic, GABAergic, or monoaminergic systems), depressing all by the same amount on some hypothetical standardized scale and to the same degree in all individuals, different individuals would still be expected to dip to below par on different functions. Which functions test as normal and which as subnormal could well depend on how far below or above average subjects were on that function to start with and would therefore be expected to differ from one person to another. The result would be the appearance of a haphazard "scattering" of the effect across tested functions, with different individuals testing abnormally low on different functions but an overall trend toward worse function in symptomatic PGW veterans than controls on many functions. This is consistent with the pattern described by some researchers.

study found that among British PGW veterans, self-reported exposure to PB was strongly and significantly related to current CDC-defined Gulf War Illness (Unwin, Blatchley, et al., 1999). However, these studies are limited by the use of self-report to determine exposure to PB because many individuals do not remember what agents they took (reducing precision and reducing the ability to detect an association) and individuals who are ill may remember use of PB differentially from individuals who are not ill (potentially producing bias). Ill individuals may have thought about it more and therefore be more likely to remember PB and other exposures (or think they remember) than do individuals who are not ill, or they may simply be more likely to respond positively, thinking an exposure must have been present. Also, the presence of serious illness may influence their thinking about how much they probably used. However, one study found that mean exposure estimates (for a set of exposures that did not include PB) in PGW veterans did not correlate with symptom scores, which militates against a strong role for recall bias. Moreover, in the British study, the observed increased risk associated with self-reported exposure to risk factors did not differ among those who had record-confirmation of exposure and the group as a whole, again suggesting that recall bias did not play a major role. In any event, no more accurate method of determining exposure to PB is currently available.

In short, there is suggestive evidence that some AChE inhibitors may cause chronic neurological changes. There is some objective evidence that chronic neurological changes exist in some ill PGW veterans compared to healthy controls. (Evidence is limited regarding whether new deficits are more common in PGW veterans—absence of relevant predeployment data renders this determination more difficult. However, whether or not this can be shown with certainty, efforts to understand the origin of deficits in those who have them are important.) Current evidence cannot rule out the possibility that long-term effects of PB might occur and might participate in production of neuropsychological deficits reported in some PGW veterans.

Finally, one chapter mentions briefly several other considerations not reviewed in detail: these include hormone and stress effects, effects on sleep, the serotonergic system, and injury from accidents. Many PGW veterans report difficulties with sleep. Sleep is prominently regulated by the ACh and serotonin/melatonin systems, both of which might be influenced by PB if PB were to gain central access. PB, in addition to augmenting ACh by inhibiting AChE, also may "mimic" serotonin by binding to a specialized site on the ACh receptor for which the "endogenous ligand"—that is, the chemical that normally binds there—is serotonin. (Just as action by PB on the ACh system may lead to altered regulation of that system, so binding by PB on a site normally bound by serotonin could possibly affect regulation of the serotonergic system.) For these reasons, an association between PB use and sleep difficulties in PGW veterans is possible, though certainly not demonstrated. Of note: A form of sleep apnea appears to be common in tested ill PGW veterans who report sleep disorders. Sleep disruption, particularly sleep apnea, has been linked to increased motor vehicle accidents, and deaths from motor vehicle accidents have been shown to be significantly increased in PGW veterans. Moreover, sleep disruption, including sleep apnea, has also been shown to have a role in production of some pain syndromes, in particular a syndrome termed "fibromyalgia," which bears much in common to pain syndromes reported by many ill PGW veterans. It is also of note that nicotine, a nicotinic ACh receptor activating drug, has been used as a treatment for sleep apnea.

On a separate note, there remain some concerns regarding the efficacy of PB in protection against nerve agent threats. For some nerve agents, such as sarin, evidence was not adequate to exclude a possible harmful effect by use of PB as a pretreatment. A modest and "militarily" unimportant reduction in efficacy of postexposure treatments is seen when PB is used in rodents, but if the reduction in protection is exaggerated in primates—as the enhancement in protection for soman is exaggerated in primates—then it is possible that a meaningful reduction in protection against death would occur. (There is no evidence that this is the case, but neither is evidence adequate to confidently exclude this possibility.) Moreover, with regard to soman, one study compared the protective efficacy of PB against soman in vitro in muscles of monkeys and humans. Ten times the dose of PB had to be applied to human muscle to produce comparable protection—although oral doses in monkey studies to produce "comparable" AChE inhibition are three to ten times as high as in people. These findings suggest by comparison that the doses given to people may be inadequate to confer benefit against lethality (and it has never been proposed that PB will enhance mission completion). Although several plausible reasons suggest that these findings might be misleading, the studies have not been done that would lay these concerns to rest.

In summary, present evidence cannot exclude a role of PB as a contributor to chronic illnesses in PGW veterans mediated through several possible pathways, individually or in concert. First, one or a combination of several factors might participate in increasing susceptibility to PB—or effective exposure to PB. These factors include increased permeability of the blood-brain barrier in conditions of stress, allowing abnormal access of PB and other chemicals to the brain; individual differences in native susceptibility to PB and/or to other exposures that interact with PB; and enhanced toxicity (effect) of PB resulting from interactions of PB with pesticides, stress, caffeine, alum adjuvant of vaccines, or other exposures. Once exposure to PB occurs, particularly central exposure, PB could conceivably produce chronic illness by engendering dysregulation in neurotransmitter systems and in particular in the ACh system. Although there is evidence that such dysregulation takes place in animals exposed to AChE inhibitors, whether some of the effects of dysregulation are chronic remains unknown. Moreover, for central dysregulation to occur, PB (or other AChE inhibitors) would (probably) need to gain access to the CNS, which would suggest that postulating PB as a plausible contributor to chronic illness would most likely require concomitant exposure to stress or other exposures that may enhance entry of PB to the brain. Alternatively, PB may enhance central entry or toxicity of other exposures, including centrally acting AChE inhibitors, such as pesticides or perhaps sarin). (Of note: The blood-brain barrier permeability is itself variable, perhaps independent of these forms of exposure.) Finally, PB could influence peripheral factors that in turn have central effects. Another form of dysregulation that has been postulated to link use of PB to later chronic illness is development of abnormal "sensitivity" of certain neurons in the brain, leading among other consequences to heightened aversive conditioning, possibly with somatic effects—that is, effects involving bodily symptoms. Evidence suggests that some parts of the brain may exhibit opposite direction effects on some aspects of the ACh system compared to other parts of the brain, so that changes consistent with both upregulation and downregulation could occur simultaneously.

LIMITATIONS AND FUTURE DIRECTIONS

The combined literature related to PB, to Persian Gulf illnesses, and particularly to acetylcholinergic function is quite extensive, and decisions were made to emphasize some factors at the expense of others. The chief "new" contribution of this report, compared to previous discussions of PB as a cause of illness in PGW veterans, is the comparatively more in-depth discussion of the acetylcholinergic system and its relation to possible mechanisms of illness. (Even in this arena, the present effort barely scratches the surface of available evidence; it is hoped that future efforts are able to build on the foundation provided here.)

Several issues important to military use of PB were reviewed but are given less attention in this report—including data on acute physiological and performance effects of PB, as well as on acute side effects, and data on alternatives to PB. These issues are relevant to military use of PB, but they were given relatively less emphasis in the current report because they do not directly address the issue of development of chronic health effects in PGW veterans.

This effort is limited, too, by the available evidence. Concern regarding PB as a possible source of chronic symptoms is relatively new, and research in this area is in its infancy. Human data regarding chronic effects are mostly epidemiological (observational—not experimental), and these epidemiological studies are complicated by lack of a consistent clinical case definition (by lack of a clear definition of which PGW veterans should be counted as "ill," or as neurologically symptomatic resulting from involvement in the PGW) and by lack of good data regarding who received which exposures, including PB. When both the exposure and the outcome are not well characterized, it is doubly difficult to clearly evaluate the connection between the exposure (here, PB) and an adverse outcome. While some experimental data are available from humans, related to fairly short-term effects of use of PB in non-war volunteers, and while these data do not suggest that short-term effects are a major concern, such studies have not looked at long-term effects and have often not entailed conditions of stress, heat, exertion, sleep disruption, and interactions with certain other exposures that may have conditioned susceptibility to PB in the PGW. Most experimental studies relating to toxic effects, and involving stress and drug interactions, are done in animals—typically rodents, but occasionally other orders, such as hens or primates—and the degree to which this evidence extrapolates to humans is uncertain. Moreover, less sensitive clinical outcome measures—such as gross neurological abnormalities or death—must be used in animals, since one cannot question them regarding self-reported symptoms. It would be expected that doses needed to produce these more dramatic abnormalities would be greater than doses needed to produce symptoms more consistent with those reported by veterans—in whom objective indices of dysfunction are difficult to identify. Indeed, substantially higher doses are used in most animal studies than those employed in PGW veterans, and different modes of administration are also employed. How the effects grade with decreasing dose—that is, whether severe symptoms with quite high doses in animals imply subtle symptoms with the *much* lower doses used in veterans—is simply not known.

CONCLUDING REMARKS

This report reviews several factors that have been postulated to contribute to heightened susceptibility or exposure to PB in PGW veterans and several proposed mechanisms by which PB may cause illness. One postulated cause is dismissed. The other postulated causes and contributors remain possible; further study is needed to assess their role, if any, in development of illnesses in PGW veterans.

Three theories propose that exposure to effects of PB may have been augmented in the conditions of the PGW in some individuals, by each of three factors: breaches in the blood-brain barrier, presence of native differences in susceptibility, and drug/chemical interactions. There is sufficient support from the literature to suggest that each of these factors *may* condition susceptibility to PB—though studies using more similar doses and conditions to those experienced by PGW veterans are needed. Several theories describe or suggest mechanisms by which PB exposure—conditioned by the above factors—may lead to subsequent illness. The evidence from the literature appears to be adequately clear on issues of dose and time-course, in humans, to allow dismissal of the theory that excessive blood levels of bromide resulting from ingestion of PB led to bromism and that symptoms in PGW veterans are the consequence. For other theories relating use of PB to illnesses in PGW veterans, particularly for cholinergic dysregulation, evidence is inadequate to foreclose them. Particularly in the case of neurotransmitter dysregulation, evidence from animal studies is sufficiently suggestive that additional research is clearly warranted. The mechanisms noted are not mutually exclusive—two or more of the postulated factors influencing susceptibility may act together. This could in turn offer conditions favorable for development of long-term problems by PB, via one or more of the proposed mechanisms or other mechanisms not yet considered. However the studies supporting these mechanisms use doses, time-courses of follow-up, and conditions sufficiently dissimilar to those in veterans that it is impossible to extrapolate directly.

Additional investigation will be required to clarify the role of these factors in the contribution of PB, if any, to illnesses in PGW veterans.

EVIDENCE FOR NEUROTRANSMITTER DYSREGULATION IDENTIFIED OR PUBLISHED SINCE THE REVIEW PROCESS

Information not included in the original discussion of neurotransmitter dysregulation is provided here. The theory of downregulation/dysregulation of ACh function, the principal theory of causation put forth by and supported in this report (other mechanisms are primarily adjunctive), was first articulated as part of this work for RAND in numerous briefings commencing in early 1997. Since then, and since much of this report was originally written, an increasing body of literature has emerged consistent with or supportive of a possible contribution of ACh dysregulation (and, as originally theorized, primarily downregulation), resulting from AChE inhibitors, and a possible contribution of such dysregulation to health conditions. Before the original draft was sent for review, acetylcholinergic dysregulation had not been articulated as a theory of illness in PGW veterans.

Both older, not-previously-discussed information and newer evidence continue to add support to the dysregulation theory, with differential effects on different receptors, enzymes (e.g., subtypes of AChE), muscles, and brain areas. The time-courses of some changes remain too small to account for truly long-term effects. Other time-courses are long-lived but have not been followed long enough to determine just how extended in time they are. Finally, it has been shown that exposure to PB may influence later response to PB (and perhaps other AChE inhibitors), although again the possible intervals between exposures that permit this effect have not been well-characterized.

Some particularly important work comes from the laboratory of Hermona Soreq and collaborators in Israel (briefed as part of a mission to the Middle East in October 1997). Prior work in animals by this group had shown that PB may penetrate the brain under stress—leading to increased ACh excitation—work that provided the conditions in which PB could exert an effect centrally. More-recent work by this group has shown that cholinergic excitation (such as that expected if PB penetrates the blood-brain barrier) leads to long-lasting changes in the brain resulting in delayed suppression of cholinergic transmission

(Friedman, Kaufer, et al., 1998) and that AChE inhibitors (of which PB is one) "induce multigenic transcriptional feedback response suppressing cholinergic neurotransmission" (Kaufer, Friedman, et al., 1999).

This work in animals, identifying mechanisms by which AChE inhibitors could exert long-lasting effects on ACh function, is complemented by epidemiological work that has suggested a relationship between PB adverse response (Haley and Kurt, 1997) and illness, or AChE exposure (PB and pesticide/insecticide exposure) and illness (Unwin, Blatchley, et al., 1999). Also critically important are clinical studies, such as those of Robert Haley and colleagues in Texas, that evaluate ill PGW veterans and controls on specific objective measures in an effort to identify subtle or marked deficits (for instance, neurological, neuropsychological, and cerebral blood flow or brain electrical activity alterations) in classes of ill PGW veterans, that may then be correlated with known aspects of cholinergic function to test and further refine (or conceivably refute) our understanding of how (and whether) disruption of the ACh system pertains to illness in some veterans. The cholinergic system has many subparts with distinct functions interacting in complicated ways, and only integration of work at many levels, including epidemiological, basic science, and clinical studies, will adequately further understanding of whether and how PB and ACh dysregulation may pertain to illness in PGW veterans.

POTENTIAL NONHOMOGENEITY OF EFFECTS

Evidence continues to mount that the impact of AChE inhibitors or other augmenters of ACh action in altering regulatory systems may be nonuniform; alterations in regulation for one area of the brain, or one muscle, may differ from those in another area of the brain, or another muscle; the impact on one type of receptor, one type of nicotinic receptor, or one type of AChE molecule may differ from the impact on another type. These observations have important implications for investigation into the possible effects of PB; quantitative and qualitative differences in different parts of the system imply that negative or positive findings for one muscle, region, receptor, or molecule are consistent with positive, negative, or different findings at another muscle, region, receptor, or molecule.

Different Nicotinic Receptors

Specifically, neuronal nicotinic receptors have been found to be functionally diverse. There exist subunits, or member of the gene family, whose functional role in neuronal nicotinic receptors remains unknown, and there may be member of the gene family not yet identified. Different genes encoding these subunits are expressed in discrete but overlapping sets of brain nuclei; almost all known members are expressed in an area of the brain termed the medial habenula. Even adjacent cells may express different alpha subunit genes, suggesting major heterogeneity in receptor phenotype even in what are usually treated as a homogenous population of cells (e.g., Purkinje's cells in the cerebellum) (Patrick, Sequela, et al., 1993). Presence of different subtypes of receptors in different brain regions may participate in accounting for different responses of different brain regions to acute and prolonged ACh stimulation.

As an example with possible clinical relevance, a study, published as an abstract, showed that "chronic" exposure of rats to the organophosphorus AChE inhibitor DFP, at a dose previously shown not to produce overt signs of toxicity (0.25 mg/kg/d for two weeks) led to sustained depression of hippocampal nicotinic receptors of a certain type, associated with sustained reduction in ability to learn a new task (Buccafusco, Prendergast, et al., 1997). Reduction of up to 50 percent was seen in the number of cortical, striatal, and hippocampal high-affinity (tritiated epibatidine) nicotinic receptors, measured by quantitative autoradiography. By three weeks after DFP withdrawal, hippocampal nicotinic receptor density did not recover significantly (but receptor densities in the other regions did). Significant impairment in learning a spatial navigation task (water maze) up to three weeks after withdrawal from DFP was seen; much less severe deficits occurred when training occurred prior to DFP administration (Buccafusco, Prendergast, et al., 1997). It was not stated whether testing beyond the three-week period was undertaken.

Different Forms of AChE

In addition, multiple forms of AChE have been found. Six to 20 cholinesterase isoenzymes have been shown in the rat, with the pattern of isoenzymes influenced by the chemical given and by the assay employed (Nagayama, Akahori, et al., 1996). (Looking crudely at red blood cell and serum cholinesterase, the latter was reduced more in comparison to control animals with administration of fenthion, chlorpyrifos, bromophos, Diazinon, propaphos, DFP, Haloxon (Nagayama, Akahori, et al., 1996).) There exist sex differences in the pattern of cholinesterase isoenzymes in rats (Nagayama, Akahori, et al., 1996). Most effects by chemicals appeared to be greater in female rats, which start with more both true and pseudocholinesterase activity (Nagayama, Akahori, et al., 1996).

Another report, from a study in guinea pigs, notes that AChE is seen as a monomer (G1), dimer (G2), and tetramer (G4), with three asymmetric forms designated A4, A8, and A12; the A12 is the functionally important form at the neuromuscular junction (Lintern, Wetherell, et al., 1998). AChE inhibitors were noted to differentially inhibit different molecular forms of AChE in human brain and rat brain and diaphragm. In untreated guinea pigs, the highest AChE activity was seen in the striatum and cerebellum, then the midbrain, medulla-pons, and cortex; the lowest activity was seen in the hippocampus. Activity in the diaphragm was in turn sevenfold lower than in the hippocampus. Differential impact of the AChE inhibitor soman (given at approximately one LD_{50}, at 27 µM/kg) on brain regions and on AChE subtypes was seen with administration of soman in guinea pigs (Lintern, Wetherell, et al., 1998). One hour after soman administration, there was a dramatic reduction in AChE activity in all tissues (since soman is an AChE inhibitor). In the muscle, the three major molecular forms of AChE (A12, G4, and G1) were similarly inhibited and manifested similar rates of recovery, with normal function by seven days. However, in the brain, the G4 form of AChE was inhibited more than the G1 form; the hippocampus, cortex, and midbrain evinced the greatest reductions in activity; at seven days, activity had recovered in the cortex, medulla-pons, and striatum but inhibition remained in the hippocampus, midbrain, and cerebellum (Lintern, Wetherell, et al., 1998).

In chickens, there is a water-soluble form and several subtypes of membrane-bound AChE that differ in such characteristics as binding characteristics (K_m), rate constant, turnover number, specificity constant, maximal velocity, and half life (the time to convert half the substrate to product) (al-Jafari and Kamal, 1994). Similarly, in humans there is a "minor form" of AChE, the water-soluble form and several subtypes of the "major form" of AChE that differ again in the kinetic properties noted above (Kamal and al-Jafari, 1996).

Existence of different species of AChE has gained importance by the finding of Israeli researchers that both stress and AChE inhibition by administration of PB (1 mM) or DFP (1 µM) led to "dramatic and persistent upregulation of AChE production in the central nervous system" (Soreq, 1999), which appears to result from calcium-dependent changes in gene expression (and alternate splicing), leading to increases in a minor, quickly migrating form of AChE (Kaufer, Friedman, et al., 1998). Studies in transgenic mice suggest that chronic increased AChE activity may delay onset of progressive deterioration in cognitive and neuromotor function (Andres, Beeri, et al., 1997; Beeri, Gnatt, et al., 1995), although whether the alterations in AChE seen in the stress/carbamate experiments would produce similar changes was not reported.

Differences Across Brain Regions

A study in rats showed that stimulation of the nicotinic classes of ACh receptors, with long-term nicotine treatment (high dose: 50 mg/kg in drinking water for nine to 41 weeks), led to no significant changes in activity of the enzyme cholineacetyltransferase (which catalyzes production of ACh) or in muscarinic binding sites (receptor sites) (Nordberg, Wahlstrom, et al., 1985). However, 24 hours after withdrawal from 41 weeks of nicotine treatment, there was a significant 46 percent increase in the number of (radiolabeled) nicotine-binding sites in the hippocampus, with a concurrent 44 percent decrease in nicotine-binding sites in the cortex, and no change in the midbrain, consistent with mixed upregulation and downregulation (Nordberg, Wahlstrom, et al., 1985). Of note, these changes had disappeared on the fourteenth day of abstinence and had not occurred when only nine weeks of nicotine treatment had occurred. Although in these conditions (with nicotine as the ACh agonist, in rats) the effects examined were not long-lasting, these effects illustrate that the impact of ACh augmentation may be regionally specific and present in one region but absent in another.

Another study (abstract) in mice, reviewed above, also supports differential impact of AChE inhibitors on different brain regions; specifically, there were differential changes in density of radiolabeled epibatidine type of high-affinity nicotinic receptors following two weeks of low-dose DFP administration; reduction in receptor number was seen in cortex, striatum, and hippocampus but was sustained only in the hippocampus (measured at three weeks post-DFP); this was accompanied by reduced performance in a water-maze learning task, both the learning and spatial elements of which would be expected to involve the hippocampus (Buccafusco, Prendergast, et al., 1997).

AChE activity in mice brain following exposure to stress (in the form of forced-swim) showed differential changes according to brain region. At 80 hours after stress, cortical AChE activity remained markedly increased, nearly double that of controls; while cerebellar AChE, which had initially dropped, was restored to control values, and hippocampal AChE, which had initially increased to approximately 75 percent over controls, was reduced to approximately 50 percent of control values. Thus, the direction and time-course of changes in AChE was markedly different from one brain region to another, potentially consistent with differential dysregulation (Kaufer, 1998). (Changes were only followed to 80 hours poststress.) Similar changes in AChE activity were reportedly seen following carbamate exposure (1 mM PB) but graphs showing the time-course of response were provided only for the instance of stress.

Another study in rats found that physostigmine (a close relative of PB that more readily crosses the blood-brain barrier) leads to opposite-direction changes in different parts of the hippocampus: using 2-deoxyglucose as an index of regional brain activity, an increase was seen in the outer zone of molecular layer of the dentate gyrus and in stratum lacunosum-moleculare of an area of the hippocampus, termed area CA3, suggesting an increase in perforant path input during theta rhythm; a decrease was seen in the hilar dentate region, felt to reflect hilar inhibition by local circuits during theta rhythm generation (Sanchez-Arroyos, Gazetlu, et al., 1993).

Differences Across Muscle Types

Studies performed in the neuromuscular junction of mice have shown that PB induces different changes in different forms of AChE, with different time-courses in different muscles (Lintern, Smith, et al., 1997). "Repeated treatment with PB in mice can have a profound delayed effect on the activity of AChE in skeletal muscle. The changes varied in magnitude, direction and time-course depending on the type of muscle examined." The differences were felt to suggest a sensitization of the metabolic pathways for synthesis of the precursor G1 form, and/or assembly of precursor forms into the functional A12 form of AChE. Oscillations in activity seen in some cases suggested possible disruption of the fine homeostatic control of the enzyme levels (Lintern, Smith, et al., 1997). A mechanism for these changes was proposed, based on prior evidence that PB can induce synthesis of beta-endorphin in motoneurons, and beta-endorphin can increase synthesis of AChE in myotubes. One source for differential responses across different muscles is the fact that ACh release is intermittent in nerve signals to "fast" muscle fibers, while the nerves to slow fibers are more continuously active. Following PB administration, the G4 and A12 forms of AChE were reduced in the diaphragm but increased in the extensor digitorum longus and soleus muscles (limb muscles); at a week later, all forms were increased in all three muscles. At two weeks, the activity had returned to normal in the diaphragm but not in the muscle of either tested limb.

DYSREGULATION AND CHRONIC EFFECTS: PB EXPOSURE MAY ALTER SENSITIVITY TO LATER EXPOSURES

Another potentially important finding was that PB treatment altered sensitivity of muscles to later exposures (Lintern, Smith, et al., 1997). A single dose of PB was given to mice that had been pretreated with PB for three weeks, then left untreated for two weeks; and to control mice. Controls showed no effect on enzyme activity in the diaphragm at up to five days, but decreases in enzyme activity in the extensor digitorum longus and increases in enzyme activity in the soleus were seen. In contrast, in the pretreated group all three examined forms of AChE were increased in the diaphragm, especially the A12 form, and the soleus and extensor digitorum longus showed prolonged decreases in all forms, although in the soleus the A12 remained above normal. Thus, the nature, direction, and time-course of changes differ according to the specific enzyme subtype and the muscle, and they depend on prior exposure.

PYRIDOSTIGMINE PHARMACOKINETIC DATA

Table A.1

Pyridostigmine Pharmacokinetic Data

Characteristic	Value	Species	Source
Onset of action after oral administration	30–45 min	Human	McEnvoy, 1991
Onset (time to initial detection in blood)	30 min	Human	Whinnery, 1984
Duration of action after oral administration	3–6 hr	Human	McEnvoy, 1991
Intravenous elimination half-life	30 min	Human ("clinical results")	Lietman, 1993
	97 min	Human	Breyer-Pfaff, 1985
	1.9 hrs		Sidell, 1990, based on Cronnelly, 1980; Breyer-Pfaff, 1985; Kornhauser, 1988
Oral elimination half-life	200 min	Human	Breyer-Pfaff, 1985
	3.7±1.0 hours	Human	Sidell, 1990, based on Cronnelly, 1980; Breyer-Pfaff, 1985; Kornhauser, 1988
	1.78±0.24 hr	Human	Whinnery, 1984, citing *Eur J Clin Pharm*, 423–428, 1980
Bioavailability	7.6±2.4%	Human	Whinnery, 1984
	14%	Human	Breyer-Pfaff, 1985
	29%	Human	Kornhauser, 1988
Mean concentration at which 50% of the red blood cell AChE activity was inhibited (IC50)	31.8 ng/ml	Human	Lietman, 1993

Table A.1—continued

Characteristic	Value	Species	Source
Time to peak plasma concentration, fasting	1.7 hr	Human	Whinnery, 1984
Time to peak plasma level after oral dosing	1.5–2.5 hrs	Human?	Kolka, 1991, citing Aquilonius 1980
Time to peak plasma concentration, with food	3.2 hr	Human	Whinnery, 1984
Plasma clearance	44.62L/hr or 744 ml/min	Human	Lietman, 1993
	0.66±0.22 l/kg[a]hr	Human	Whinnery, 1984
Time at which 95% of the drug is eliminated	8–10 hours	Human	Kolka, 1991, citing Aquilonius 1980
Total clearance	8.5 (SD 8.7) (ml/min/kg)	Human	Sidell, 1990, based on Cronnelly, 1980; Breyer-Pfaff, 1985; Kornhauser, 1988
Volume of distribution	1.1 (SD 0.3) L/kg	Human	Sidell, 1990, based on Cronnelly, 1980; Breyer-Pfaff, 1985; Kornhauser, 1988
Mean rate constant of elimination	1.365/hr	Human	Lietman, 1993
Urinary excretion	80–90% (SD 0.3)		Sidell, 1990, based on Cronnelly, 1980; Breyer-Pfaff, 1985; Kornhauser, 1988

[a]Whinnery: from 5 males given 120 mg PB orally.

Table A.2

Animal Data

Characteristic	Value	Species	Source
Urinary Excretion	90%	rat	Yamamoto, Sawada, et al., 1995
Metabolite, 3-hydroxy-N-methylpyridium, as fraction of excreted dose	1/3	rat	Yamamoto, Sawada, et al., 1995
Plasma elimination half life (iv)	19 min	rat	Yamamoto, Sawada, et al., 1995

Additional information derived from rats:

- No dose dependence in pharmacokinetic behavior in the range of 0.5–2 μmol/kg of PB in rats (Yamamoto, Sawada, et al., 1995).

• Elimination: role of liver and kidneys. Contrary to rapid elimination, high accumulations are found in liver and kidney. Tissue: plasma partition coefficients (Kp) of cholinesterase inhibitors are about eight for liver and 15 for kidney at 20 minutes, suggesting these must be concentratively uphill transported into these tissues like other quaternary ammonium compounds. Though about 50 percent of the dose is distributed into liver and kidney at 20 minutes after intravenous administration, distribution volumes at steady state are relatively small—0.3–0.7 l/kg—larger than the extracellular space and similar to the muscle/plasma concentration ratio. Once in the liver and kidney, PB may not be able to return to plasma compartment; uptake to these tissues may be regarded as an elimination process, and uptake to liver and kidneys may be the major determinant of total body clearance (Yamamoto, Sawada, et al., 1995).

EFFECTS OF PB IN HUMANS

Table B.1

Physiological Findings

Author	Sample Size	Sample/Study Characteristics	Dose	Findings
Wenger, 1993	7	Healthy male soldiers age 22±2.8 Placebo controlled partial-double-blind crossover with 7 d phases after heat acclimation	30 mg q8 hr for 19 doses, or placebo	PB caused a modest increase in whole-body sweating and reduced skin temperature on the chest during exercise by 0.5–0.9° C. Trend toward increased rectal temperature "Near lack of adverse effects"
Wenger, 1992; Wenger, 1992	6	Healthy male soldiers, age 25.6±9.6: test outcomes with heat, exercise, and hypohydration	PB 30 mg tab or placebo	"PB had only minor effects on tolerance to moderate exercise-heat stress and did not aggravate the strain of hypohydration" Rectal temperature: PB reduced rise in Tre but significant only during hypohydration Skin temperature on chest: decreased with exercise at 20% rh, more with PB, significant only in condition 2 Skin temperature on upper arm: no difference? Skin temperature on calf: No difference Heart rate: lowered 3 beats/min (p = .004) PB decreased expansion of plasma volume that occurred during heat exposure: significant only at 75% rh
Roberts, 1994	7	Healthy male		No change in thermoregulation during exercise in cold air
Roach, 1991	30	10 nonsmokers, 10 smokers, and 10 mild asthmatics Double-blind placebo-controlled crossover with PB or placebo before bronchoprovocation	30 mg q8 hr	No effect of PB on nonspecific bronchial hyperreactivity in normals, smokers, or asthmatics

Table B.1—continued

Author	Sample Size	Sample/Study Characteristics	Dose	Findings
Ram, 1991	25	12 healthy and 13 asthmatic	60 mg once	Statistically but not physiologically significant decrease in FEV1 at rest (p < .015) and with exercise (p < .05), strongly correlated to degree of AChE inhibitor (p < .00001)
			30 mg	AChE inhibition: 28% with 60 mg; 23% with 30 mg Pulse: significantly reduced (p < .005) Respiratory function: no change Cannot preclude more vulnerable subpopulation of asthmatics
Arad, 1992	8	Hypertensive patients on beta-blockers Randomized double-blind crossover PB or placebo for 2 days	30 mg tid for 2 days	No clinical adverse effects of PB No significant effect on heart rate, plasma catecholamine level, or resting blood pressure Lower diastolic blood pressure with PB with exercise (average decrease 5 mm Hg versus placebo, p < .01)
Epstein, 1990	8	Male heat-acclimatized volunteers, age 23.5±1.1 Randomized double-blind crossover with subjects exposed to 170 min of exercise heat stress (relative humidity 60%, Tdb 33° C)	30 mg q8 hr for 4 doses versus placebo	Average 33% whole blood cholinesterase inhibition 4 hr after last tablet Higher non-evaporative heat exchange with PB (p < .03) No difference in heart rate, rectal temperature, heat storage, and sweat rate with PB versus placebo
Levine, 1991	10	Healthy male soldiers Counterbalanced drug and control: 2 days tested with drug, 2 with placebo Not stated to be blinded	PB 30 mg tab once, or placebo; test days separated by = 48 hr	No change in pulmonary function tests with PB: FEV1, FVC, maximum voluntary ventilation in 15 seconds, carbon dioxide sensitivity, or maximum inspiratory or expiratory flow rates
Levine, 1991	7	Healthy male soldiers Counterbalanced drug and control: 2 days tested with drug, 2 with placebo Not stated to be blinded	PB 30 mg tab once or placebo test days separated by = 48 hr	No significant change in skeletal muscle strength (peak hand-grip strength and 60% peak hand-grip endurance time, peak torque for leg extension), and muscle tissue damage by serum enzymes

Table B.1—continued

Author	Sample Size	Sample/Study Characteristics	Dose	Findings
Kolka, 1991		Placebo-controlled crossover	PB 30 mg po tid	PB lowers esophageal temperature and HR in hot environment; HR in warm environment
	5	Healthy males age 20±2 tested at rest, 2 hr after PB, and 2 hr p seventh PB tab in hot environment		Reduced resting esophageal temperature and heart rate with PB (p < .05) no change in arterial blood pressure, forearm blood flow and forearm skin blood flow; *74 hr data presented for a mean of only 3 of the 5 subjects because PB was discontinued in 2 due to high red blood cell AChE inhibition
	4	Healthy males age 19.4±0.5 tested (a) control at sea level (b) control at 10,000 feet; (c) 2 hr after first PB at 10,000 feet; (d) 26 hr after first and 2 hr after fourth PB tab; (e) sea level 2 hr after tenth tab Tested in warm environment at sea level and 10,000 feet		Lower esophageal temperature (trend only) at sea level HR lower at sea level 74 hr after PB
Stephenson, 1989; Stephenson, 1990; Kolka, 1990	5 4	Healthy adult males	PB 30 mg po or no drug, 150 min before	40% decrease red blood cell AChE (329%±7) PB decreased skin blood flow; PB decreased heart rate at rest and in exercise Esophageal temperature: increased with exercise only with PB 8-site mean skin temperature Forearm blood flow (venous occlusion plethysmography): no change Cutaneous perfusion (laser doppler velocimetry): reduced 37% after PB (p = .05) with higher temperature threshold for initiation of cutaneous perfusion of PB (p = .01) Slope of LDV: esophageal temperature was reduced 35% with PB (p = 0.22) Metabolic rate (indirect calorimetry)

Table B.2

Performance

Author	Sample Size	Sample/Study Characteristics	Dose	Findings
Arad, 1992	8	Healthy males	30 mg q8 hr for 4 doses	No significant effect of PB, protective gear, or interactions on performance of vertical addition, reaction time, or perceptual speed
Forster, 1994	5	Healthy male members of human centrifuge acceleration pattern; age 26±3; weight 80±4 kg	30 mg q8 hr or placebo	PB level range: 6–31 ng/ml AChE inhibitor range: 12–45% No significant differences in ratings for fatigue, symptoms, and work effort; grip strength; tapping task Sternberg memory search; critical tracking, Dual Sternberg, and tracking pulmonary function tests; Acceleration tolerance; heart rate, QT interval, PR interval
Borland, 1985	4	Healthy male 19-27 years Crossover; double-blind crossover	PB 30 mg q8 hr for 3 days or placebo	"Minimal if any effects" Increased mean critical flicker fusion; impaired visuomotor coordination performance; no changes in mood, mean choice reaction time; grating contrast sensitivity; macular thresholds, digit symbol substitution, symbol copying; quantitative kinetic perimetry, EEG during mental arithmetic
Wiley, 1992	4	Healthy aviators	PB 30 mg q8 hr for 3 days after baseline measurements	Visual ability "not significantly compromised"; refractive error and pupil diameter significantly different, but no change in lateral phoria, fusional vergence, accommodative amplitude with PB

Table B.2—continued

Author	Sample Size	Sample/Study Characteristics	Dose	Findings
Izraeli, 1990	10	Pilots experienced in actual and simulated A-4 flights Double-blind placebo-controlled crossover	PB 30 mg q8 hr	No decrement in performance under treatment with PB
Brooks, 1992	24	A-10 pilots Crossover counterbalanced double-blind trial of performance with PB versus placebo	PB 30 mg tid versus placebo	No operationally significant effects of PB. No clear interference of PB with performance

Table B.3
Side Effects

Author	Sample Size	Sample/Study Characteristics	Dose	Findings
Sharabi, Danon, et al., 1991	213	Male Israeli soldiers 18–22, retro-spective cohort	30 mg q3 hr	No correlation between AChE inhibition and type or severity of symptoms Malaise: 53% Fatigue, numbness: 37% Headache: 29% Dizziness, imbalance: 19% Moodiness: 18% Restlessness: 18% Heavy extremities: 10% Excessive sweating: 9% Altered mood: 8% Sense of fear: 6% GI: Dry mouth: 71% Nausea: 22% Abdominal pain: 20% Lack of appetite: 14% Diarrhea: 6% Other: Hot flushes: 20% Rhinorrhea: 10% Rapid heart beats: 8% Frequent urination: 11%
Keeler, 1991	"Approx-imately 30"	Retrospective survey of proxy recollection by medical support personnel involved with 41,650 soldiers in PGW	30 mg q3 hr	GI symptoms: 50% Urinary: 5–30% Headache, rhinorrhea, diaphoresis, tingling of extremities: < 5% Need for medical visit: 1% Discontinuation on medical advice: < 0.1%

Table B.3—continued

Author	Sample Size	Sample/Study Characteristics	Dose	Findings
Kennedy, 1991	1	Case report of PGW medical officer (letter to editor)	30 mg q8 hr	Esophageal spasm with chest pain and trouble swallowing. Reports of others' abdominal and skeletal muscle cramps, increased bowel gas, blurred vision, and one claim of a 36-hour erection
Almog, 1991	9	Observational report of 9 cases of PB overdose	13 to 39 PB tabs	Muscarinic: abdominal cramps, diarrhea, nausea, vomiting, salivation, urinary incontinence (lacrimation and sweating not prominent) Nicotinic symptoms: transient fasciculations and muscle weakness Central symptoms: (not seen: ataxia, confusion, psychosis, respiratory or cardiovascular depression, seizure, coma) No relation between symptoms and AChE inhibition; major symptoms resolved in several hours while cholinesterase returned to normal in 1–2 days

FURTHER DISCUSSION OF THE
ACETYLCHOLINE-SEROTONIN RELATIONSHIP

PB, in addition to affecting the cholinergic system by inhibiting acetyl-cholinesterase (AChE), exerts an effect by directly binding to a site on the acetylcholine (ACh) receptor, distinct from the site that binds ACh itself (Albuquerque, Alkondon, et al., 1997; Albuquerque, Pereira, et al., 1997). It is believed that the "endogenous ligand" for this site—that is, the substance that "normally" binds here to exert an effect—is serotonin, so that PB is mimicking serotonin in this role (Albuquerque, Alkondon, et al., 1997; Albuquerque, Pereira, et al., 1997). Whether consequences of serotonergic dysregulation might ensue is not known. Other evidence exists to connect the serotonin and acetylcholine systems.

Carbamates related to PB (namely, physostigmine) have been shown to simul-taneously increase platelet counts and reduce the maximum velocity of platelet serotonin uptake in humans (without changing the affinity constant for platelet serotonin uptake) (Rausch, Shah, et al., 1982; Rausch, Janowsky, et al., 1985). Platelet serotonin is often used as a marker of central serotonin function at the synapse (Rausch, Janowsky, et al., 1985; Rotman, 1983; Sneddon, 1973), though the effects may not correspond exactly. Because depression and pain are asso-ciated both with low serotonin and with high ACh function (indeed, depressive effect can occur quickly after administration of drugs like physostigmine (Rausch, Janowsky, et al., 1985) and nerve agents), it is speculated that platelet serotonin uptake may be reduced in depressed patients by cholinergic mech-anisms (Rausch, Shah, et al., 1982; Rausch, Janowsky, et al., 1985). Reduced platelet serotonin uptake with physostigmine is similar to the reduced platelet serotonin uptake reported in drug-free depressed patients in several studies (Tuomisto, Tukiainen, and Ahlfors, 1979; Scott, Reading, and Louden, 1979; Meltzer, Arora, et al., 1981; Coppen, Swade, and Wood, 1978; Rausch, Janowsky, et al., 1985).

It has also been noted, in this vein, that cholinergic receptors control serotonin release in hypothalamic slices of rat brain; and that striatal cholinergic interneurons are modulated via serotonergic projections from the raphe (Rausch, Shah, et al., 1982; Vizi, Harsing, and Zsilla, 1981; Hery, Burgoin, et al., 1977).

Both serotonin and physostigmine have been reported to inhibit cell membrane AChE activity (Rausch, Janowsky, et al., 1985).

Cholinergic agonists have been shown to cause a release of serotonin in canine platelets, an effect blocked by muscarinic antagonists (Rausch, Janowsky, et al., 1985).

Serotonin nerve endings in rat brain are sensitive to cholinergic stimulation (Hery, Burgoin, et al., 1977; Rausch, Janowsky, et al., 1985).

Physostigmine can inhibit serotonin uptake in hypothalamic synaptosomes and can increase extracellular serotonin in rat cortex and hypothalamic slices (Aiello-Malmberg, Bartolini, et al., 1979; Hery, Burgoin, et al., 1977; Rausch, Janowsky, et al., 1985) probably through the special ACh receptor, since this effect does not arise from the anticholinesterase effect (Aiello-Malmberg, Bartolini, et al., 1979) but does appear to be via nicotinic cholinergic stimulation (Westfall, Grant, and Perry, 1983; Hery, Burgoin, et al., 1977; Rausch, Janowsky, et al., 1985).

Brain serotonin turnover is increased following administration of cholinesterase inhibitors, including carbamates (physostigmine) as well as organophosphates (OPs) (including soman) (Prioux-Guyonneau, Coudray-Lucas, et al., 1982; Pscheidt, Votava, and Himwich, 1967; Kleinrok, Jagiello-Wojtowicz, and Sieklucka, 1975; Haubrich and Reid, 1972; Rausch, Janowsky, et al., 1985). These effects differed in different parts of the brain, being strongest in the striatum, present in most areas of the brain, but absent in the hypothalamus in one study (Prioux-Guyonneau, Coudray-Lucas, et al., 1982).

Increased levels of serotonin may be seen with some AChE-inhibiting agents, e.g., soman, but not with others, e.g., DFP. These levels return to normal before restoration of AChE activity, while the serotonin turnover, gauged by levels of the serotonin metabolite 5-HIAA, remains high (Prioux-Guyonneau, coudray-Lucas, et al., 1982). There is no proportional relationship between increased turnover and either AChE activity or ACh levels—the serotonin effect continues after ACh levels are expected to have returned to normal (though AChE remains inhibited), and continues to increase while AChE inhibition remains constant or is decreasing (Prioux-Guyonneau, Coudray-Lucas, et al., 1982). Although this effect has been termed "long-lasting," effects were only evaluated up to 24 hours after administration of soman or paraoxon.

AChE inhibitors (namely the OP insecticide parathion) have been shown to enhance the nighttime rise in serotonin "N-acetyltransferase" in the pineal gland, an area involved in production of melatonin and regulation of sleep, and have been shown to increase nighttime serum melatonin levels (Attia, Mostafa, et al., 1995a). This effect is blocked by ß adrenergic blockers and has been speculated to occur at the level of the ß adrenergic receptor or via sympathetic innervation to the pineal gland (Attia, Mostafa, et al., 1995b).

The selective serotonin 1D receptor agonist, sumatriptan (used clinically to abort migraine headaches), has been shown to increase growth hormone (a pituitary hormone) released in response to growth hormone releasing hormone (a hypothalamic hormone)—the same effect that PB has on growth hormone. It has been postulated that this may occur by inhibition of hypothalamic somatostatin release—the same mechanism by which PB is thought to influence growth hormone release (see Chapter Fifteen, "Other Effects," section on hormones (Mota, Bento, et al., 1995). It is tempting to speculate on the relation or possible equivalence between the 5HT1D (serotonin 1D) receptor and the specialized receptor on ACh to which PB and serotonin bind. (No information related to this has been uncovered in the present literature review.)

The serotonin-3 antagonist ondansetron did not produce inhibition of AChE by itself when given to guinea pigs (a common animal model for the benefit of PB versus nerve agent); however ondansetron (10 or 20 mg/kg) added to PB increased the inhibition of AChE produced by PB alone (0.94 mg/kg given orally) at all times evaluated, from 30 to 240 minutes (Capacio, Byers, et al., 1993; Capacio, Koplovitz, et al., 1996). (The increases averaged 12 percent (range 10–17 percent) for 10 mg/kg and 16 percent (14–20 percent) for 20 mg/kg of ondansetron; moreover, the slope of recovery of AChE function was slowed when ondansetron was given.

Non–peer reviewed reports circulating on the Internet state that treatment with a combination of the serotonergic agent fenfluramine (now pulled from the market because of adverse effects) and the adrenergic agent phentermine, a drug combination formerly popular in the treatment of obesity, produced 50–100 percent benefit in symptoms in ill PGW veterans as well as in other individuals with symptoms of fibromyalgia (Hitzig, 1997). These were open label trials and this work has in no way been subjected to peer review.

Abdulla, F. A., E. Bradbury, et al., "Relationship Between Up-Regulation of Nicotine Binding Sites in Rat Brain and Delayed Cognitive Enhancement Observed After Chronic or Acute Nicotinic Receptor Simulation," *Psychopharmacol*, 124(4), 1996, pp. 323–331.

Abou-Donia, M., "Metabolism and Toxicokinetics of Xenobiotics," in Derelanko and Hollinger, eds., *CRC Practical Handbook of Toxicology*, Boca Raton, Fla.: CRC Press, 1995, pp. 282–289.

Abou-Donia, M., "Organophosphorus-Induced Delayed Neurotoxicity," *Ann Rev Pharmacol Toxicol*, 21, 1981, pp. 511–548.

Abou-Donia, M., personal communication, 1998.

Abou-Donia, M., and D. M. Lapadula, "Mechanisms of Organophosphorus Ester-Induced Delayed Neurotoxicity: Type I and Type II," *Ann Rev Pharmacol Toxicol*, 30, 1990, pp. 405–440.

Abou-Donia, M., and S. Preissig, "Delayed Neurotoxicity from Continuous Low-Dose Oral Administration of Leptophos in Hens," *Toxicol Appl Pharmacol*, 38, 1976, pp. 595–608.

Abou-Donia, M. B., A. A. Abdel-Rahman, et al., "Stress with Exposure to Pyridostigmine Bromide (PB), DEET, and Permethrin Increases Rat Blood-Brain Barrier (BBB) Permeability," *FASEB Journal*, 11(3), 1997, Abstract 3617.

Abou-Donia, M., K. Wilmarth, et al., "Increased Neurotoxicity Following Concurrent Exposure to Pyridostigmine Bromide (PB), Deet, and Chlorpyrifos," *Fundam Appl Toxicol*, 34, 1996a, pp. 201–222.

Abou-Donia, M., K. Wilmarth, et al., "Neurotoxicity Resulting from Coexposure to Pyridostigmine Bromide, DEET, and Permethrin: Implications of Gulf War Chemical Exposures," *J of Toxicol and Environmental Health*, 48, 1996b, pp. 35–56.

Abou-Donia, M., K. Wilmarth, et al., "Increased Neurotoxicity Following Simultaneous Exposure to Pyridostigmine Bromide (PB), Deet, and Chlorpyrifos,"

Joint Meeting of the American Society for Biochemistry and Molecular Biology, American Society for Investigative Pathology, and the American Association of Immunologists, *FASEB Journal*, 1996c.

Adler, M., D. Hinman, et al., "Role of Muscle Fasciculations in the Generation of Myopathies in Mammalian Skeletal Muscle," *Brain Research Bulletin*, 29, 1992, pp. 179–187.

Adler, M., D. Maxwell, et al., *In Vivo and in Vitro Pathophysiology of Mammalian Skeletal Muscle Following Acute and Subacute Exposure to Pyridostigmine. Studies on Muscle Contractility and Cellular Mechanisms*, Aberdeen Proving Ground, Md.: 4th Annual Chemical Defense Bioscience Review, 1984.

Adler, S., M. Lam, et al., *A Pocket Manual of Differential Diagnosis*, Boston: Little Brown and Company, 1994.

Agnati, L., M. Zoli, et al., "Intercellular Communication in the Brain: Wiring Versus Volume Transmission," *Neuroscience*, 69, 1995, p. 711.

Agnoli, A., N. Martucci, et al., "Effect of Cholinergic and Anticholinergic Drugs on Short Term Memory in Alzheimer's Dementia: A Neuropsychological and Computerized Electroencephalographic Study," *Clin Neuropharmacol*, 6, 1983, pp. 311–323.

Aiello-Malmberg, P., A. Bartolini, et al., "Effects of Morphine, Physostigmine and Raphe Nuclei Stimulation on 5-Hydroxytryptamine Release from the Cerebral Cortex of the Cat," *Brit J Pharmacol*, 65(4), 1979, pp. 547–555.

Akaike, A., S. Ikeda, et al., "The Nature of the Interactions of Pyridostigmine with the Nicotinic Acetylcholine Receptor-Ionic Channel Complex II. Patch Clamp Studies," *Mol Pharmacol*, 25, 1984, pp. 102–112.

Akiyama, N., K. Okumura, et al., "Altered Acetylcholine and Norepinephrine Concentrations in Diabetic Rat Hearts. Role of Parasympathetic Nervous System in Diabetic Cardiomyopathy," *Diabetes*, 38, 1989, pp. 231–236.

Albright, J., and R. Goldstein, "Is There Evidence of an Immunologic Basis for Multiple Chemical Sensitivity," *Toxicol Ind Health*, 8, 1992, pp. 215–219.

Albuquerque, E., "The Molecular Targets of Selected Organophosphorus Compounds at Nicotinic, Muscarinic, GABA, and Glutamate Synapses: Acute and Chronic Studies Including Prophylactic and Therapeutic Approaches," Fort Detrick, Md.: U.S. Army Medical Research and Development Command, 1985.

Albuquerque, E., M. Alkondon, et al., "Properties of Neuronal Nicotinic Acetylcholine Receptors: Pharmacological Characterization and Modulation of Synaptic Function," *J Pharmacol Exp Therapeutics*, 280(1-3), 1997, pp. 1117–1136.

Albuquerque, E., A. Boyne, et al., "Molecular and Behavioral Studies of Anti-cholinesterase Agents on Various Receptor Targets in the Peripheral and Central Nervous System: Acute and Chronic Studies Using Biophysical, Biochemical, Histological and Therapeutic Approaches," Fort Detrick, Md.: U.S. Army Medical Research and Development Command. Contract DAMD17-81-C-1279, 1983.

Albuquerque, E., A. Boyne, et al., "The Molecular Targets of Selected Organophosphorus Compounds at Nicotinic, Muscarinic, GABA, and Gluta-mate Synapses: Acute and Chronic Studies Using Biophysical, Biochemical, Histological and Therapeutic Approaches," Fort Detrick, Md.: U.S. Army Medical Research and Development Command, annual report, Contract DAMD17-81-C-1279, 1995.

Albuquerque, E., A. Costa, et al., "Functional Properties of the Nicotinic and Glutamatergic Receptors," J of Receptor Research, 11, 1991, pp. 1–4.

Albuquerque, E., S. Deshpande, et al., "Multiple Actions of Anticholinesterase Agents on Chemosensitive Synapses: Molecular Basis for Prophylaxis and Treatment of Organophosphate Poisoning," Fundam Appl Toxicol, 5, 1985, S182–S203.

Albuquerque, E., E. Pereira, et al., "Nicotinic Receptor Function in the Mammalian Central Nervous System," Ann NY Acad Sci, 757, 1995, pp. 48–72.

Albuquerque, E., E. Pereira, et al., "Nicotinic Acetylcholine Receptors on Hippocampal Neurons: Distribution on the Neuronal Surface and Modulation of Receptor Activity," J of Receptor and Signal Transduction Research, 17(1-3), 1997, pp. 243–266.

Alisoglu, R., J. Nagelhout, et al., "Reversal of Pipecuronium Bromide with Pyridostigmine," Clinical Forum for Nurse Anesthetists, 6(1), 1995, pp. 43–45.

al-Jafari, A. A., and M. A. Kamal, "The Preparation and Kinetic Analysis of Multiple Forms of Chicken Brain Acetylcholinesterase," Cell Biochem Funct, 12(1), 1994, pp. 29–35.

Alkondon, M., and E. Albuquerque, "Diversity of Nicotinic Acetylcholine Receptors in Rat Hippocampal Neurons. I. Pharmacological and Functional Evidence for Distinct Structural Subtypes," J Pharmacol Exp Therapeutics, 265(3), 1993, pp. 1455–1473.

Alkondon, M., E. Rocha, et al., "Diversity of Nicotinic Acetylcholine Receptors in Rat Brain V. Alpha Bungarotoxin-Sensitive Nicotinic Receptors in Olfactory Bulb Neurons and Presynaptic Modulation of Glutamate Release," J Pharmacol Exp Therapeutics, 278, 1996, pp. 1460–1471.

Allan, W., "Bromism and Iodism in Gulf War and Other Illness," Internet report, www.teleport.com, accessed 1997.

Allen, C., and E. Albuquerque, "Conductance Properties of GABA-Activated Chloride Currents Recorded from Cultured Hippocampal Neurons," *Brain Res,* 410, 1987, pp. 159–163.

Alles, G., and R. Hawes, "Cholinesterases in the Blood of Man," *J Biol Chem,* 133, 1940, p. 375.

Almog, S., E. Winkler, et al., "Acute Pyridostigmine Overdose: A Report of Nine Cases," *Isr J Med Sci,* 27, 1991, pp. 659–663.

Altland, K., H. Goedde, et al., "New Biochemical and Immunological Data on Quantitative and Qualitative Variability of Human Pseudocholinesterase," *Humangenetik,* 14, 1971, pp. 56–60.

Amato, A., A. McVey, et al., "Evaluation of Neuromuscular Symptoms in Veterans of the Persian Gulf War," *Neurology,* 48, 1997, pp. 4–12.

American Hospital Formulary Service, "Pyridostigmine Bromide," in G. McEvoy, ed., *AHFS Drug Information,* Bethesda, Md.: American Society of Hospital Pharmacists, Inc., 1991, pp. 680–682.

Ames, R., K. Steenland, et al., "Chronic Neurologic Sequelae to Cholinesterase Inhibition Among Agricultural Pesticide Applicators," *Archives of Environmental Health,* 50(6), 1995, pp. 440–444.

Amr, M., M. Allam, et al., "Neurobehavioral Changes Among Workers in Some Chemical Industries in Egypt," *Environ Res,* 63, 1993, pp. 295–300.

Anderson, D., L. Harris, et al., "The Effect of Pyridostigmine Pretreatment on Oxime Efficacy Against Intoxication by Soman or VX in Rats," *Drug Chem Toxicol,* 15, 1992, pp. 285–294.

Anderson, R., W. Chamberlain, et al., "Decreased Tetanic Contracture of Rat Skeletal Muscle Induced by Pyridostigmine," *J Toxicol Environ Health,* 18, 1986, pp. 221–230.

Andres, C., R. Beeri, et al., "Cholinergic Drug Resistance and Impaired Learning in Transgenic Mice Overexpressing Brain Acetylcholinesterase," section in unclassified document, "Studies on the Molecular Dissection of the Human Cholinesterase Variants and their Genomic Origins," Jerusalem, Israel: Hebrew University, 1996.

Andres, C., R. Beeri, et al., "Cholinergic Drug Resistance and Impaired Spatial Learning in Transgenic Mice Overexpressing Human Brain Acetylcholinesterase," *Prog Brain Res,* 109, 1996, pp. 265–272.

Andres, C., et al., "Acetylcholinesterase-Transgenic Mice Display Embryonic Modulations in Spinal Cord Choline Acetyltransferase and Neurexin Ibeta Gene Expression Followed by Late-Onset Neuromotor Deterioration," *Proc Natl Acad Sci USA,* 94, 1997, pp. 8173–8178.

Antelman, S., "Time-Dependent Sensitization as the Cornerstone for a New Approach to Pharmacotherapy: Drugs as Foreign/Stressful Stimuli," *Drug Devel Res,* 14, 1988, pp. 1–30.

Antelman, S., A. Eichler, et al., "Interchangeability of Stress and Amphetamine in Sensitization," *Science,* 207, 1980, pp. 329–331.

Antelman, S., D. Kocan, et al., "One Brief Exposure to a Psychological Stressor Induces Long-Lasting, Time-Dependent Sensitization of Both the Cataleptic and Neurochemical Responses to Haloperidol," *Life Sci,* 51, 1992, pp. 261–266.

Antelman, S., S. Knopf, et al., "One Stressful Event Blocks Multiple Actions of Diazepam for at Least a Month," *Brain Res,* 445, 1988, pp. 380–385.

Antonini, G., S. Morino, et al., "Myasthenia Gravis in the Elderly: A Hospital Based Study," *Acta Neurol Scand,* 93, 1996, pp. 260–262.

Aquilonius, S., S. Eckernas, et al., "A Pharmacokinetic Study of Neostigmine in Man Using Gas Chromatography-Mass Spectrometry," *Eur J Clin Pharmacol,* 15(5), 1979, pp. 367–371.

Aquilonius, S., S. Eckernas, et al., "Pharmacokinetics and Oral Bioavailability of Pyridostigmine in Man," *Eur J Clin Pharmacol,* 18, 1980, pp. 428–432.

Aracava, Y., S. Deshpande, et al., "The Molecular Basis of Anticholinesterase Actions," *Ann NY Acad Sci,* 505, 1987, pp. 226–255.

Arad, M., A. Roth, et al., "Safety of Pyridostigmine in Hypertensive Patients Receiving Beta Blockers," *The Am J Cardiology,* 69, 1992, pp. 518–522.

Arad, M., R. Arnon, et al., "Effects of Heat-Exercise Stress, NBC Clothing, and Pyridostigmine Treatment on Psychomotor and Subjective Measures of Performance," *Military Medicine,* 157, 1992, pp. 210–214.

Araneta, M. R. G., C. A. Moore, et al., "Goldenhar Syndrome Among Infants Born in Military Hospitals to Gulf War Veterans," *Teratology,* 56, 1997, pp. 244–251.

Arendash, G. W., P. R. Sanberg, and G. J. Sengstock, "Nicotine Enhances the Learning and Memory of Aged Rats," *Pharmacol Biochem Behav,* 52(3), 1995, pp. 517–523.

Arendash, G. W., G. J. Sengstock, et al., "Improved Learning and Memory in Aged Rats with Chronic Administration of the Nicotinic Receptor Agonist GTS-21," *Brain Res,* 674(2), 1995, pp. 252–259.

Ariens, A., E. Meeter, et al., "Reversible Necrosis at the End-Plate Region in Striated Muscle of the Rat Poisoned with Cholinesterase Inhibitors," *Experientia,* 25, 1969, pp. 57–59.

Arvat, E., L. Gianotti, et al., "The Enhancing Effect of Pyridostigmine on the GH Response to GHRH Undergoes an Accelerated Age-Related Reduction in Down Syndrome," *Dementia*, 7, 1996, pp. 288–292.

Åsberg, M., "Monoamine Neurotransmitters in Human Aggressiveness and Violence: A Selective Review," *Criminal Behaviour and Mental Health*, 4, 1994, pp. 303–327.

Attia, A. M. M. H. Mostafa, et al., "Changes in Nocturnal Pineal Indoleamine Metabolism in Rats Treated with Parthion Are Prevented by Beta-Adrenergic Antagonist Administration," Toxicol, 97(1-3), 1995a, pp. 183–189.

Attia, A. M., M. H. Mostafa, et al., "Night-Time Rise in Rat Pineal N-Acetyltransferase Due to Carbaryl Administration is Reduced by Propranolol Treatment," *Biomed and Environ Sci*, 8(1), 1995b, pp. 45–53.

Augerson, W., "Chemical Casualty Treatment Protocol Development. Phase I: Treatment Approaches. Chapter 5: Nerve Agents," final report to Aerospace Medical Division, Air Force Systems Command, USAF, Arthur D. Little, Inc., 1986.

Augerson, W., *A Review of the Scientific Literature As It Pertains to Gulf War Illnesses*, Vol. 5: *Chemical and Biological Warfare Agents*, Santa Monica, Calif.: RAND, MR-1018/5, forthcoming.

Avlonitou, E., and R. Elizondo, "Effects of Atropine and Pyridostigmine in Heat-Stressed Patas Monkeys," *Aviat Space Environ Med*, 59, 1988, pp. 544–548.

Axelrod, B. N., and I. B. Milner, "Neuropsychological Findings in a Sample of Operation Desert Storm Veterans," *J Neuropsychiatry Clin Neurosci*, 9(1), 1997, pp. 23–28.

Bagchi, D., G. Bhattacharya, et al., "In Vitro and in Vivo Induction of Heat Shock (Stress) Protein (Hsp) Gene Expression by Selected Pesticides," *Toxicology*, 112, 1996, pp. 57–68.

Bajgar, J., "Biological Monitoring of Exposure to Nerve Agents," *Brit J Industrial Medicine*, 49, 1992, pp. 648–653.

Baker, D., and E. Sedgwick, "Single Fibre Electromyographic Changes in Man After Organophosphate Exposure," *Hum & Exp Toxicol*, 15(5), 1996, pp. 369–375.

Baker, E., "Organic Solvent Neurotoxicity," *Ann Rev Public Health*, 9, 1988, pp. 223–232.

Baldinger, S. L., and D. J. Schroeder, Nicotine Therapy in Patients with Alzheimer's Disease, *Ann Pharmacother*, 29(3), 1995, pp. 314–315.

Barnes, J., and F. Denz, "Experimental Demyelination with Organophosphorus Compounds," *J Pathol Bacteriol*, 65, 1974, pp. 597–606.

Banks, W., and A. Kastin, "Aluminium Increases Permeability of the Blood-Brain Barrier to Labeled DSIP and Beta-Endorphin: Possible Implications for Senile and Dialysis Dementia," *Lancet*, 2, 1983, pp. 1237–1239.

Bannon, A. W., K. L. Gunther, et al., "Is Epibatidine Really Analgesic? Dissociation of the Activity, Temperature, and Analgesic Effects of (+/-)-Epibatidine," *Pharmacol Biochem Behav*, 51(4), 1995, pp. 693–698.

Barkai, E., and M. H. Hasselmo, "Acetylcholine and Associative Memory in the Piriform Cortex," *Mol Neurobiol*, 15(1), 1997, pp. 17–29.

Barker, W. W., D. Loewenstein, et al., "Effects of Physostigmine on Cerebral Glucose Metabolism (CMRglc) Measured by 18FDG/PET Studies in Normals," *Soc Neurosci Abstr*, 13, 1987, p. 1716.

Barlocco, D., G. Cignarella, et al., "Mono- and Disubstituted-3,8-Diazabicyclo[3.2.1]Octane Derivatives as Analgesics Structurally Related to Epibatidine: Synthesis, Activity, and Modeling," *J Med Chem*, 41(5), 1998, pp. 674–681.

Barnaby, F., "Iran-Iraq War: The Use of Chemical Weapons Against the Kurds," *Ambio*, 17(6), 1985, pp. 407–408.

Barnes, J., and F. Denz, "The Reaction of Rats to Diets Containing Octamethyl Pyrophosphoramide (Schradan) and O,O Diethyl-S-Ethyl-Mercaptoethanol Thiophosphate (Systox)," *Brit J Ind Med*, 11, 1954, pp. 11–19.

Baron, J. A., "Beneficial Effects of Nicotine and Cigarette Smoking: The Real, the Possible and the Spurious," *Br Med Bull*, 52(1), 1996, pp. 58–73.

Baron, R., "Delayed Neurotoxicity and Other Consequences of Organophosphate Esters," *Ann Rev Entomol*, 26, 1981, pp. 29–48.

Barrett, D., and F. Oehme, "A Review of Organophosphorus-Induced Delayed Neurotoxicity," *Vet Hum Toxicol*, 27, 1985, pp. 22–37.

Bartels, C. F., F. S. Jensen, et al., "DNA Mutation Associated with the Human Butyrylcholinesterase K-Variant and Its Linkage to the Atypical Variant Mutation and Other Polymorphic Sites," *Am J Hum Genet*, 50, 1992, pp. 1086–1103.

Bascom, R., "Multiple Chemical Sensitivity: A Respiratory Disorder?" *Toxicol Ind Health*, 8, 1992, pp. 221–228.

Bassant, M. H., F. Jazat, and Y. Lamour, "Tetrahydroaminoacridine and Physostigmine Increase Cerebral Glucose Utilization in Specific Cortical and Subcortical Regions in the Rat," *J Cereb Blood Flow and Metab*, 13(5), 1995, pp. 855–864.

Battin, D., and T. Varkey, "Neuropsychiatric Manifestations of Bromide Ingestion," *Postgraduate Medical Journal,* 58, 1982, pp. 523–524.

Baumsweiger, W., personal communication, 1998.

Baynes, R. E., K. B. Halling, et al., "The Influence of Diethyl-m-Toluamide (DEET) on the Percutaneous Absorption of Permethrin and Carbaryl," *Toxicol Appl Pharmacol,* 144(2), 1997, pp. 332–339.

Beach, J., A. Spurgeon, et al., "Abnormalities on Neurological Examination Among Sheep Farmers Exposed to Organophosphorous Pesticides," *Occup Environ Med,* 53, 1996, pp. 520–525.

Beale, P., "Gulf Illness," *BMJ,* 308(6943), 1994, p. 1594.

Beatty, W., N. Butters, et al., "Patterns of Memory Failure After Scopolamine Treatment: Implications for Cholinergic Hypotheses of Dementia," *Behav Neural Biol,* 45, 1986, pp. 196–211.

Beekman, R., J. B. Kuks, et al., "Myasthenia Gravis: Diagnosis and Follow-Up of 100 Consecutive Patients," *J Neurol,* 244(2), 1997, pp. 112–118.

Beeri, R., A. Gnatt, et al., "Testicular Amplification and Impaired Transmission of Human Butyrylcholinesterase cDNA in Transgenic Mice," *Human Reproduction,* 9(2), 1994, pp. 284–292.

Beeri, R., et al., "Transgenic Expression of Human Acetylcholinesterase Induces Progressive Cognitive Deterioration in Mice," *Curr Biol,* 5(2), 1995, pp. 1063–1071.

Bell, I., C. Miller, et al., "An Olfactory-Limbic Model of Multiple Chemical Sensitivity Syndrome: Possible Relationships to Kindling and Affective Spectrum Disorders," *Biol Psychiatry,* 32, 1992, pp. 218–242.

Bell, I., G. Schwartz, et al., "Self-Reported Illness from Chemical Odors in Young Adults Without Clinical Syndromes or Occupational Exposures," *Archives of Environmental Health,* 48(1), 1993a, pp. 6–13.

Bell, I., G. Schwartz, et al., "Symptom and Personality Profiles of Young Adults from a College Student Population with Self-Reported Illness from Foods and Chemicals," *J Am Coll Nutrition,* 12(6), 1993b, pp. 693–702.

Bell, I., G. Schwartz, et al., "Sensitization to Early Life Stress and Response to Chemical Odors in Older Adults," *Biol Psychiatry,* 35, 1994, pp. 857–863.

Belova, I., and G. Jonsson, "Blood-Brain Barrier Permeability and Immobilization Stress," *Acta Physiol Scand,* 116, 1982, pp. 21–29.

Ben-Nathan, D., S. Lustig, et al., "Stress-Induced Neuroinvasiveness of a Neurovirulent Noninvasive Sindbis Virus in Cold or Isolation Subjected Mice," *Life Sci,* 48, 1991, pp. 1493–1500.

Bennett, R., "Fibromyalgia: The Commonest Cause of Widespread Pain," *Comprehensive Therapy*, 21(6), 1995, pp. 269–275.

Benowitz, N. L., "Pharmacology of Nicotine: Addiction and Therapeutics," *Ann Rev Pharmacol Toxicol*, 36, 1996, pp. 597–613.

Benwell, M., D. Balfour, et al., "Evidence That Tobacco Smoking Increases the Density of (-)-[3H]nicotine Binding Sites in Human Brain," *J Neurochemistry*, 50, 1988, pp. 1243–1247.

Berenbaum, M., "The Expected Effect of a Combination of Agents: The General Solution," *J Theoretical Biology*, 114, 1985, pp. 413–431.

Berezuk, G., and G. McCarty, "Investigational Drugs and Vaccines Fielded in Support of Operation Desert Storm," *Milit Med*, 157, 1992, pp. 404–406.

Berglund, M., S. Nielsen, et al., "Regional Cerebral Blood Flow in a Case of Bromide Psychosis," *Arch Psychiat Nervenkr*, 223, 1977, pp. 197–201.

Berkowitz, A., L. Sutton, et al., "Pilocarpine, an Orally Active Muscarinic Cholinergic Agonist, Induces REM Sleep and Reduces Delta Sleep in Normal Volunteers," *Psychiatry Res*, 33, 1990, pp. 113–119.

Berman, P., and J. Patrick, "Experimental Myasthenia Gravis," *J Exp Med*, 151, 1980, pp. 204–223.

Berry, W., and D. Davies, "The Use of Carbamates and Atropine in the Protection of Animals Against Poisoning by 1.2.1-Trimethylpropylmethyl Phosphonofluoridate," *Biochem Pharmacol*, 19(1), 1970, pp. 927–934.

Birchall, J., and J. Chappell, "Aluminium, Chemical Physiology, and Alzheimer's Disease," *Lancet*, 2, 1988, pp. 1008–1010.

Birtley, R., J. Toberts, et al., "Excretion and Metabolism of (14C)-Pyridostigmine in the Rat," *Br J Pharmacol*, 26, 1966, pp. 393–402.

Birtwistle, J., "Quitting Smoking Could Increase Your Risk of Surgery for Ulcerative Colitis," *Br J Theatre Nurs*, 5(6), 1995, pp. 27–28.

Birtwistle, J., "The Role of Cigarettes and Nicotine in the Onset and Treatment of Ulcerative Colitis," *Postgrad Med J*, 72(854), 1996, pp. 714–718.

Bishop, C., *Neural Networks for Pattern Recognition*, Oxford, England: Oxford University Press, 1995.

Blackhall, M., G. Buckley, et al., "Drug-Induced Neonatal Myasthenia," *J Obstet Gynaec Brit Cwlth*, 76, 1969, pp. 157–162.

Blake, P., R. Gleadle, et al., "Evaluation of Pyridostigmine Bromide as a Pretreatment for Nerve Agent Poisoning (External Studies)," Porton Down, U.K.: Chemical Defence Establishment, 1985.

Blick, D., S. Kerenyi, et al., "Behavioral Toxicity of Anticholinesterases in Primates: Chronic Pyridostigmine and Soman Interactions," *Pharmacol Biochem Behav,* 38, 1991, pp. 527–532.

Blick, D. W., M. R. Murphy, et al., "Acute Behavioral Toxicity of Pyridostigmine or Soman in Primates," *Toxicol and Appl Pharmacol,* 126, 1994, pp. 311–318.

Blick, D., M. Murphy, et al., "Effects of Carbamate Pretreatment and Oxime Therapy on Soman-Induced Performance Decrements and Blood Cholinesterase Activity in Primates," *Soc Neurosci Abstr,* 13, 1987, p. 1716.

Blick, D. W., F. Weathersby, et al., "Behavioral Toxicity of Anticholinesterases in Primates: Effects of Daily Repeated Soman Exposure," *Pharmacology Biochemistry and Behavior,* 48(3), 1994, pp. 643–649.

Blin, J., P. Mazetti, et al., "Does the Enhancement of Cholinergic Neurotransmission Influence Brain Glucose Kinetics and Clinical Symptomatology in Progressive Supranuclear Palsy?" *Brain,* 118(Pt 6), 1995, pp. 1485–1495.

Blomquist, L., and W. Thorsell, "Distribution and Fate of the Insect Repellent 14C-*N,N*-Diethyl-*m*-Toluamide in the Animal Body. II. Distribution and Excretion After Cutaneous Application," *Acta Pharmacol Toxicol,* 41, 1977, pp. 235–243.

Blumberg, A., and W. Nelp, "Total Body Bromide Excretion in a Case of Prolonged Bromide Intoxication," *Helvetica Medica Acta,* 1966, pp. 330–333.

Bokina, A., N. Eksler, et al., "Investigation of the Mechanism of Action of Atmospheric Pollutants on the Central Nervous System and Comparative Evaluation of Methods of Study," *Environ Health Prospect,* 13, 1976, pp. 37–42.

Bombinski, T., and K. DuBois, "Toxicity and Mechanism of Action of Disyston," *AMA Arch Ind Health,* 17, 1958, pp. 192–199.

Bonapace, C. R., and D. A. Mays, "The Effect of Mesalamine and Nicotine in the Treatment of Inflammatory Bowel Disease," *Ann Pharmacother,* 31(7-8), 1997, pp. 907–913.

Borges, M., R. Castro, et al., "Different Effects of Pyridostigmine on Growth Hormone (GH) Response to GH-Releasing Hormone in Endogenous and Exogenous Hypercortisolemic Patients," *Brazilian J Med Biol Res,* 26, 1993, pp. 1191–1200.

Borland, R., D. Brennan, et al., "Studies on the Possible Central and Peripheral Effects in Man of a Cholinesterase Inhibitor (Pyridostigmine)," *Hum Toxicol,* 4, 1985, pp. 293–300.

Bowers, M., E. Goodman, et al., "Some Behavioral Changes in Man Following Anticholinesterase Administration," *J Nerv Ment Dis,* 138, 1964, p. 383.

Bowman, P., S. Schuschereba, et al., "Myopathic Changes in Diaphragm of Rats Fed Pyridostigmine Bromide Subchronically," *Fundam Appl Toxicol,* 13, 1989, pp. 110–117.

Bradbury, M., J. Burden, "Stimulation Electrically and by Acetylcholine of the Rat Hypothalamus in Vitro," *J Physiol (Lond),* 239, 1974, p. 269.

Braga, M., E. Rowan, et al., "Prejunctional Action of Neostigmine on Mouse Neuromuscular Preparations," *Brit J Anesthesia,* 70, 1993, pp. 405–410.

Braham, J., "Drop Attacks in the Elderly: Effect of Pyridostigmine," *Postgraduate Medical Journal,* 70(829), 1994, p. 848.

Brake, B., response to inquiry, 1997.

Breyer-Pfaf, U., U. Maier, et al., "Pyridostigmine Kinetics in Healthy Subjects and Patients with Myasthenia Gravis," *Clin Pharmacol Ther,* 37, 1985, pp. 495–501.

Briggs, G., R. Freeman, et al., eds., *Drugs in Pregnancy and Lactation,* Baltimore: Williams and Wilkins, 1990.

Brodeur, J., and K. DuBois, "Studies of the Mechanism of Acquired Tolerance by Rats to O,O Diethyl S-2-(ethylthio)ethyl Phosphorodithioate (Di-Syston)," *Arch Int Pharmacodyn,* 149, 1964, pp. 560–570.

Brooks, R., D. Hubbard, et al., "Effects of Pyridostigmine Bromide on A-10 Pilots During Execution of a Simulated Mission: Performance," Fort Detrick, Md.: U.S. Army Medical R&D Command, 1992.

Brown, D., "Slow Cholinergic Excitation—A Mechanism for Increasing Neuronal Excitability," *Trends Neurosci,* 6, 1983, pp. 302–306.

Brown, G., and F. Goodwin, "Cerebrospinal Fluid Correlates of Suicide Attempts and Aggression," *Psychobiology of Suicide,* 487, 1986a, pp. 175–188.

Brown, G., and F. Goodwin, "Human Aggression and Suicide," *Suicide and Life-Threatening Behavior,* 16, 1986b, pp. 141–161.

Brown, G., F. Goodwin, et al., "Aggression in Humans Correlates with Cerebrospinal Fluid Amine Metabolites," *Psychiatry Research,* 1, 1979, pp. 131–139.

Brown, G., F. Goodwin, et al., "Human Aggression and Suicide: Their Relationship to Neuropsychiatric Diagnoses and Serotonin Metabolism," in B. Ho, J. Schoolar, and E. Usdin, eds., *Serotonin in Biological Psychiatry: Advances in Biochemical Psychopharmacology,* New York: Raven Press, 1982.

Brown, G., M. Ebert, et al., "Aggression, Suicide and Serotonin: Relationships to CSF Amine Metabolites," *Am J Psychiat,* 139, 1982, pp. 741–716.

Brown, H., "Electroencephalographic Changes and Disturbance of Brain Function Following Human Organophosphate Exposure," *Northwest Med,* 70, 1971, pp. 845–846.

Brugada, R., N. Wenger, et al., "Changes in Plasma Cholesterol Levels After Hospitalization for Acute Coronary Events," *Cardiology,* 87(3), 1986, pp. 194–199.

Brust, P., "Blood-Brain-Barrier Transport Under Different Physiological and Pathophysiological Circumstances Including Ischemia," *Exp Pathol,* 42, 1991, pp. 213–219.

Buccafusco, J., M. Prendergast, et al., "A Rate Model for Gulf War Illness-Related Selective Memory Impairment and the Loss of Hippocampal Nicotinic Receptors," *Society for Neuroscience Abstracts,* 23, 1997, part 1, p. 90.19.

Burchfiel, J. L., and F. H. Duffy, "Organophosphate Neurotoxicity: Chronic Effects of Sarin on the Electroencephalogram of Monkey and Man," *Neurobehavioral Toxicology and Teratology,* 4, 1982, pp. 767–778.

Butterfield, P. G., B. G. Valanis, et al., "Environmental Antecedents of Young-Onset Parkinson's Disease," *Neurology,* 43(6), 1993, pp. 1150–1158.

Cain, D., and M. Corcoran, "Epileptiform Effects of Met-enkephalin, ß-Endorphin, and Morphine: Kindling of Generalized Seizures and Potentiation of Epileptiform Effects by Handling," *Brain Res* 338, 1985, pp. 327–336.

Callender, T. J., L. Morrow, and K. Subramanian, "Evaluation of Chronic Neurological Sequelae After Acute Pesticide Exposure Using SPECT Brain Scans," (published erratum appears in *J Toxicol Environ Health,* 44(2), 1995, pp. vii–viii), *J Toxicol Environ Health,* 41(3), 1994, pp. 275–284.

Campbell, S., J. Gillin, et al., "Lithium Delays Circadian Phase of Temperature and REM Sleep in a Bipolar Depressive: A Case Report," *Psychiatry Res,* 27, 1989, pp. 23–29.

Canadian Department of National Defence, "Health Study of Canadian Forces Personnel Involved in the 1991 Conflict in the Persian Gulf, Volumes I and II, prepared for the Gulf War Illness Advisory Committee, Department of National Defence, by Goss Gilroy, Inc., Management Consultants, Ottawa, April 20, 1998, *http://www.DND.ca/menu/press/reports/health/health_study_e_vol1_TOC.htm.*

Capacio, B., C. Byers, et al., "Drug Interaction Studies of Pyridostigmine with the 5HT3 Receptor Antagonist Ondansetron and Granisetron in Guinea Pigs," Aberdeen Proving Ground, Md.: U.S. Army Medical Research Institute of Chemical Defense, 1993.

Capacio, B., I. Koplovitz, et al., "Drug Interaction Studies of Pyridostigmine with the 5HT3 Receptor Antagonist Ondansetron and Granisetron in Guinea

Pigs," Aberdeen Proving Ground, Md.: U.S. Army Medical Research Institute of Chemical Defense, 1995.

Cappa, M., A. Grossi, et al., "Effect of the Enhancement of the Cholinergic Tone by Pyridostigmine on the Exercise-Induced Growth Hormone Release in Man," *J Endocrinol Invest*, 16, 1993, pp. 421–424.

Carney, M., "Bromism—A Clinical Chameleon," *Nursing Times*, July 5, 1973, pp. 859–861.

Carney, M., "Five Cases of Bromism," *Lancet*, II, 1971, pp. 523–524.

Casida, J., D. Gamman, et al., "Mechanisms of Selective Actions of Pyrethroid Insecticides," *Ann Rev Pharmacol Toxicol*, 23, 1983, pp. 413–438.

Cassel, W., T. Ploch, et al., "Risk of Traffic Accidents in Patients with Sleep-Disordered Breathing: Reduction with Nasal CPAP," *European Respiratory Journal*, 9(12), 1986, pp. 2606–2611.

Centers for Disease Control and Prevention (CDC), "Unexplained Illness Among Persian Gulf War Veterans in an Air National Guard Unit: Preliminary Report—August 1990–March 1995," *MMWR*, 44, 1995, pp. 443–447.

Chaney, L., J. Moss, et al., "Toxic Interactions Between Pyridostigmine (PB), N,N-Diethyl-m-Toluamide (DEET), Adrenergic Agents and Caffeine (Abstract)," *SOT 1997 Annual Meeting*, 1997.

Chang, H., and E. Neumann, "Dynamic Properties of Isolated Acetylcholine Receptor Proteins: Release of Calcium Ion Caused by Acetylcholine Binding," *Proc Natl Acad Sci USA*, 73(10), 1976, pp. 3364–3368.

Changeux, J.-P., A. Bessis, et al., "Nicotinic Receptors and Brain Plasticity," *Cold Spring Harbor Symposia on Quantitative Biology*, 66, 1996, pp. 343–362.

Chiappa, S., S. Padilla, et al., "Slow Accumulation of Acetylcholinesterase in Rat Brain During Enzyme Inhibition by Repeated Dosing with Chlorpyrifos," *Biochemical Pharmacology*, 49(7), 1995, pp. 955–963.

Christie, J. E., A. Shering, et al., "Physostigmine and Arecoline: Effects of Intravenous Infusions in Alzheimer Presenile Dementia," *Br J Psychiatry*, 138, 1981, pp. 46–50.

Chubb, I. W., A. J. Hodgson, and G. H. White, "Acetylcholine Hydrolyzes Substance P," *Neuroscience*, 5, 1980, pp. 2065–2072.

Clawson, R., personal communication, 1997, 1998, and 1999.

Clark, G., "Organophosphate Insecticides and Behavior: A Review," *Aerosp Med*, 4, 1971, pp. 735–740.

Clement, J. G., D. G. Bailey, et al., "The Acetylcholinesterase Oxime Reactivator HI-6 in Man: Pharmacokinetics and Tolerability in Combination with Atropine," *Biopharm Drug Dispos,* 16(5), 1995, pp. 415–425.

Clement, J., "Hormonal Consequences of Organophosphate Poisoning," *Fund Appl Toxicol,* 5, 1985, pp. S61–S77.

Clement, J., "Distribution of Pyridostigmine in Rats and Guinea Pigs," Suffield Technical Paper 464, 1977.

Coccaro, E. F., "Central Serotonin and Impulsive Aggression," *BJP,* December (8), 1989, Supplement, pp. 52–62.

Coccaro, E. F., L. J. Siever, et al., "Serotonergic Studies in Patients with Affective and Personality Disorders. Correlates with Suicidal and Impulsive Aggressive Behavior" (published erratum appears in *Arch Gen Psychiatry,* 47(2), 1990, p. 124), *Arch Gen Psychiatry,* 46(7), 1989, pp. 587–599.

Cohan, S., K. Drettchen, et al., "Malabsorption of Pyridostigmine in Patients with Myasthenia Gravis," *Neurology,* 27, 1977, pp. 299–301.

Cohan, S. L., J. L. Pohlmann, et al., "The Pharmacokinetics of Pyridostigmine," *Neurology,* 26, 1976, pp. 536–539.

Coiro, V., R. Volpi, et al., "Different Effects of Pyridostigmine on the Thyrotropin Response to Thyrotropin-Releasing Hormone in Endogenous Depression and Subclinical Thyrotoxicosis," *Metabolism,* 47(1), 1998, pp. 50–53.

Collins, A., and M. Marks, "Regulation of Behavioral and Physiological Sensitivity to Nicotine by Brain Nicotinic Receptors," in F. Clement, ed., *Nicotinic Acetylcholine Receptors in the Nervous System,* New York: Springer-Verlag, 1988.

Committee on Veterans Affairs, "Is Military Research Hazardous to Veterans' Health? Lessons from World War II, The Persian Gulf, and Today," hearing U.S. Senate, Washington, D.C., 1994.

Committee to Review the Health Consequences of Service During the Persian Gulf War (IOM), *Health Consequences of Service During the Persian Gulf War: Recommendations for Research and Information Systems,* Washington, D.C.: National Academy Press, 1996.

Committee to Study the Interactions of Drugs, Biologics, and Chemicals in US Military Forces, *Interactions of Drugs, Biologics, and Chemicals in US Military Forces,* Washington, D.C.: National Academy Press, 1996.

Conti-Fine, B., and R. Horton, "A 'Neuronal' Nicotinic Acetylcholine Receptor Regulating Cell Adhesion Is Expressed in Human Epidermal Keratinocytes," *International Symposium on the Cholinergic Synapse: Structure, Function, and Regulation (3rd),* Baltimore: University of Maryland, 1994.

Cook, J., M. Kolka, et al., "Chronic Pyridostigmine Bromide Administration: Side Effects Among Soldiers Working in a Desert Environment," *Military Medicine*, 157, 1992, pp. 250–254.

Coppen, A., C. Swade, and K. Wood, "Platelet 5-Hydroxytryptamine Accumulation in Depressive Illness," *Clinica Chimica Acta*, 87(1), 1978, pp. 165–168.

Corringer, P.-H., S. Bertrand, et al., "Critical Elements Determining Diversity in Agonist Binding and Desensitization of Neuronal Nicotinic Acetylcholine Receptors," *J of Neuroscience*, 18(2), 1998, pp. 648–657.

Corsello, S., A. Tofani, et al., "Effects of Sex and Age on Pyridostigmine Potentiation of Growth Hormone-Releasing Hormone-Induced Growth Hormone Release," *Neuroendocrinology*, 56, 1991, pp. 208–213.

Costa, L., et al., "Species Differences in Serum Paraoxonase Activity Correlate with Sensitivity to Paraoxon Toxicity, in L. Costa et al., eds., *Toxicology of Pesticides: Experimental, Clinical, and Regulatory Aspects, NATO ASI series*, Berlin: Springer-Verlag, 1987, H13, pp. 263–266.

Costa, L., et al., "Serum Paraoxonase and Its Influence on Paraoxon and Chlorpyrifos-Oxon toxicity in Rats," *Toxicol Appl Pharmacol*, 103, 1990, pp. 66–76.

Costa, L., B. Schwab, et al., "Reduced [3Hquinuclidinyl Benzilate Binding to Muscarinic Receptors in Disulfoton-Tolerant Mice," *Toxicol Appl Pharmacol*, 60, 1981, pp. 441–450.

Costa, L., B. Schwab, et al., "Differential Alterations of Cholinergic Muscarinic Receptors in Chronic and Acute Tolerance to Organophosphorus Insecticides," *Biochem Pharmacol*, 31, 1982a, pp. 3407–3413.

Costa, L., B. Schwab, et al., "Tolerance to Anticholinesterase Compounds in Mammals," *Toxicology*, 25, 1982b, pp. 79–97.

Cowan, D. N., R. F. De Fraites, et al., "The Risk of Birth Defects Among Children of Persian Gulf War Veterans," *New Engl J Med*, 336, 1997, pp. 1650–1656.

Cronnelly, R., D. Stanski, et al., "Pyridostigmine Kinetics with and Without Renal Function," *Clin Pharmacol Ther*, 28, 1980, pp. 78–81.

Cullen, M., "The Worker with Multiple Chemical Sensitivities: An Overview," *Occupational Medicine*, 2(4), 1987, pp. 655–661.

Cupler, F. J., C. Otero, et al., "Acetylcholine Receptor Antibodies as Markers of Treatable Fatigue in HIV-1 Infected Individuals," *Muscle and Nerve*, 19, 1996, pp. 1186–1188.

Currie, E., "The Gulf War Syndrome (letter)," *BMJ*, 310(6990), 1995, pp. 1334–1335.

Dagan, Y., P. Lavie, et al., "Elevated Awakening Thresholds in Sleep Stage 3-4 in War-Related Post-Traumatic Stress Disorder," *Biol Psychiatry*, 30, 1991, pp. 618–622.

Damaj, M. I., K. R. Creasy, et al., "Pharmacological Effects of Epibatidine Optical Enantiomers," *Brain Res*, 664(1-2), 1994, pp. 34–40.

Damaj, M. I., and B. R. Martin, "Tolerance to the Antinociceptive Effect of Epibatidine After Acute and Chronic Administration in Mice," *Eur J Pharmacol*, 300(1-2), 1996, pp. 51–57.

Daniell, W., S. Barnhart, et al., "Neuropsychological Performance Among Agricultural Pesticide Applicators," *Environ Res*, 59(1), 1992, pp. 217–228.

Davidoff, A., and P. Keyl, "Symptoms and Health Status in Individuals with Multiple Chemical Sensitivities Syndrome from Four Reported Sensitizing Exposures and a General Population Comparison Group," *Archives of Environmental Health*, 51(3), 1996, pp. 201–213.

Davies, D., P. Holland, et al., "The Relationship Between the Chemical Structure and Neurotoxicity of Alkyl Organophosphorus Compounds," *Br J Pharmacol*, 23, 1960, pp. 295–304.

Davies, H., R. Richter, et al., "The Effect of the Human Serum Paraoxonase Polymorphism Is Reversed with Diazonon, Soman, and Sarin," *Nature Genetics*, 14, 1996, pp. 334–336.

Davies, J., "Neurotoxic Concern of Human Pesticide Exposures," *Am J Ind Med*, 18, 1990, pp. 327–331.

Davila, D. G., R. D. Hurt, et al., "Acute Effects of Transdermal Nicotine on Sleep Architecture, Snoring, and Sleep-Disordered Breathing in Nonsmokers," *Am J Respir Crit Care Med*, 150(2), 1994, pp. 469–474.

Davis, B., and K. Davis, "Acetylcholine and Anterior Pituitary Hormone Secretion," in K. Davis and P. Berger, eds., *Brain Acetylcholine and Neuropsychiatric Disease*, New York: Plenum Press, 1979, pp. 445–458.

Davis, D., "Reduced Ratio of Male to Female Births in Several Industrial Countries: A Sentinel Health Indicator?" *JAMA*, 279, 1998, pp. 1018–1023,

Davis, K., K. Faull, et al., "Physostigmine Related Changes in Cerebrospinal Fluid Neurotransmitter Metabolites in Man," in K. Davis and P. Berger, eds., *Brain Acetylcholine and Neuropsychiatric Disease*, New York: Plenum Press, 1979, pp. 435–443.

Davis, K. L., R. C. Mohs, et al., "Physostigmine: Improvement of Long-Term Memory Processes in Normal Humans," *Science*, 201(4352), 1978, pp. 272–274.

Davis, K. L., and H. I. Yamamura, "Cholinergic Underactivity in Human Memory Disorders," *Life Sci,* 23(17-18), 1978, pp. 1729–1733.

Davis, K. L., J. A. Yesavage, et al., "Single Case Study. Possible Organophosphate-Induced Parkinsonism," *J Nerv Ment Dis,* 166(3), 1978, pp. 222–225.

De Bleecker, J. L., "Intermediate Syndrome: Prolonged Cholinesterase Inhibition" (letter), *J Toxicol Clin Toxicol,* 31(1), 1993, pp. 197–199.

De Bleecker, J., K. Van Den Neucker, et al., "The Intermediate Syndrome in Organophosphate Poisoning: Presentation of a Case and Review of the Literature" (published erratum appears in *J Toxicol Clin Toxical,* 30(4), 1992, p. 697), *J Toxicol Clin Toxicol,* 30(3), 1992, pp. 321–329, pp. 331–332 (discussion).

Defense Science Board Task Force on Persian Gulf War Health Effects, "Report of the Defense Science Board Task Force on Persian Gulf War Health Effects," Washington, D.C., Office of the Under Secretary of Defense for Acquisition and Technology, 1994.

De Fraites, R., "Pyridostigmine Bromide (PB) Use in Operations Desert Shield and Desert Storm (ODS)," information paper, DASG-HS-PM, 1996.

De Fraites, R., E. I. Wanat, et al., "Investigation of a Suspected Outbreak of an Unknown Disease Among Veterans of Operation Desert Shield/Storm 123rd Army Reserve Command, Fort Benjamin Harrison, Indiana, April 1992," Washington, D.C.: Walter Reed Army Institute of Research, 1992.

De Garbino, J. P., and A. Laborde, "Toxicity of an Insect Repellent: N-N-Diethyltoluamide," *Veterinary and Human Toxicology,* 25(6), 1983, pp. 422–423.

Department of Defense. comments on Public Citizen Litigation Group's Petition to Repeal Interim Rule on the Treatment Use Without Informed Consent of Investigational New Drugs in Military Combat Exigency, 1996.

Department of Defense, "Comprehensive Clinical Evaluation Program for Persian Gulf War Veterans: CCEP Report on 18,598 Participants," 1996.

Dettbarn, W.-D., "Pesticide Induced Muscle Necrosis: Mechanisms and Prevention," *Fundam Appl Toxicol,* 4, 1984, pp. S18–S26.

Deutsch, J., and J. Roger, "Cholinergic Excitability and Memory: Animal Studies and Their Clinical Implications," in K. Davis and P. Berger, eds., *Brain Acetylcholine and Neuropsychiatric Disease,* New York: Plenum Press, 1979, pp. 175–204.

Devinsky, O., J. Kernan, et al., "Aggressive Behavior Following Exposure to Cholinesterase Inhibitors," *J Neuropsychiatry and Clin Neurosciences*, 4, 1992, pp. 189–194.

Deyi, X., W. Limxiu, et al., "The Inhibition and Protection of Cholinesterase by Physostigmine and Pyridostigmine Against Soman Poisoning in Vivo," *Fundam Appl Toxicol*, 1, 1981, pp. 217–221.

Didier, M., S. Bursztajn, et al., "DNA Strand Breaks Induced by Sustained Glutamate Excitotoxicity in Primary Neuronal Cultures," *J of Neurosci*, 16(7), 1996, pp. 2238–2250.

Dietrich, W. D., M. D. Ginsburg, et al., "Effects of Physostigmine on Local Glucose Utilization in the Rat," *Ann Neurol*, 16(1), 1984, pp. 117–118 (abstract).

Dille, J., and P. Smith, "Central Nervous System Effects of Chronic Exposure to Organophosphate Insecticides," *Aerosp Med*, 35, 1964, p. 475.

Dimsdale, J., and J. Herd, "Variability of Plasma Lipids in Response to Emotional Arousal," *Psychosom Med*, 44, 1982, pp. 413–430.

Dinan, T., V. O'Keane, et al., "Pyridostigmine Induced Growth Hormone Release in Mania: Focus on the Cholinergic/Somatostatin System," *Clinical Endocrinology*, 40, 1994, pp. 93–96.

Dirnhuber, P. and M. C. French, "Effectiveness of Pyridostigmine in Reversing the Neuromuscular Blockade Produced by Soman," *J Pharm Pharmacol*, 30, 1978, pp. 419–425.

Dirnhuber, P., M. C. French, et al., "The Effect of Chronic Administration of Pyridostigmine in the Rat, Guinea Pig, and Rhesus Monkey," Chemical Defence Establishment Technical Paper 218, Porton Down, U.K., 1977.

Dirnhuber, P., M. French, et al., "The Protection of Primates Against Soman Poisoning by Pretreatment with Pyridostigmine," *J Pharm Pharmacol*, 31, 1979, pp. 295–299.

Dirnhuber, P. and D. M. Green, "Effectiveness of Pyridostigmine in Reversing the Neuromuscular Blockade Produced by GD," Chemical Defence Establishment Technical Paper 231, Porton Down, U.K., 1977.

Dirnhuber, P., D. M. Green, et al., "Comparison Between the Bromide and Methane Sulphonate Salts of Pyridostigmine as Pretreatmetn against Nerve Agent Poisoning," Chemical Defense Establishment, Porton Down, U. K., 1978.

D'Mello, G., "Behavioral Toxicity of Anticholinesterases in Humans and Animals—A Review," *Hum Exp Toxicol*, 12, 1993, pp. 3–7.

D'Mello, G., N. Cross, et al., "A Novel Method to Enable Evaluation of Relative Effect—Application to the Comparison of Different Medical Counter-measures for Nerve Agent Poisoning (U)," Chemical and Biological Defence Establishment. Porton Down, U.K., 1994.

D'Mello, G., S. Miles, et al., "Protection Against Nerve Agent Poisoning: An Overview of Animal Behavioural Toxicological Studies and Their Implications for Man," Chemical and Biological Defence Establishment, Porton Down, U.K., 1988.

D'Mello, G., and E. Scott, "Relative Efficacy of Pretreatment with Physostigmine and Hyoscine Against GB and GD in Marmosets: Evaluation Using Clinical Signs and Eye-Hand Co-ordination Performance as Indices of Residual Toxicity," Chemical and Biological Defence Establishment, Porton Down, U.K., 1990.

Doctor, B., D. Blick, et al., "Cholinesterases as Scavengers for Organophosphorus Compounds: Protection of Primate Performance Against Soman Toxicity," *Chem Biol Interact*, 87, 1993, pp. 285–293.

Dominguez, R. A., and P. J. Goodnick, "Adverse Events After the Abrupt Discontinuation of Paroxetine," *Pharmacotherapy*, 15(6), 1995, pp. 778–780.

Donnay, A., personal communication, 1999.

Donnelly-Roberts, D. L., P. S. Puttfarcken, et al., "ABT-594 [(R)-5-(2-Azetidinyl-methoxy)-2-Chloropyridine]: A Novel, Orally Effective Analgesic Acting via Neuronal Nicotinic Acetylcholine Receptors: I. In Vitro Characterization," *J Pharmacol Exp Ther*, 285(2), 1998, pp. 777–786.

Dorner, G., K. Hecht, et al., "Teratopsychogenetic Effects Apparently Produced by Nonphysiological Neurotransmitter Concentrations During Brain Differentiation," *Endokrinologie*, 68(1), 1976, pp. 1–5.

Dorner, G., and G. Hinz, "Apparent Effects of Neurotransmitters on Sexual Differentiation of the Brain Without Mediation of Sex Hormones," *Endokrinologie*, 71(1), 1978, pp. S104–S108.

Dorner, G., J. Staudt, et al., "Further Evidence of Teratogenic Effects Apparently Produced by Neurotransmitters During Brain Differentiation," *Endokrinologie*, 70(3), 1977, pp. S326–S330.

Doty, R., et al., "Olfactory Sensitivity, Nasal Resistance, and Autonomic Function in Patients with Multiple Chemical Sensitivities," *Arch Otolaryngol-Head and Neck Surg*, 144, 1988, pp. 1422–1427.

Doyle, P., E. Roman, et al., "Birth Defects Among Children of Persian Gulf War Veterans (letter)," *New Engl J Med*, 337, 1997, p. 1175.

Drachman, D., "Memory and Cognitive Function in Man: Does the Cholinergic System Have a Specific Role?" *Neurology*, 27, 1977, p. 783.

Drachman, D., "Myasthenia Gravis," *New Engl J Med*, 330(25), 1994, pp. 1797–1810.

Drachman, D., and J. Leavitt, "Human Memory and the Cholinergic System," *Arch Neurol*, 30, 1974, p. 113.

Drenth, J., I. Ensberg, et al., "Neuromuscular Function in Agricultural Workers Using Pesticides," *Arch Envir Health*, 25, 1972, pp. 395–398.

Dringenberg, H. C., M. A. De Souza-Silva, et al., "Histamine H1 Receptor Antagonists Produce Increases in Extracellular Acetylcholine in Rat Frontal Cortex and Hippocampus," *J Neurochem*, 70(4), 1998, pp. 1750–1758.

Duffy, F., and J. Burchfiel, "Long Term Effects of the Organophosphate Sarin on EEGs in Monkeys and Humans," *Neurotoxicology*, 1, 1980, pp. 667–689.

Duffy, F., J. Burchfiel, et al., "Long Term Effects of an Organophosphate upon the Human Electroencephalogram," *Toxicol Appl Pharmacol*, 46, 1979, pp. 161–176.

Duggan, A., and D. Smith, "Physiological Aspects of an Investigation into the Effects of Pyridostigmine Bromide Pretreatment on Work Capacity in the Heat," Institute of Naval Medicine (U.K.), 1982.

Dummer, S., A. Lee, et al., "Investigation of Cytomegalovirus Infection as a Risk Factor for Coronary Atherosclerosis in the Explanted Hearts of Patients Undergoing Heart Transplantation," *J Med Virol*, 44(3), 1994, pp. 305–309.

Duna, G., and W. Wilke, "Diagnosis, Etiology and Therapy of Fibromyalgia," *Comprehensive Therapy*, 19(2), 1993, pp. 60–63.

Dunn, M., B. Hackley, et al., "Chapter 6: Pretreatment for Nerve Agent Exposure," in R. Bellamy, F. Sidell, E. Takafuji, and D. Franz, eds., *Textbook of Military Medicine. Part I. Medical Aspects of Chemical and Biological Warfare*, Office of the Surgeon General, Department of the Army, 262, 1997, pp. 649–652.

Dunn, M., and F. Sidell, "Progress in Medical Defense Against Nerve Agents," *JAMA*, 262(5), pp. 649–652.

Durham, W., H. Wolfe, et al., "Organophosphorous Insecticides and Mental Alertness," *Arch Environ Health*, 10, 1965, pp. 55–66.

Duvoisin, R., E. Deneris, et al., "The Functional Diversity of the Neuronal Nicotinic Acetylcholine Receptors Is Increased by a Novel Subunit: ß4," *Neuron*, 3, 1989, pp. 487–496.

Dvorska, I., et al., "On the Blood-Brain Barrier to Peptides: Effects of Immobilization Stress on Regional Blood Supply and Accumulation of Labeled Peptides in the Rat Brain," *Endocr Res,* 26, 1992, pp. 77–82.

Dwyer, J., USC Department of Research, personal communication, 1998.

Eakman, G., J. Dallas, et al., "The Effects of Testosterone and Dihydrotestosterone on Hypothalamic Regulation of Growth Hormone Secretion," *J Clin Endocrinol and Metabolism,* 81(3), 1996, pp. 1217–1223.

Eastwood, J., G. Levine, et al., "Aluminium Deposition in Bone After Contamination of Drinking Water," *Lancet,* 2, 1990, pp. 462–464.

Eaton, L., and E. Lambert, "Electromyography and Electrical Stimulation of Nerve in Diseases of Motor Units," *JAMA,* 163, 1957, pp. 1117–1124.

Eberly, R., and B. Engdahl, "Prevalence of Somatic and Psychiatric Disorders Among Foreign Prisoners of War," *Hospital and Community Psychiatry,* 42(8), 1991, pp. 807–813.

Ecobichon, D., J. Davies, et al., "Neurotoxic Effects of Pesticides, in S. Baker and C. Wilkinson, eds., *The Effect of Pesticides on Human Health,* Princeton, N. J.: Princeton Scientific Publishers, 1990, pp. 131–199.

Edwards, D., and C. Johnson, "Insect-Repellent-Induced Toxic Encephalopathy in a Child," *Clin Pharmacol,* 6, 1987, pp. 496–498.

Ehlert, F., N. Kokka, et al., "Altered (3H)-Quinuclidinyl Benzilate Binding in the Striatum of Rats Following Chronic Cholinesterase Inhibition with Diisopropylfluorophosphate," *Mol Pharmacol,* 17, 1980, pp. 24–30.

Ehlert, F., N. Kokka, et al., "Muscarinic Subsensitivity in the Longitudinal Muscle of the Rat Ileum Following Anticholinesterase Treatment with Diisopropylfluorophosphate," *Biochem Pharmacol,* 29, 1980, pp. 1391–1397.

Ehrich, M., L. Shell, et al., "Short-Term Clinical and Neuropathologic Effects of Cholinesterase Inhibitors in Rats," *J Am Coll Toxicol,* 12, 1993, pp. 55–67.

Eichelman, B., "Role of Biogenic Amines in Aggressive Behavior," in M. Sandler, ed., *Psychopharmacology of Aggression,* New York: Raven Press, 1979, pp. 61–93.

Eiermann, B., N. Sommer, et al., "Renal Clearance of Pyridostigmine in Myasthenia Patients and Volunteers Under the Influence of Ranitidine and Pirenzepine," *Xenobiotica,* 23, 1993, pp. 1263–1175.

El-Fakahany, E., and E. Richelson, "Involvement of Calcium Channels in Short-Term Desensitization of Muscarinic Receptor-Mediated Cyclic G<P Formation in Mouse Neuroblastoma Cells," *Proc Nat Acad Sci USA,* 77, 1980, pp. 6897–6901.

El-Fakahany, E., and E. Richelson, "Phenoxybenzamine and Dibenamine Interactions with Calcium Channel Effectors of the Muscarinic Receptor," *Mol Pharmacol*, 20, 1981, pp. 519–525.

Elgoyen, A., D. Johnson, et al., *Alpha 9: A New Acetylcholine Receptor with Novel Pharmacological Properties*, International Symposium on the Cholinergic Synapse: Structure, Function and Regulation (3rd), Baltimore: University of Maryland, 1994.

Elin, R., E. Robertson, et al., "Bromide Interferes with Determination of Chloride by Each of Four Methods," *Clin Chem*, 27, 1981, pp. 778–779.

Ellenhorn, M., S. Schonwald, et al., *Ellenhorn's Medical Toxicology*, Baltimore: Williams and Wilkins, 1997.

Ellman, G., K. Coortney, et al., "A New and Rapid Colorimetric Determination of Acetylcholinesterase Activity," *Biochem Pharmacol*, 7, 1961, pp. 88–95.

Ellman, P., D. King, et al., "Preictal Headache as a Potential Red Flag for Non-epileptic Seizures," American Epilepsy Society meeting, Boston, Mass., December 7–10, 1997, *Epilepsia*, 38, 1997, Supplement 8, p. 50.

Elsmore, T., "Circadian Susceptibility to Soman Poisoning," *Fund Appl Toxicol*, 1, 1981, pp. 238–241.

Elson, E., "Report on Possible Effects of Organophosphate 'Low-Level' Nerve Agent Exposure," *Health Affairs*, 1996.

El-Yousef, M., D. Janowsky, et al., "Induction of Severe Depression by Physostigmine in Marihuana Intoxicated Individuals," *Br J Addict Alcohol Other Drugs*, 68(4), 1973, pp. 321–325.

Engel, A., E. Lambert, and T. Santa, "Study of Long-Term Anticholinesterase Therapy," *Neurology*, 23, 1973, p. 1273.

Engel, A., E. Lambert, et al., "A New Myasthenic Syndrome with End-Plate Acetylcholinesterase Deficiency, Small Nerve Terminals and Reduced Acetylcholine Release," *Ann Neurol*, 1, 1977, pp. 315–330.

Engel, A., E. Lambert, et al., "A Newly Recognized Congenital Myasthenic Syndrome Attributed to a Prolonged Open Time of the Acetylcholine-Induced Ion Channel," *Ann Neurol*, 11, 1981, pp. 553–569.

Epstein, Y., D. Seidman, et al., "Heat-Exercise Performance of Pyridostigmine-Treated Subjects Wearing Chemical Protective Clothing," *Aviat Space Environ Med*, 61, 1990, pp. 310–313.

Eriksson, P. U. Johansson, et al., "Neonatal Exposure to DDT Induces Increased Susceptibility to Pyrethroid (Bioallethrin) Exposure at Adult Age—Changes in

Cholinergic Muscarinic Receptor and Behavioural Variables," *Toxicol*, 77(1-2), 1993, pp. 21–30.

Ernest, K., M. Thomas, et al., "Delayed Effects of Exposure to Organo-phosphorus Compounds," *Indian J Med Res*, 101, 1995, pp. 81–84.

Fagerstrom, K., O. Pomerleau, et al., "Nicotine May Relieve Symptoms of Parkinson's Disease," *Psychopharmacology*, 116, 1994, pp. 117–119.

Falk, J., and K. Halmi, "Amenorrhea in Anorexia Nervosa: Examination of the Critical Body Weight Hypothesis," *Biol Psychiatry*, 17, 1982, pp. 799–806.

Farrington, C., J. Nash, et al., "Case Series Analysis of Adverse Reactions to Vac-cines: A Comparative Evaluation," *Am J Epidemiology*, 143, 1996, pp. 1165–1173.

Fatranska, M., M. Vargova, et al., "Circadian Susceptibility Rhythms to Some Organophosphate Compounds in the Rat," *Chronobiologia*, 5, 1978, pp. 39–44.

FDA, personal communication with Stuart Nightingale, Brian Malkin, and oth-ers regarding PB, 1997.

Federal Register, "Accessibility to New Drugs for Use in Military and Civilian Exigencies When Traditional Human Efficacy Studies Are Not Feasible; Determination Under the Interim Rule That Informed Consent Is Not Feasi-ble for Military Exigencies; Request for Comments," *Federal Register*, 62(147), 1997, pp. 40996–41001.

Feldt-Rasmussen, B., K. Gefke, et al., "Effect of a Mixture of Pyridostigmine and Atropine on Forced Expiratory Volume and Serum Cholinesterase Activity in Normal Subjects," *Br J Anaesth*, 57, 1985, pp. 204–207.

Felix, R., and E. D. Levin, "Nicotinic Antagonist Administration into the Ventral Hippocampus and Spatial Working Memory in Rats," *Neuroscience*, 81(4), 1997, pp. 1009–1017.

Feng, H., A. Rogers, et al., "Recovery of Esterases at Muscle Endplates Inacti-vated by DFP," *J Cell Biol*, 59, 1973, p. 98a.

Fenichel, G., W.-D. Dettbarn, et al., "An Experimental Myopathy Secondary to Excessive Acetylcholine Release," *Neurology*, 24, 1974, pp. 41–45.

Fenichel, G., W. Kibler, et al., "Chronic Inhibition of Cholinesterase as a Cause of Myopathy," *Neurology*, 22, 1972, pp. 1026–1033.

Fenichel, G., W. Kibler, et al., "The Effect of Immobilization and Exercise on Acetylcholine-Mediated Myopathies," *Neurology*, 24, 1974, pp. 1086–1090.

Fiedler, N., H. Kipen, et al., "Chemical Sensitivities and the Gulf War: Depart-ment of Veterans Affairs Research Center in Basic and Clinical Science Studies of Environmental Hazards," *Regulatory Toxicology and Pharmacology*, 24, 1996, pp. S129–S138.

Field, L., "Toxic Alopecia Caused by Pyridostigmine Bromide," *Arch Dermatol*, 116, 1980, p. 1103.

Field Manual: Treatment of Chemical Agent Casualties and Conventional Military Chemical Injuries, Washington, D. C.: Departments of the Army, the Navy, and the Air Force, 1990.

Field Manual: Treatment of Chemical Agent Casualties and Conventional Military Chemical Injuries, Washington, D. C.: Departments of the Army, the Navy, and the Air Force, and Commandant, Marine Corps, 1995.

Findley, L., M. Fabrizio, et al., "Severity of Sleep Apnea and Automobile Crashes," *New Engl J Med*, 320(13), 1989, pp. 868–869.

Findley, L., M. Unverzagt, et al., "Vigilance and Automobile Accidents in Patients with Sleep Apnea or Narcolepsy," *Chest*, 108(3), 1995, pp. 619–624.

Findley, L., M. Unverzagt, et al., "Automobile Accidents Involving Patients with Obstructive Sleep Apnea," *Am Rev of Respiratory Disease*, 138(2), 1988, pp. 337–340.

Findley, L., J. Weiss, et al., "Drivers with Untreated Sleep Apnea. A Cause of Death and Serious Injury," *Arch of Intern Med* 151(7), 1991, pp. 1451–1452.

Fischer, G., "Inhibierung und Restitution der Azetylcholinesterase an der motorischen Endplatte im Zwerchfell der Ratte nach Intoxikation mit Soman," *Histochemie*, 16, 1968, pp. 144–149.

Fischler, B., H. D'Haenen, et al., "Comparison of 99m Tc HMPAO SPECT Scan Between Chronic Fatigue Syndrome, Major Depression and Healthy Controls: An Exploratory Study of Clinical Correlates of Regional Cerebral Blood Flow," *Neuropsychobiology*, 34(4), 1996, pp. 175–183.

Fleming, N., S. Macres, et al., "Neuromuscular Blocking Action of Suxamethonium After Antagonism of Vecuronium by Edrophonium, Pyridostigmine or Neostigmine," *Brit J Anaesth*, 77, 1996, pp. 492–495.

Flemons, W., and W. Tsai, "Quality of Life Consequences of Sleep-Disordered Breathing," *J Allergy and Clin Immunology*, 99(2), 1997, pp. S750–S756.

Flores, C., S. Rogers, et al., "A Subtype of Nicotinic Cholinergic Receptor in Rat Brain Is Composed of Alpha4 and ß2 Subunits and Is Up-Regulated by Chronic Nicotine Treatment," *Mol Pharmacol*, 41, 1992, pp. 31–37.

Forbes, A., "Smoking and Inflammatory Bowel Disease," *Eur J Gastroenterol Hepatol*, 8(8), 1996, pp. 761–763.

FORSCOM Operations Support Directive, "Pyridostigmine Pretreatment for Nerve Agents," FORSCOM, 1990.

Forster, E. M., J. A. Barber, et al., "Effect of Pyridostigmine Bromide on Acceleration Tolerance and Performance," *Aviat Space Environ Med,* February 1994, pp. 110–116.

Foulds, J., J. Stapleton, et al., "Cognitive Performance Effects of Subcutaneous Nicotine in Smokers and Never-Smokers," *Psychopharmacology,* 127(1), 1996, pp. 31–38.

Fraga, C., P. Oteiza, et al., "Effects of Aluminium on Brain Peroxidation," *Toxicol Lett,* 51, 1990, pp. 213–219.

Francesconi, R., M. Bosselaers, et al., "Pyridostigmine, 2-PAM and Atropine: Effects on the Ability to Work in the Heat," U.S. Army Research Institute of Environmental Medicine, 1987.

Francesconi, R., R. Hubbard, and M. Mager, "Effects of Pyridostigmine on Ability of Rats to Work in the Heat," *J Appl Physiol,* 56(4), 1984, pp. 891–895.

Freedman, A., H. Kaplan, et al., *Comprehensive Text Book of Psychiatry,* Baltimore: Williams and Wilkins, 1978, Vol. 1, pp. 1110–1111.

French, J., American Epilepsy Society meeting, Boston, Mass., 1997.

French, M., J. Wetherell, et al., "The Reversal by Pyridostigmine of Neuromuscular Block Produced by Soman," *J Pharm Pharmacol,* 31, 1979, pp. 290–294.

Fried, F., and P. Malek-Ahmadi, "Bromism: Recent Perspectives," *South Med J,* 68, 1975, pp. 220–222.

Friedman, A., D. Kaufer, et al., "Pyridostigmine Brain Penetration Under Stress Enhances Neuronal Excitability and Induces Early Immediate Transcriptional Response," *Nature Medicine,* 2, 1996, pp. 1382–1384.

Friedman, A., D. Kaufer, et al., "Cholinergic Excitation Induces Activity-Dependent Electrophysiological and Transcriptional Responses in Hippocampal Slices," *Journal de Physiologie,* 92(3-4), 1998, pp. 329–335.

Friedman, M., letter regarding breach of conditions for waiver of informed consent, Washington, D. C.: FDA, 1997.

Fukuda, K., R. Nisenbaum, et al., "Chronic Multisystem Illness Affecting Air Force Veterans of the Gulf War," *JAMA,* 280, 1998, pp. 981–988.

Furlong, C., R. Richter, et al., "Spectrophotometric Assays for the Enzymatic Hydrolysis of the Active Metabolites of Chlorpyrifos and Paration by Plasma Paraoxonase/Arylesterase," *Analyt Biochem,* 180, 1989, pp. 242–247.

Gaff, G., M. Rand, et al., "A Rapid Screening Test for Bromism," *Medical J of Australia*, 1969, pp. 967–969.

Gall, D., "The Use of Therapeutic Mixtures in the Treatment of Cholinesterase Inhibition," *Fundam Appl Toxicol*, 1, 1981, pp. 214–216.

Galynker, I. I., J. Weiss, et al., "ECT Treatment and Cerebral Perfusion in Catatonia," *J Nucl Med*, 38(2), 1997, pp. 251–254.

Gawron, V., "The Effect of Pyridostigmine Bromide on Inflight Aircrew Performance," USAF School of Aerospace Medicine, Brooks AFB, Tex., 1987.

Gebbers, J., M. Lotscher, et al., "Acute Toxicity of Pyridostigmine in Rats: Histological Findings," *Arch Toxicol*, 58, 1986, pp. 271–275.

Geldmacher–von Mallinckrodt, M., and T. Diepgen, "The Human Serum Paraoxonase-Polymorphism and Specificity," *Toxicol Environ Chem*, 18, 1988, pp. 79–196.

Geller, I., R. Hartmann, et al., "Acute Soman Effects in the Juvenile Baboon: Effects on a Match-to-Sample Discrimination Task and on Total Blood Acetylcholinesterase," *Pharmacol Biochem Behav*, 22, 1985, pp. 961–966.

Gentry, M., "The Metabolism of Proposed Nerve Agent Pretreatment, Pyridostigmine Bromide," in J. King, ed., *Medical Defense Bioscience Review: Proceedings*, U.S. Army Medical Research and Materiel Command, 1996, Vol. 2, pp. 1272–1283.

Gentry, M., N. Bitsko, et al., *Pyridostigmine Inhibition of Acetylcholinesterase and Phenotyping of Butyrylcholinesterase: A Comparison in Gulf War Veterans and Normal Controls*, CB Medical Treatment Symposium, Spiez, Switzerland: NC-Laboratory, 1996.

Gentry, M., S. Powell, et al., "In Vitro Pyridostigmine Inhibition of Red Cell Acetylcholinesterase: A Comparison in Gulf War Veterans and Normal Controls," *Medical Defense Bioscience Review*, U.S. Army Medical Research and Materiel Command, 1992.

George, S., and A. Balasubramanian, "The Aryl Acylamidases and Their Relationship to Cholinesterases in Human Serum, Erythrocyte and Liver," *Eur J Biochem*, 2, 1981, pp. 177–186.

Georguieff, M., M. Lefloch, et al., "Nicotinic Effect of Acetylcholine on the Release of Newly Synthesized 3H Dopamine in Rat Striatal Slices and Cat Caudate Nucleus," *Brain Res*, 106, 1976, p. 117.

Gerner, R., "Bromism from Over-the-Counter Medications," *Am J Psychiatry*, 135, 1978, p. 1428.

Gershon, S., and F. Shaw, "Psychiatric Sequelae of Chronic Exposure to Organophosphorus Insecticides," *Lancet*, i, 1961, pp. 1371–1374.

Geschwind, S., and B. A. Golomb, *A Review of the Scientific Literature As It Pertains to Gulf War Illnesses*, Vol. 8: *Pesticides*, Santa Monica, Calif.: RAND, MR-1018/8, forthcoming.

Ghatan, P. H., M. Ingvar, et al., "Cerebral Effects of Nicotine During Cognition in Smokers and Non-Smokers," *Psychopharmacol*, 136(2), 1998, pp. 178–189.

Ghigo, E., M. Nicolosi, et al., "Growth Hormone Secretion in Alzheimer's Disease: Studies with Growth Hormone-Releasing Hormone Alone and Combined with Pyridostigmine or Arginine," *Dementia*, 4, 1993, pp. 315–320.

Ghigo, E., S. Goffi, et al., "A Neuroendocrinological Approach to Evidence an Impairment of Central Cholinergic Function in Aging," *J Endocrinol Invest*, 15, 1992, pp. 665–670.

Ghoneim, M., and S. Mewaldt, "Effects of Diazepam and Scopolamine on Storage, Retrieval and Organizational Processes in Memory," *Psychopharmacologia (Berl)*, 44, 1975, p. 257.

Ghoneim, M., and S. Mewaldt, "Studies on Human Memory: The Interactions of Diazepam, Scopolamine, and Physostigmine," *Psychopharmacology*, 52, 1977, p. 1.

Gillies, J., and J. Allen, "Effects of Neostigmine and Pyridostigmine at the Neuromuscular Junction," *Clin Exp Neurol*, 14, 1977, pp. 271–279.

Gillin, J., L. Sutton, et al., "The Cholinergic Rapid Eye Movement Induction Test with Arecoline in Depression," *Arch Gen Psychiatry*, 48, 1991, pp. 264–270.

Girgis, M., "Biochemical Patterns in Limbic System Circuitry: Biochemical-Electrophysiological Interactions Displayed by Chemitrode Techniques," *The Limbic System: Functional Organization and Clin Disorders*, New York: Raven Press, 1986, pp. 55–65.

Giustina, A., S. Bossoni, et al., "Effect of Pretreatment with Pyridostigmine on the Thyrotropin Response to Thyrotropin-Releasing Hormone in Patients with Cushing's Disease," *Horm Metab Res*, 24, 1992, pp. 248–250.

Giustina, A., E. Bresciani, et al., "Effect of Pyridostigmine on the Growth Hormone Response to Growth-Hormone-Releasing Hormone in Lean and Obese Type II Diabetic Patients," *Metabolism*, 43(7), 1994, pp. 893–898.

Gizurarson, S., "Optimal Delivery of Vaccines. Clinical Pharmacokinetic Considerations," *Clinical Pharmacokinetics*, 30, 1996, pp. 1–15.

Glass-Marmor, L., and R. Beitner, "Effects of Carbamylcholine and Pyridostigmine on Mitochondrial-Bound Hexokinase in Skeletal Muscle and Heart," *Biochemical and Molecular Medicine*, 57, 1996, pp. 67–70.

Gleadle, R., K. Kemp, and A. Wetherell, "A Study of the Effects of Three Weeks' Treatment with Pyridostigmine Bromide on Men Undergoing Moderate to Strenuous Physical Exercise," Technical Note 568, Chemical Defence Establishment, Porton Down, U.K., March 1983a.

Gleadle, R., K. Kemp, and A. Wetherell, "Three Studies of the Effects of Four Weeks' Treatment with Pyridostigmine Bromide 3x30 mg Daily," Technical Note 585, Chemical Defence Establishment, Porton Down, U.K., September 1983b.

Gleadle, R., K. Kemp, et al., "The Effect on Man of Four Weeks' Treatment of Pyridostigmine Bromide (3x30 mg p.o. Daily)," Technical Note 682 (formerly restricted), Chemical Defence Establishment, Porton Down, U.K., 1985.

Glickson, M., A. R. Achiron, Z., et al., "The Influence of Pyridostigmine Administration on Human Neuromuscular Functions—Studies in Healthy Human Subjects," *Fundam Appl Toxicol*, 16, 1991, pp. 288–298.

Glover, V., J. Jarman, and M. Sandler, "Migraine and Depression: Biological Aspects," *J Psychiatric Res*, 27(2), 1993, pp. 223–231.

Gold, D., S. Rogacz, et al., "Rotating Shift Work, Sleep, and Accidents Related to Sleepiness in Hospital Nurses," *Am J Public Health*, 82(7), 1992, pp. 1011–1014.

Goldman, G., S. Evans, et al., "Neural Regulation of Acetylcholine Receptor Gene Expression," *Ann NY Acad Sci*, 505, 1987, pp. 286–300.

Goldstein, G., S. Beers, et al., "A Preliminary Neuropsychological Study of Persian Gulf Veterans," *JINS*, 2, 1996, pp. 001–004.

Golomb, B., "Are Placebos Bearing False Witness?" *Chemistry and Industry*, 1995, p. 900.

Golomb, B., *A Review of the Scientific Literature As It Pertains to Gulf War Illnesses*, Vol. 3: *Immunizations*, Santa Monica, Calif.: RAND, MR-1018/3, forthcoming.

Goodman, J., F. Kellogg, et al., "Decrease in Serum Cholesterol with Surgical Stress," *Cal Med*, 97(5), 1962, pp. 278–280.

Gordon, J., R. Inns, et al., "The Delayed Neuropathic Effects of Nerve Agents and Some Other Organophosphorus Compounds," *Arch Toxicol*, 52, 1983, pp. 71–82.

Gordon, J., L. Leadbeater, et al., "The Protection of Animals Against Organo-phosphate Poisoning by Pretreatment with a Carbamate," *Toxicol Appl Pharmacol*, 43, 1978, pp. 207–216.

Gordon, J., M. Maidment, and L. Leadbeater, "Carbamate Prophylaxis in the Treatment of Nerve Agent Poisoning," Chemical Defence Establishment, Porton Down, U.K., 1974.

Gordon, V., "Identification of Gulf War Syndrome: Methodological Issues and Medical Illnesses (letter)," *JAMA*, 278(5), 1997, p. 383.

Gots, R., T. Hamosh, et al., "Multiple Chemical Sensitivities: A Symposium on the State of the Science," *Regulatory Toxicology and Pharmacology*, 18, 1993, pp. 61–78.

Gouge, S., D. Daniels, et al., "Exacerbation of Asthma After Pyridostigmine During Operation Desert Storm," *Military Medicine*, 159, 1994, pp. 108–111.

Grabenstein, J., "Drug Interactions Involving Immunologic Agents. Part I. Vaccine-Vaccine, Vaccine-Immunoglobulin, and Vaccine-Drug Inter-actions," *Drug Intelligence and Clin Pharmacy*, 24, 1990, pp. 67–81.

Grady, E., M. Carpenter, et al., "Rheumatic Findings in Gulf War Veterans," *Arch Intern Med*, 158, 1998, pp. 367–371.

Graham, C., *Oral Dose Effects of Pyridostigmine on Human Performance*, 4th Annual Chemical Defense Bioscience Review, Fort Detrick, Md., 1984.

Granacher, R., and R. Baldessarini, "Physostigmine: Its Use in Acute Anti-cholinergic Syndrome with Antidepressant and Antiparkinson Drugs," *Arch Gen Psychiatry*, 32, 1975, p. 375.

Grando, S., R. Horton, et al., "A Nicotinic Acetylcholine Receptor Regulating Cell Adhesion and Motility Is Expressed in Human Keratinocytes," *J Investigative Dermatology*, 105(6), 1995, pp. 774–781.

Grant, L., D. Coscina, et al., "Muricide After Serotonin-Depleting Lesions of Midbrain Raphe Nuclei," *Pharmacol Biochem Behav*, 1, 1973, pp. 77–80.

Grauer, E., D. Ben Nathan, et al., *Cholinesterase Inhibitors Increase Blood-Brain Barrier (BBB) Permeability: Neuroinvasion of a Noninvasive Sindbis Virus as a Marker for BBB Integrity*, 1996 Medical Defense Bioscience Review, U.S. Army Medical Research and Materiel Command, 1996.

Gray, G. C., B. D. Coate, et al., "The Postwar Hospitalization Experience of U.S. Veterans of the Persian Gulf War," *New Engl J Med*, 335(20), 1996, pp. 1505–1513.

Grayston, J. T., C. C. Kuo, et al., "Chlamydia Pneumoniae, Strain TWAR and Atherosclerosis," *Eur Heart J*, 14, 1993, Supplement K, pp. 66–71.

Green, J. T., G. A. Thomas, et al., "Nicotine Enemas for Active Ulcerative Colitis—A Pilot Study," *Aliment Pharmacol Ther,* 11(5), 1997, pp. 859–863.

Greig, M., and W. Holland, "Increased Permeability of Hemoencephalic Barrier Produced by Physostigmine and Acetylcholine," *Science,* 110, 1949, p. 237.

Griffel, L., and K. M. Das, "Nicotine and Ulcerative Colitis," *Natl Med J India,* 7(5), 1994, pp. 222–223.

Grob, D., and A. Harvey, "The Effects and Treatment of Nerve Gas Poisoning," *Am J Med,* 24, 1953, pp. 52–63.

Gryboski, J., D Weinstein, et al., "Toxic Encephalopathy Apparently Related to Use of an Insect Repellent," *New Engl J Med,* 264, 1961, pp. 289–291.

Gulflink, "U.S. Troop Exposure During Khamisiyah Demolitions Not Found at Dangerous Levels," http://www.gulflink.osd.mil/news/na_plume_081997.htm, 1997.

Gunderson, C., C. Lehmann, et al., "Nerve Agents: A Review," *Neurology,* 42, 1992, pp. 946–950.

Gupta, R., G. Patterson, et al., "Mechanisms of Toxicity and Tolerance to Diisopropylphosphorofluoridate at the Neuromuscular Junction of the Rat," *Toxicol Appl Pharmacol,* 84, 1986, pp. 541–550.

Gurba, P., and R. Richardson, "Partial Characterization of Neurotoxic Esterase of Human Placenta," *Toxicol Lett,* 15, 1983, pp. 13–17.

Gurfinkel, E., G. Bozovich, et al., "Randomized Trial of Roxithromycin in Non-Q-Wave Coronary Syndromes: ROXIS Pilot Study," *Lancet,* 350, 1997, pp. 404–407.

Guslandi, M., and A. Tittobello, "Steroid-Sparing Effect of Transdermal Nicotine in Ulcerative Colitis," *J Clin Gastroenterol,* 18(4), 1994, pp. 347–348.

Guslandi, M., and A. Tittobello, "Pilot Trial of Nicotine Patches as an Alternative to Corticosteroids in Ulcerative Colitis," *J Gastroenterol,* 31(4), 1996, pp. 627–629.

Gutmann, L., and R. Besser, "Organophosphate Intoxication: Pharmacologic, Neurophysiologic, Clinical and Therapeutic Considerations," *Seminars in Neurology,* 10(1), 1990, pp. 46–51.

Gutteridge, J., G. Quinlan, et al., "Aluminium Salts Accelerate Peroxidation of Membrane Lipids Stimulated by Iron Salts," *Biochim Biophys Acta,* 835, 1985, pp. 441–447.

Haddad, P., "Newer Antidepressants and the Discontinuation Syndrome," *J of Clin Psychiatry,* 58, 1997, Supplement 7, pp. 17–22.

Haley, R., personal communication, 1997 and 1998a.

Haley, R., "Point: Bias from the 'Healthy Warrior Effect' and Unequal Follow-Up in Three Government Studies of Health Effects of the Gulf War," *Am J Epidemiol,* 148(4), 1998b, pp. 334–338.

Haley, R., "Counterpoint: Haley Replies," *Am J Epidemiol,* 148(4), 1998c, pp. 334–338.

Haley, R., and T. Kurt, "Self-Reported Exposure to Neurotoxic Chemical Combinations in the Gulf War: A Cross-Sectional Epidemiologic Study," *JAMA,* 277(3), 1997, pp. 231–237.

Haley, R., J. Hom, et al., "Evaluation of Neurologic Function in Gulf War Veterans," *JAMA,* 277(3), 1997, pp. 223–230.

Haley, R., T. Kurt, and J. Hom, "Is There a Gulf War Syndrome? Searching for Syndromes by Factor Analysis of Symptoms," *JAMA,* 277(3), 1997, pp. 215–222.

Hallak, M., and E. Giacobini, "Physostigmine, Tacrine and Metrifonate: The Effect of Multiple Doses on Acetylcholine Metabolism in Rat Brain," *Neuropharmacology,* 28, 1989, pp. 199–206.

Halliwell, B., and J. Gutteridge, "Oxygen Radicals and the Nervous System," *TINS,* 8, 1985, pp. 22–26.

Hamden, J., open letter to Gen. H. Norman Schwarzkopf, 1997.

Handbook on the Medical Aspects of NBC Defensive Operations, Section V, "Nerve Agent Pyridostigmine Pretreatment," accessed from Internet, 1997.

Handforth, A., C. M. DeGiorgio, et al., "Vagus Nerve Stimulation Therapy for Partial-Onset Seizures: A Randomized Active-Control Trial," *Neurology,* 51(1), 1998, pp. 48–55.

Hane, D., "Acute Toxicity Studies in Mice, Rats, Rabbits, and Dogs with Pyridostigmine Bromide (Ro 1-5130) and Ro1-5237/000," Nutley, N.J., Roche Laboratories (internal report), 1977.

Hanes, F., and A. Yates, "An Analysis of 400 Instances of Chronic Bromide Intoxication," *Southern Med J,* 31, 1938, pp. 667–671.

Hanin, I., "The Gulf War, Stress and a Leaky Blood-Brain Barrier," *Nature Medicine,* 2(12), 1996, pp. 1307–1308.

Haraldsson, P., C. Carenfelt, et al., "Clinical Symptoms of Sleep Apnea Syndrome and Automobile Accidents," *J of Oto-Rhino-Laryngology and Its Related Specialties,* 52(1), 1990, pp. 57–62.

Haraldsson, P., C. Carenfelt, et al., "Does Uvulopalatopharyngoplasty Inhibit Automobile Accidents?" *Laryngoscope,* 105(6), 1995, pp. 657–661.

Harden, C., American Epilepsy Society meeting, Boston, Mass., 1997.

Harden, C. L., A. Jacobs, et al., "Effect of Menopause on Epilepsy," American Epilepsy Society meeting, Boston, Mass., December 7–10, 1997, *Epilepsia,* 38, Supplement 8, 133–134.

Harder, J. A., H. F. Baker, et al., "The Role of the Central Cholinergic Projections in Cognition: Implications of the Effects of Scopolamine on Discrimination Learning by Monkeys," *Brain Res Bull,* 45(3), 1998, pp. 319–326.

Hardman, J., L. Limbird, et al., eds., *Goodman & Gilman's the Pharmacological Basis of Therapeutics*, New York: McGraw-Hill, 1996.

Harenko, A., "Irreversible Cerebello-Bulbar Syndrome as the Sequela of Bromisovalum Poisoning," *Ann Med Int Fenn,* 56, 1967, pp. 29–36.

Harik, S., and R. Kalaria, "Blood-Brain-Barrier Abnormalities in Alzheimer's Disease," *Ann NY Acad Sci,* 640, 1991, pp. 47–52.

Harris, L., B. Talbot, et al., "Oxime Induced Decarbamylation of Pyridostigmine Inhibited Acetylcholinesterase," *Proc West Pharmacol Soc,* 28, 1985, pp. 281–285.

Harris, L., B. Talbot, et al., "Oxime-Induced Decarbamylation and Atropine/Oxime Therapy of Guinea Pigs Intoxicated with Pyridostigmine," *Life Sci,* 40, 1987, pp. 577–583.

Harris, L., W. Lennox, et al., "Toxicity of Anticholinesterases: Interaction of Pyridostigmine and Physostigmine with Soman," *Drug Chem Toxicol,* 7, 1984, pp. 507–526.

Harris, L. W., B. G. Talbot, et al., "The Relationship Between Oxime-Induced Reactivation of Carbamylated Acetylcholinesterase and Antidotal Efficacy against Carbamate Intoxication," *Toxicol Appl Pharmacol,* 98(1), 1989, pp. 128–133.

Haubrich, D. R., and W. D. Reid, "Effects of Pilocarpine or Arecoline Administration on Acetylcholine Levels and Serotonin Turnover in Rat Brain," *J Pharmacol and Exp Therapeutics,* 181(1), 1972, pp. 19–27.

Hawkins, R., D. Kripke, et al., "Circadian Rhythm of Lithium Toxicity in Mice," *Psychopharmacology (Berl),* 56, 1978, pp. 113–114.

Hayward, I., H. Wall, et al., "Decreased Brain Pathology in Organophosphate Exposed Rhesus Monkeys Following Benzodiazepine Therapy," *J Neurological Sci,* 98, 1990, pp. 99–106.

Health Services, Office of the Surgeon General, "Pyridostigmine Bromide (PB) Use in Operations Desert Shield and Desert Storm (ODS)," October, 2, 1996.

Heick, H., R. Shipman, et al., "Reye-Like Syndrome Associated with Use of Insect Repellent in a Presumed Heterozygote for Ornithine Carbaryl Transferase Deficiency," *J Pediatr*, 97, 1980, pp. 471–473.

Hein, H., D. Kirsten, et al., "Nicotine as Therapy of Obstructive Sleep Apnea?" *Pneumologie*, 49, 1995, Supplement 1, pp. 185–186.

Heinemann, S., G. Asouline, et al., "Molecular Biology of the Neural and Muscle Nicotinic Acetylcholine Receptors," in S. Heinemann and J. Patrick, eds., *Molecular Neurobiology: Recombinant DNA Approaches*, New York: Plenum Press, 1987.

Hennis, P., R. Cronnelly, et al., "Metabolites of Neostigmine and Pyridostigmine Do Not Contribute to Antagonism of Neuromuscular Blockade in the Dog," *Anesthesiology*, 61, 1984, pp. 534–539.

Hery, F. S. Burgoin, et al., "Control of the Release of Newly Synthesized 3H-5-Hydroxytryptamine by Nicotinic and Muscarinic Receptors in Rat Hypothalmic Slices, *Naunyn-Schmiedeberg's Archives of Pharmacol*, 296(2), 1977, pp. 91–97.

Heuser, G., I. Mena, et al., "Neurospect Findings in Patients Exposed to Neurotoxic Chemicals," *Toxicol Ind Health*, 10(4/5), 1994, pp. 561–571.

Hide, D., S. Matthews, et al., "Allergen Avoidance in Infancy and Allergy at 4 Years of Age," *Allergy*, 51, 1996, pp. 89–93.

Hilborne, L., and B. Golomb, *A Review of the Scientific Literature As It Pertains to Gulf War Illnesses, Vol. 1: Infectious Diseases*, Santa Monica, Calif.: RAND, MR-1018/1, forthcoming.

Hill, D., and N. Thomas, "Reactivation by 2-PAM Cl of Human Red Blood Cell Cholinesterase Poisoned in Vitro by Cyclohexylmethylphosphonofluoridate (GF)," Edgewood Arsenal, Md.: Medical Research Laboratory, 1969.

Hillhouse, E., J. Burden, et al., "The Effect of Various Putative Neurotransmitters on the Release of Corticotrophin Releasing Hormone from the Hypothalamus of the Rat in Vitro. I. The Effect of Acetylcholine and Noradrenaline," *Neuroendocrinology*, 17, 1975, p. 1.

Hitzig, P., "Fen/Phen and Gulf War Syndrome," http://www.fenphen.com/gulfwar-experiences.html., accessed 1997.

Holinger, P., and E. Klemen, "Violent Deaths in the United States, 1900–1975: Relationships Between Suicide, Homicide and Accidental Deaths," *Soc Sci Med*, 16(22), 1982, pp. 1929–1938.

Holladay, M. W., J. T. Wasicak, et al., "Identification and Initial Structure-Activity Relationships of (R)-5-(2-Azetidinylmethoxy)-2-Chloropyridine (ABT-594), a Potent, Orally Active, Non-Opiate Analgesic Agent Acting Via Neuronal Nicotinic Acetylcholine Receptors," *J Med Chem*, 41(4), 1998, pp. 407–412.

Holmes, J., "Organophosphorus Insecticides in Colorado," *Arch Environ Health*, 9, 1964, pp. 445–453.

Hood, L., "Myasthenia Gravis: Regimens and Regime-Associated Problems in Adults," *J Neurosci Nurs*, 22, 1990, pp. 358–364.

Hom, J., R. Haley, et al., "Neuropsychological Correlates of Gulf War Syndrome," *Arch Clin Neuropsychol*, 12(6), 1997, pp. 531–544.

Horowitz, B., "Bromism from Excessive Cola Consumption," *Clinical Toxicology*, 35(3), 1997, pp. 315–320.

Hubble, J. P., T. Cao, et al., "Risk Factors for Parkinson's Disease," *Neurology*, 43(9), 1993, pp. 1693–1697.

Hubert, M., and D. Lison, "Study of Muscular Effects of Short-Term Pyridostigmine Treatment in Resting and Exercising Rats," *Human and Experimental Toxicology*, 14, 1995, pp. 49–54.

Hudson, C., "The Effects of Pyridostigmine and Physostigmine on the Cholinergic Synapse," Fort Detrick, Md.: U.S. Army Medical Research and Development Command, 1985.

Hudson, C., J. Rash, et al., "Neostigmine-Induced Alterations at the Mammalian Neuromuscular Junction. II. Ultrastructure," *J of Pharmacol Exp Therapeutics*, 205(2), 1978, pp. 340–356.

Hudson, C., and R. Foster, "Ultrastructural Pathology in Mammalian Skeletal Muscle Following Acute and Subacute Exposure to Pyridostigmine. Studies of Dose-Response and Recovery," *4th Annual Chemical Defense Bioscience Review*, 1984, pp. 131–171.

Hudson, C., R. Foster, et al., "Neuromuscular Toxicity of Pyridostigmine Bromide in the Diaphragm, Extensor Digitorum Longus, and Soleus Muscles of the Rat," *Fundam Appl Toxicol*, 5, 1985, pp. S260–S269.

Hulihan-Giblin, B., M. Lumpkin, et al., "Acute Effects of Nicotine on Prolactin Release in the Rat: Agonist and Antagonist Effects of a Single Injection of Nicotine," *J Pharmacol Exp Therapeutics*, 252(1), 1990, pp. 15–20.

Hulihan-Giblin, B., M. Lumpkin, et al., "Effects of Chronic Administration of Nicotine on Prolactin Release in the Rat: Inactivation of Prolactin Response by Repeated Injections of Nicotine," *J Pharmacol Exp Therapeutics*, 252(1), 1990, pp. 21–25.

Husain, K., R. Vijayaraghavan, et al., "Delayed Neurotoxic Effect of Sarin in Mice after Repeated Inhalation Exposure," *J Appl Toxicol*, 13(2), 1993, pp. 143–145.

Hussain, A., and W. Ritschel, "Influence of Dimethylacetamine, *N, N*-Diethyl-m-Toluamide, and 1-Dodecylazacycloheptan-2-One on ex Vivo Permeation of Phosphonoformic Acid Through Rat Skin," *Methods Fundam Exp Clin Pharmacol*, 10, 1988, pp. 691–694.

Hyams, K., F. Hanson, et al., "The Impact of Infectious Diseases on the Health of U.S. Forces Deployed to the Persian Gulf During Operations Desert Shield and Desert Storm," *Clin Infect Dis*, 20(6), 1995, pp. 1497–1504.

Hyams, K., F. Wignall, et al., "War Syndromes and Their Evaluation: From the U.S. Civil War to the Persian Gulf War," *Annals of Internal Medicine*, 125(5), 1996, pp. 398–405.

Hyams, K. C., and F. S. Wignall, "Identification of Gulf War Syndrome: Methodological Issues and Medical Illnesses" (letter, comment), *JAMA*, 278(5), 1997, p. 384, pp. 385–387 (discussion).

Idriss, M., L. Aguayo, et al., "Organophosphate and Carbamate Compounds Have Pre- and Post-Junctional Effects at the Insect Glutamatergic Synapse," *J Pharmacol Exp Therapeutics*, 239(1), 1986, pp. 279–285.

Iidaka, T., T. Nakajima, et al., "Quantitative Regional Cerebral Flow Measured by Tc-99M HMPAO SPECT in Mood Disorder," *Psychiatry Res*, 68(2-3), 1997, pp. 143–154.

Inns, R., and L. Leadbeater, "The Efficacy of Bispyridinium Derivatives in Treatment of Organophosphate Poisoning in the Guinea-Pig," *J Pharm Pharmacol*, 35, 1983, pp. 427–433.

Institute of Medicine: Division of Health Promotion and Disease Prevention, Committee on the Evaluation of the Department of Defense Comprehensive Clinical Evaluation Program, *Adequacy of the Comprehensive Clinical Evaluation Program: Nerve Agents*, Washington, D.C.: National Academy Press, 1997.

Iowa Persian Gulf Study Group, "Self-Reported Illness and Health Status Among Gulf War Veterans: A Population-Based Study," *JAMA*, 277, 1997, pp. 238–245.

Ito, H., R. Kawashima, et al., "Hypoperfusion in the Limbic System and Prefrontal Cortex in Depression: SPECT with Anatomic Standardization Technique [see comments]," *J Nucl Med*, 37(3), 1996, pp. 410–414.

Ito, T., N. Akiyama, et al., "Changes in Myocardial Mitochondrial Electron Transport Activity in Rats Administered with Acetylcholinesterase Inhibitor," *Biochem Biophys Res Commun*, 164, 1989, pp. 997–1002.

Iwasaki, Y., N. Wakata, et al., "Parkinsonism Induced by Pyridostigmine," *Acta Neurol Scand,* 78, 1988, p. 236.

Izraeli, S., D. Avgar, et al., "The Effect of Repeated Doses of 30 Mg Pyridostigmine Bromide on Pilot Performance in an A-4 Flight Simulator," *Aviat Space Environ Med,* 61, 1990, pp. 430–432.

Jacobs, D., M. Tang, et al., "Cognitive Function in Nondemented Women Who Took Estrogen After Menopause," *Neurology,* 50(2), 1998, pp. 368–373.

Jamal, G., "Long Term Neurotoxic Effects of Chemical Warfare Organophosphate Compounds (Sarin)," *Adverse Drug React Toxicol Rev,* 14(2), 1995a, pp. 83–84.

Jamal, G., "Long Term Neurotoxic Effects of Organophosphate Compounds," *Adverse Drug React Toxicol Rev,* 14(2), 1995b, pp. 85–99.

Jamal, G., S. Hansen, et al., "The 'Gulf War Syndrome.' Is There Evidence of Dysfunction in the Nervous System?" *J of Neurology, Neurosurgery, and Psychiatry,* 60, 1996, pp. 449–451.

Janowsky, D., personal communication, 1997.

Janowsky, D., A. Abrams, et al., "Lithium Administration Antagonizes Cholinergic Behavioral Effects in Rodents," *Psychopharmacology (Berl),* 63, 1979, pp. 147–150.

Janowsky, D., K. El-Yousef, et al., "Parasympathetic Suppression of Manic Symptoms by Physostigmine," *Arch Gen Psychiatry,* 28, 1973, pp. 542–547.

Janowsky, D., K. El-Yousef, et al., "Acetylcholine and Depression," *Psychosomatic Medicine,* 36(3), 1974, pp. 248–257.

Janowsky, D., and D. Overstreet, "Cholinergic Dysfunction in Depression," *Pharmacol Toxicol,* 66, 1990, pp. 100–111.

Janowsky, D., and D. Overstreet, "The Role of Acetylcholine Mechanisms in Mood Disorders," Chapter 82, in F. Bloom and D. Kupfer, eds., *Psychopharmacology: The Fourth Generation of Progress,* New York: Raven Press, Ltd., 1995.

Janowsky, D., D. Overstreet, et al., "Is Cholinergic Sensitivity a Genetic Marker for the Affective Disorders?" *Am J Medical Genetics,* 54(3), 1994, pp. 335–344.

Janowsky, D., and S. C. Risch, "Cholinomimetic and Anti Cholinergic Drugs Used to Investigate an Acetylcholine Hypothesis of Affective Disorders and Stress," *Drug Dev Res,* 1984, pp. 125–142.

Janowsky, D., and S. C. Risch, "Adrenergic-Cholinergic Balance and Affective Disorders," in A. Rush and K. Altschuler, eds., *Depression: Basic Mechanisms, Diagnosis, and Treatment,* New York: The Guilford Press, 1986.

Janowsky, D., and S. C. Risch, "Role of Acetylcholine Mechanisms in the Affective Disorders," in H. Meltzer, ed., *Psychopharmacology: The Third Generation of Progress,* New York: Raven Press, Ltd., 1987.

Janowsky, D., S. C. Risch, et al., "Increased Vulnerability to Cholinergic Stimulation in Affective Disorder Patients," *Psychopharmacol Bull,* 16, 1980, pp. 29–31.

Janowsky, D., S. C. Risch, et al., "Adrenergic-Cholinergic Balance and the Treatment of Affective Disorders," *Prog Neuropsychopharmacol Biol Psychiatry,* 7, 1983, pp. 297–307.

Janowsky, D., S. C. Risch, et al., "Central Cardiovascular Effects of Physostigmine in Humans," *Hypertension,* 7, 1985, pp. 140–145.

Janowsky, D., S. C. Risch, et al., "Effects of Physostigmine on Pulse, Blood Pressure and Serum Epinephrine Levels," *Am J Psychiatry,* 142, 1985, pp. 738–740.

Janowsky, D., S. C. Risch, et al., "Physostigmine-Induced Epinephrine Release in Patients with Affective Disorder," *Am J Psychiatry,* 143, 1986, pp. 919–921.

Janowsky, D., S. C. Risch, et al., "Cholinergic Involvement in Affective Illness," in A. Sen and T. Lee, eds., *Intercellular and Intracellular Communications, 3. Receptors and Ligands in Psychiatry,* New York: Cambridge University Press, 1988.

Janowsky, D., S. C. Risch, et al., "Increased Vulnerability to Cholinergic Stimulation in Affect Disorder Patients," *Psychopharmacol Bull,* 16, 1980, pp. 29–31.

Janowsky, D., S. C. Risch, et al., "Cholinergic Supersensitivity in Affect Disorder Patients: Behavioral and Neuroendocrine Observations," *Psychopharmacol Bull,* 17, 1981, pp. 129–132.

Javoy, F., Y. Agid, et al., "Changes in Neostriatal Dopamine Metabolism After Carbachol or Atropine Microinjections into the Substantia Nigra," *Brain Res,* 68, 1974, p. 253.

Jenson, F., L. Nielsen, et al., "Detection of the Plasma Cholinesterase K Variant Using an Amplification-Created Restriction Site," *Hum Heredity,* 46, 1996, pp. 26–31.

Johansson, M., E. Hellstrom-Lindahl, et al., "Steady-State Pharmacokinetics of Tacrine in Long-Term Treatment of Alzheimer Patients," *Dementia,* 7(2), 1996, pp. 111–117.

Johansson, U., A. Fredriksson, and P. Eriksson, "Bioallethrin Causes Permanent Changes in Behavioural and Muscarinic Acetylcholine Receptor Variables in Adult Mice Exposed Neonatally to DDT, *Eur J Pharmacol,* 293(2), 1995, pp. 159–166.

Johnson, M., "A Phosphorylation Site in Brain and the Delayed Neurotoxic Effect of Some Organophosphorus Compounds," *Biochem J,* 111, 1969, pp. 487–495.

Johnson, M., "Organophosphorus Esters Causing Delayed Neurotoxic Effects," *Arch Toxicol,* 34, 1975, pp. 259–288.

Johnson, M., "Improved Assay of Neurotoxic Esterase for Screening Organophosphates for Delayed Neurotoxicity Potential," *Arch Toxicol,* 37, 1977, pp. 113–115.

Johnson, M., "The Target for Initiation of Delayed Neurotoxicity by Organophosphorus Esters: Biochemical Studies and Toxicological Applications," *Rev Biochem Toxicol,* 4, 1982, p. 141.

Johnson, M., and R. Richardson, "Biochemical End Points: Neurotoxic Esterase Assay," *Neurotoxicology,* 4, 1983, pp. 311–320.

Joiner, R., G. Dill, et al., "Evaluating the Efficacy of Antidote Drug Combinations Against Soman or Tabun Toxicity in the Rabbit," Columbus, Ohio: Battelle Memorial Institute, 1989.

Jolly, E., R. Gleadle, et al., "Investigation of Possible Interaction Between Pyridostigmine Pretreatment and a Thermally Stressful Environment," Institute of Naval Medicine (UK), 1981.

Jones, D., W. J. Carter, et al., "Assessing Pyridostigmine Efficacy by Response Surface Modeling," *Fundam Appl Toxicol,* 5, 1985, pp. S242–S251.

Joo, F., and T. Varkonyi, "Correlation Between the Cholinesterase Activity of Capillaries and the Blood-Brain Barrier in the Rat," *Acta Biol Acad Sci Hung,* 20, 1969, pp. 359–372.

Joseph, S., "A Comprehensive Clinical Evaluation of 20,000 Persian Gulf War Veterans," *Military Medicine,* 162(3), 1997, pp. 149–155.

Jusko, W. J., and H. C. Ko, "Physiologic Indirect Response Models Characterize Diverse Types of Pharmacodynamic Effects" (see comments), *Clin Pharmacol Therapeutics,* 56(4), 1994, pp. 406–419.

Kalow, W., and N. Staron, "On Distribution and Inheritance of Atypical Forms of Human Serum Cholinesterase, as Indicated by Dibucaine Number," *Can J Biochem Physiol,* 35, 1957, p. 1305.

Kamal, M. A., and A. A. al-Jafari, "The Preparation and Kinetic Analysis of Multiple Forms of Human Erythrocyte Acetylcholinesterase," *Prep Biochem Biotechnol,* 26(2), 1996, pp. 105–119.

Kang, H., and T. Bullman, *A Mortality Follow-Up Study of Persian Gulf War Veterans (Abstr)*, 123rd Annual Meeting of the American Public Health Association, 1995.

Kang, H., and T. Bullman, "Mortality Among US Veterans of the Persian Gulf War," *New Engl J Med*, 335(20), 1996, pp. 1498–1504.

Kantak, K., L. Hegstrand, et al., "Dietary Tryptophan Modulation and Aggressive Behavior in Mice," *Pharmacol Biochem Behav*, 12, 1980, pp. 675–679.

Kao, K. P., S. Y. Kwan, et al., "Coexistence of Parkinson's Disease and Myasthenia Gravis: A Case Report," *Clin Neurol Neurosurg*, 95(2), 1993, pp. 137–139.

Kaplan, J., J. Kessler, et al., "Sensory Neuropathy Associated with Dursban (Chlorpyrifos) Exposure," *Neurology*, 43, 1993, pp. 2193–2196.

Kare, M., "Direct Pathways to the Brain," *Science*, 163, 1968, pp. 952–953.

Karler, R., K. Finnegan, et al., "Blockade of Behavioral Sensitization to Cocaine and Amphetamine by Inhibitors of Protein Synthesis," *Brain Res*, 603, 1993, pp. 19–24.

Kato, T., S. Sugiyama, et al., "Role of Acetylcholine in Pyridostigmine-Induced Myocardial Injury: Possible Involvement of Parasympathetic Nervous System in the Genesis of Cardiomyopathy," *Arch Toxicol*, 63, 1989, pp. 137–143.

Kaube, H., K. L. Hoskin, and P. J. Goadsby, "Inhibition by Sumatriptan of Central Trigeminal Neurones Only After Blood-Brain Barrier Disruption," *Brit J Pharmacol*, 109(3), 1993, pp. 788–792.

Kaufer, D., A. Friedman, et al., "Acute Stress Facilitates Long-Lasting Changes in Cholinergic Gene Expression [see comments]," *Nature*, 393(6683), 1998, pp. 373–377.

Kaufer, D., A. Friedman, et al., "Anticholinesterases Induce Multigenic Transcriptional Feedback Response Suppressing Cholinergic Neurotransmission," *Chemico-Biologic Interactions*, 120, 1999, pp. 249–360.

Kawabuchi, M., "Neostigmine Myopathy Is a Calcium Ion-Mediated Myopathy Initially Affecting the Motor End-Plate," *J Neuropathol Exp Neurol*, 41, 1982, pp. 298–314.

Kawabuchi, M., M. Osame, et al., "Myopathic Changes at the End-Plate Region Induced by Neostigmine Methylsulfate," *Experientia*, 32, 1976, pp. 623–625.

Kayadjanian, N., S. Retaux, et al., "Stimulation by Nicotine of the Spontaneous Release of [3H]Gamma-Aminobutyric Acid in the Substantia Nigra and in the Globus Pallidus of the Rat," *Brain Res*, 649(1-2), 1994, pp. 129–135.

Keeler, J., "Drug Interactions of Combined Use of Nerve Agent Pretreatment with Anesthetics, Analgesics, and Other Battlefield Medications," Aberdeen Proving Ground, Md,: U.S. Army Medical Research Institute of Chemical Defense, 1988.

Keeler, J., "Interactions Between Nerve Agent Pretreatment and Drugs Commonly Used in Combat Anesthesia," *Military Medicine*, 155, 1990, pp. 527–533.

Keeler, J. R., C. G. Hurst, et al., "Pyridostigmine Used as a Nerve Agent Pretreatment Under Wartime Conditions," *JAMA*, 266(5), 1991, pp. 693–695.

Kemp, R., and A. Wetherell, "A Lab Study of the Performance of Men Taking Pyridostigmine Bromide Orally for Two Weeks," Chemical Defence Establishment, Porton Down, U.K., 1981.

Kennedy, B., D. Janowsky, et al., "Central Cholinergic Stimulation Causes Adrenal Epinephrine Release," *J Clin Invest*, 74, 1984, pp. 972–975.

Kennedy, P., "Oesophageal Spasm as a Side Effect of Nerve Agent Pretreatment System (letter)," *J Royal Army Medical Corps*, 137, 1991, pp. 152–153.

Kerenyi, S., M. Murphy, et al., "Toxic Interactions Between Repeated Soman and Chronic Pyridostigmine in Rodents," *Pharmacology Biochemistry and Behavior*, 37, 1990, pp. 267–271.

Ketchum, J., F. Sidell, et al., "Atropine, Scopolamine, and Ditran: Comparative Pharmacology and Antagonists in Man," *Psychopharmacologia (Berl)*, 28, 1973, p. 121.

Khan, I. M., T. L. Yaksh, et al., "Epibatidine Binding Sites and Activity in the Spinal Cord," *Brain Res*, 753(2), 1997, pp. 269–282.

Kisters, K., C. Spieker, et al., "Clinical Aspects of Aluminium Metabolism and Aluminium Containing Drugs," in P. Collery, L. Poirier, et al., eds., *Metal Ions in Biology and Medicine*, Paris: John Libbey, 1990, pp. 320–322.

Kleinrok, Z., E. Jagiello-Wojtowicz, and M. Sieklucka, "Influence of Fluorostigmine on Some Parameters of the Catecholaminergic and Serotoninergic Systems in the Mouse Brain," *Archivum Immunologiae et Therapiae Experimentalis*, 23(6), 1975, pp. 769–776.

Kluwe, W., J. Chinn, et al., "Efficacy of Pyridostigmine Pretreatment Against Acute Soman Intoxication in a Primate Model," *Sixth Medical Chemical Defense Bioscience Review*, Aberdeen Proving Ground, Md.: U.S. Army Medical Research Institute of Chemical Defense, 1987, pp. 227–234.

Koelle, G., "Protection of Cholinesterase Against Irreversible Activation by DFP in Vitro," *J Pharmacol Exp Therapeutics*, 88, 1946, pp. 232–237.

Koelle, G., "Histochemical Localization of Cholinesterases in the Central Nervous System of the Rat," *J Pharmacol Exp Therapeutics,* 106, 1952, p. 401.

Kohler, E. C., L. V. Riters, et al., "The Muscarinic Acetylcholine Antagonist Scopolamine Impairs Short-Distance Homing Pigeon Navigation," *Physiol Behav,* 60(4), 1996, pp. 1057–1061.

Kok, A., "REM Sleep Pathways and Anticholinesterase Intoxication: A Mechanism for Nerve Agent–Induced Central Respiratory Failure," *Medical Hypotheses,* 41, 1993, pp. 141–149.

Kolka, M., and L. Stephenson, "Human Temperature Regulation During Exercise After Oral Pyridostigmine Administration," *Aviat Space Environ Med,* 61, 1990, pp. 220–224.

Kolka, M., P. Burgoon, et al., "Multiple Dose Pyridostigmine Administration: Cardiovascular Effects at Rest During Acute Heat and Altitude Exposure," U.S. Army Research Institute of Environmental Medicine, 1991a.

Kolka, M., P. Burgoon, et al., "Red Blood Cell Cholinesterase Activity and Plasma Pyridostigmine Concentration During Single and Multiple Dose Studies," U.S. Army Research Institute of Environmental Medicine, 1991b.

Kondo, S., T. Mizuno, et al., "Effects of Penetration Enhancers on Percutaneous Absorption of Nifedipine. Comparison Between Deet and Azone," *J Pharmacobiodyn,* 11(2), 1988, pp. 88–94.

Koplovitz, I., "U.S. Strategy for the Evaluation of Nerve Agent Countermeasures," NATO Unclassified, undated.

Koplovitz, I., V. Gresham, et al., "Evaluation of the Toxicity, Pathology, and Treatment of Cyclohexylmethylphosphono-Fluoridate (CMFF) Poisoning in Rhesus Monkeys," *Arch Toxicol,* 66, 1992, pp. 622–628.

Koplovitz, I., L. Harris, et al., "Reduction by Pyridostigmine Pretreatment of the Efficacy of Atropine and 2-PAM Treatment of Sarin and VX Poisoning in Rodents," *Fundam Appl Toxicol,* 18, 1992, pp. 102–106.

Koplovitz, I., and J. Stewart, "A Comparison of the Efficacy of HI6 and 2-PAM Against Soman, Tabun, Sarin, and VX in the Rabbit," *Toxicol Lett,* 70, 1994, pp. 269–279.

Kornfeld, P., A. Samuels, et al., "Metabolism of 14C-Labeled Pyridostigmine in Myasthenia Gravis," *Neurology,* 20, 1970, pp. 634–641.

Kornhauser, D., B. Petty, et al., unpublished data on safety, tolerance, pharmacokinetics, and pharmacodynamics of intravenous pyridostigmine and oral doses of standard and sustained-release pyridostigmine in healthy men and influence of food on oral pyridostigmine, cited in Sidell (1990).

Korpela, M., and H. Tahti, "Effect of Organic Solvents on Human Erythrocyte Membrane Acetylcholinesterase Activity in Vitro: Toxic Interfaces of Neurones, Smoke, and Genes," *Arch Toxicol Suppl,* 9, 1986, pp. 320–323.

Korpela, M., H. Tahti, et al., "The Effect of Selected Organic Solvents on Intact Human Red Cell Membrane Acetylcholinesterase in Vitro," *Toxicol Appl Pharmacol,* 85, 1986, pp. 257–262.

Korsak, R., and M. Sato, "Effects of Chronic Organophosphate Pesticide Exposure on the Central Nervous System," *Clin Toxicol,* 11, 1977, pp. 83–95.

Koster, R., "Synergisms and Antagonisms Between Physostigmine and Di-Isopropyl Fluorophosphate in Cats," *J Pharmacol Exp Therapeutics,* 88, 1946, pp. 39–46.

Kostka, G., D. Palut, et al., "The Effect of Permethrin and DDT on the Activity of Cytochrome P-450 1A and 2B Molecular Forms in Rat Liver," *Rocz Panstw Zakl Hig,* 48(3), 1997, pp. 229–237.

Kostowski, W., and L. Valzelli, "Biochemical and Behavioral Effects of Lesions of Raphe Nuclei in Aggressive Mice," *Pharmacol Biochem Behav,* 2, 1974, pp. 277–280.

Kotler-Cope, S., J. Milby, et al., "Neuropsychological Deficits in Persian Gulf War (PGW) Veterans. A Preliminary Report (abstract)," *J of the International Neuropsychological Society,* 2, 1996, p. 63.

Kramer, P., and C. McClain, "Depression of Aminopyrine Metabolism by Influenza Vaccine," *New Engl J Med,* 305, 1981, pp. 1262–1264.

Krausz, Y., O. Bonne, et al., "Brain SPECT Imaging of Neuropsychiatric Disorders," *Eur J Radiol,* 21(3), 1996, pp. 183–187.

Kuffler, S., and D. Yoshikami, "The Number of Transmitter Molecules in a Quantum: An Estimate from Iontophoretic Application of Acetylcholine at the Neuromuscular Junction," *J Physiol,* 251, 1975, pp. 465–482.

Kuffler, S., J. Nicholls, et al., *From Neuron to Brain.* Sunderland, Mass.: Sinauer Associates, Inc., 1984.

Kulkarni, A., "Muricidal Block Produced by 5-Hydroxytryptophan and Various Other Drugs," *Life Sci,* 7, 1968, pp. 125–128.

Kunze, U., "Chronic Bromide Intoxication with a Severe Neurological Deficit," *J Neurol,* 213, 1976, pp. 149–152.

Laine-Cessac, P., A. Turcant, et al., "Inhibition of Cholinesterases by Histamine 2 Receptor Antagonist Drugs," *Res Commun in Chem Pathol and Pharmacol,* 79(2), 1993, pp. 185–193.

Lallement, G., A. Foquin, et al., "Heat Stress, Even Extreme, Does Not Induce Penetration of Pyridostigmine into the Brain of Guinea-Pigs (abstract)," *U.S. Army Medical Research and Materiel Command, Bioscience Review Program Book*, 1998, p. 201.

Landauer, W., "Cholinomimetic Teratogens: Studies with Chicken Embryos," *Teratology*, 12, 1975, pp. 125–146.

Landrigan, P., D. Graham, et al., "Environmental Neurotoxic Illness: Research for Prevention," *Environmental Health Perspectives*, 102, 1994, Supplement 2, pp. 117–120.

Lange, G., L. Tiersky, et al., *The Relationship Between Psychiatric Diagnoses and Fatiguing Illness in Gulf War Veterans*, Conference on Federally Sponsored Gulf War Veterans' Illnesses Research, June 17–19, 1998a, Pentagon City, Va.

Lange, G., L. Tiersky, et al., *Pattern of Cognitive Function in Registry Gulf War Veterans: A Preliminary Study [abstract]*, Conference on Federally Sponsored Gulf War Veterans' Illnesses Research, June 17–19, 1998b, Pentagon City, Va.

Langenberg, J., L. De Jong, et al., "Protection of Guinea Pigs Against Soman Poisoning by Pretreatment with P-Nitrophenyl Phosphoramidates," *Toxicol Appl Pharmacol*, 140, 1996, pp. 444–450.

Lashner, B. A., S. B. Hanauer, and M. D. Silverstein, "Testing Nicotine Gum for Ulcerative Colitis Patients. Experience with Single-Patient Trials," *Digestive Diseases and Sci*, 35(7), 1990, pp. 827–832.

Laskowski, M., W. Olson, et al., "Ultrastructural Changes at the Motor End-Plate Produced by an Irreversible Cholinesterase Inhibitor," *Exp Neurol*, 47, 1975, pp. 290–306.

Laskowski, M., W. Olson, et al., "Initial Ultrastructural Abnormalities at the Motor End Plate Produced by a Cholinesterase Inhibitor," *Exp Neurol*, 57, 1977, pp. 13–33.

Lasseter, K., and D. Garg, "A Study to Evaluate the Safety, Tolerance, Pharmacokinetics and Pharmacodynamics of Pyridostigmine When Given in Single and Multiple Doses to Males and Females in Different Weight Groups," Department of the Army, 1996.

Latven, A., and A. Sloane, "A Toxicologic Appraisal of Mestinon Bromide," Darby, Pa.: Pharmacology Research, Inc. (internal report), 1954.

Leadbeater, L., R. Inns, et al., "Treatment of Poisoning by Soman," *Fundam Appl Toxicol*, 5, 1985, pp. S225–S231.

Leber, P., letter from Director, Division of Neuropharmacological Drug Products, Office of Drug Evaluation I, Center for Drug Evaluation and Research, to

Dr. Ronald E. Clawson, Office of the Surgeon General, Department of the Army, Human Use Review and Regulatory Affairs, Fort Detrick, Md., 1994.

Lederberg, J., "Report of the Defense Science Board (DSB) Task Force on Persian Gulf War Health Effects," Washington, D.C.: Office of the Secretary of Defense, 1994.

Lee, B., T. Stelly, et al., "Inhibition of Acetylcholinesterase by Hemicholiniums, Conformationally Constrained Choline Analogues. Evaluation of Aryl and Alkyl Substituents. Comparisons with Choline and (3-Hydroxyphenyl) Trimethylammonium," *Chem Res Toxicol*, 5(3), 1992, pp. 411–418.

Lees-Haley, P., and R. Brown, "Biases in Perception and Reporting Following a Perceived Toxic Exposure," *Perceptual and Motor Skills*, 75, 1992, pp. 531–544.

Lehmann, D., C. Johnston, et al., "Synergy Between the Genes for Butyrylcholinesterase K Variant and Apolipoprotein E4 in Late-Onset Confirmed Alzheimer's Disease," *Hum Mol Genet*, 6, 1997, pp. 1933–1936.

Lejoyeux, M., and J. Ades, "Antidepressant Discontinuation: A Review of the Literature," *J of Clin Psychiatry*, 58, 1997, Supplement 7, pp. 11–16.

Lemmer, B., "Clinical Chronopharmacology: The Importance of Time in Drug Treatment," *Ciba Found Symp*, 183, 1995, pp. 235–247; discussion pp. 247–253.

Lena, C., and J.-P. Changeux, "Pathological Mutations of Nicotinic Receptors and Nicotine-Based Therapies for Brain Disorders," *Current Opinion in Neurobiology*, 7, 1997, pp. 674–682.

Lena, C., J.-P. Changeux, et al., "Evidence for 'Preterminal' Nicotinic Receptors on GABAergic Axons in the Rat Interpeduncular Nucleus," *J Neurosci*, 13, 1993, pp. 2680–2688.

Lennox, W., L. Harris, et al., "Relationship Between Reversible Acetylcholinesterase Inhibition and Efficacy Against Soman Lethality," *Life Sci*, 37, 1985, pp. 793–798.

Leo, K., and J. Grace, "The Metabolism of Proposed Nerve Agent Pretreatment, Pyridostigmine Bromide," in J. King, ed., *Medical Defense Bioscience Review: Proceedings*, U.S. Army Medical Research and Materiel Command, 2, 1996, pp. 1272–1283.

Leonard, J., and M. Salpeter, "Agonist Induced Myopathy at the Neuromuscular Junction Is Mediated by Calcium," *J Cell Biol*, 82, 1979, pp. 811–819.

Leon-S, F., G. Pradilla, and Vezga, "Neurological Effects of Organophosphate Pesticides," *BMJ*, 313, 1996, pp. 690–691.

Leon-S, F., G. Pradilla, et al., "Multisystem Failure Atrophy, Intermediate Syndrome, Anticholinesterase Treatment and Congenital Acetylcholinesterase Deficiency: The Linkage Is Puzzling," *J Toxicol Clin Toxicol*, 34, 1996a, pp. 245–246.

Leon-S, F., G. Pradilla, et al., "Multiple System Organ Failure, Intermediate Syndrome, Congenital Myasthenic Syndrome, and Anticholinesterase Treatment: The Linkage Is Puzzling" (letter, comment), *J Toxicol Clin Toxicol*, 34(2), 1996b, pp. 245–247.

Leopold, I. H., and P. R. McDonald, "Diisopropyl Fluorophosphate (DFP) in Treatment of Glaucoma. Further Observations," *Arch Ophthalmol*, 40, 1948, pp. 176–186.

Lester, A., and J. Dani, *Desensitization by Nicotine of Central Acetylcholine Receptors*, International Symposium on the Cholinergic Synapse: Structure, Function and Regulation (3rd), University of Maryland, Baltimore, 1994.

Levey, A. I., "Muscarinic Acetylcholine Receptor Expression in Memory Circuits: Implications for Treatment of Alzheimer Disease," *Proc Natl Acad Sci USA*, 93(24), 1996, pp. 13541–13546.

Levi, F., S. Giacchetti, et al., "Chronomodulation of Chemotherapy Against Metastatic Colorectal Cancer. International Organization for Cancer Chronotherapy," *Eur J Cancer*, 31A(7-8), pp. 1264–1270.

Levin, A., and V. Byers, "Multiple Chemical Sensitivities: A Practicing Clinician's Point of View. Clinical and Immunological Research Findings," *Toxicol Ind Health*, 8, 1992, pp. 95–109.

Levin, E., C. Conners, et al., "Nicotine Effects on Adults with Attention-Deficit/Hyperactivity Disorder," *Psychopharmacology*, 123, 1996, pp. 55–63.

Levin, E. D., D. Torry, et al., "Is Binding to Nicotinic Acetylcholine and Dopamine Receptors Related to Working Memory in Rats?" *Brain Res Bull*, 43(3), 1997, pp. 295–304.

Levin, H., R. Rodnitzky, et al., "Anxiety Associated with Exposure to Organophosphate Compounds," *Arch Gen Psychiatry*, 33, 1976, pp. 225–228.

Levin, M., "Eye Disturbances in Bromide Intoxication," *Amer J Ophthalmol*, 50, 1960, pp. 478–483.

Levine, B., and R. Parker, "Reproductive and Developmental Toxicity Studies of Pyridostigmine Bromide in Rats," *Toxicology*, 69(3), 1991, pp. 291–300.

Levine, L., M. Kolka, et al., "Respiratory and Skeletal Muscle Function After Acute Pyridostigmine Bromide Administration," U.S. Army Research Institute of Environmental Medicine, 1991.

Levitzki, A., "Bacterial Adaptation, Visual Adaptation, Receptor Desensitization—A Common Link?" *Trends Pharmacol Sci,* 7, 1986, pp. 3–6.

Li, W.-F., L. Costa, et al., "Serum Paraoxonase Status: A Major Factor in Determining Resistance to Organophosphates," *J Tox Envir Hlth,* 40, 1993, pp. 337–346.

Lieske, C., R. Gepp, et al., "Cholinesterase Studies with (R) (+)-and (S) (-)-5-(1,3,3-Trimethylindolinyl)-N- (1-Phenylethyl)Carbamate," *J Enzyme Inhibition,* 6, 1993, pp. 283–291.

Lietman, P., and B. Petty, "Phase I Clinical Pharmacology Studies," Fort Detrick, Md.: U.S. Army Medical Research and Development Command, 1993.

Ligget, S., and C. Daughaday, "Ipratropium in Patients with COPD Receiving Cholinesterase Inhibitors," *Chest,* 94, 1988, pp. 210–212.

Lintern, M., M. Smith, et al., "Effect of Repeated Treatment with Pyridostigmine on Acetylcholinesterase in Mouse Muscles," *Human and Experimental Toxicology,* 16, 1997, pp. 158–165.

Lintern, M., M. Smith, et al., "The Effect of Repeated Treatment with Pyridostigmine on the Activity of Acetylcholinesterase Molecular Forms in Mouse Skeletal Muscle," *Br J Pharmacol,* 116, 1995, p. 81P.

Lintern, M., M. Smith, et al., "Effects of Pyridostigmine on Acetylcholinesterase in Different Muscles of the Mouse," *Human and Experimental Toxicology,* 16, 1996, pp. 18–24.

Lintern, M., J. Wetherell, et al., "Differential Recovery of AChE in Guinea Pig Muscle and Brain Regions After Soman Treatment," *Human and Experimental Toxicology* 17, 1998, pp. 157–161.

Lipp, J., "Effect of Diazepam upon Soman-Induced Seizure Activity and Convulsions," *Electroencephalog Clin Neurophysiol,* 32, 1972, pp. 557–560.

Lipp, J., "Effect of Benzodiazepine Derivatives on Soman-Induced Seizure Activity and Convulsions in the Monkey," *Arch Inte Pharmacodyn,* 202, 1973, pp. 244–251.

Liu, W.-F., "Acute Effects of Oral Low Doses of Pyridostigmine on Simple Visual Discrimination and Unconditioned Consummatory Action," *Pharmachol Biochem Behav,* 41, 1991, pp. 251–254.

Llorente, I., F. Lizcano, et al., "Cholinergic Modulation of Spontaneous Hypothalamic-Pituitary–Adrenal Activity and Its Circadian Variation in Man," *J Endocrinol Metab,* 81(8), 1996, pp. 2902–2907.

Loewenstein-Lichtenstein, Y., M. Schwarz, et al., "Genetic Predisposition to Adverse Consequences of Anti-Cholinesterases in 'Atypical' BCHE Carriers," *Nature Medicine,* 1(10), 1995, pp. 1082–1084.

Lotti, M., "The Pathogenesis of Organophosphate Polyneuropathy," *Crit Rev Toxicol,* 21(6), 1991, pp. 465–487.

Lotti, M., S. Caroldi, et al., "Promotion of Organophosphate-Induced Delayed Polyneuropathy by Phenylmethanesulfonyl Fluoride [see comments]," *Toxicol Appl Pharmacol,* 108(2), 1991, pp. 234–241.

Lotti, M., and A. Moretto, "The Search for the Physiological Functions of NTE; Is NTE a Receptor?" *Chem Biol Interact,* 87(1-3), 1993, pp. 407–416.

Lotti, M., and A. Moretto, "Cholinergic Symptoms and Gulf War Syndrome," *Nature Medicine,* 1, 1995, pp. 1225–1226.

Lotti, M., A. Moretto, et al., "Inhibition of Lymphocytic Neuropathy Target Esterase Predicts the Development of Organophosphate-Induced Polyneuropathy," *Arch Toxicol,* 59, 1986, pp. 176–179.

Lotti, M., A. Moretto, et al., "Interactions Between Neuropathy Target Esterase and its Inhibitors and the Development of Polyneuropathy," *Toxicol Appl Pharmacol,* 122(2), 1993, pp. 165–171.

Lucey, J., G. Butcher, et al., "Elevated Growth Hormone Responses to Pyridostigmine in Obsessive-Compulsive Disorder: Evidence of Cholinergic Supersensitivity," *Am J Psychiatry,* 150(6), 1993, pp. 961–962.

Luetje, C., J. Patrick, et al., "Nicotine Receptors in the Mammalian Brain," *The FASEB Journal,* 4, 1990, pp. 2753–2760.

MacDonald, T., and R. Martin, "Aluminium Ion in Biological Systems," *TIBS,* 13, 1988, pp. 15–19.

Machade, S., and G. Robinson, "A Direct, General Approach Based on Isobolograms for Assessing the Joint Action of Drugs in Pre-Clinical Experiments," *Statistics in Medicine,* 13, 1994, pp. 2289–2309.

Maes, V., L. Huyghens, et al., "Acute and Chronic Intoxication with Carbromal Preparations," *Clinical Toxicology,* 23(4-6), 1985, pp. 341–346.

Mager, P., *Multidimensional Pharmacochemistry,* San Diego, Calif.: Academic Press, 1984, pp. 52–53.

Maizlish, N., "A Behavioral Evaluation of Pest Control Workers with Short Term Low Level Exposure to Organophosphate Diazinon," *Am J Ind Med,* 12, 1987, pp. 153–172.

Mani, A., M. S. Thomas, and A. P. Abraham, "Type II Paralysis or Intermediate Syndrome Following Organophosphorus Poisoning," *J Assoc Physicians of India,* 40(8), 1992, 542–544.

Marino, M., B. Schuster, et al., "Population Kinetics and Dynamics of Pyridostigmine Bromide in Man: Implications for Effectiveness in Field Units," in J. M. King, ed., *US Medical Defense Bioscience Review. Proceedings,* 2, Fort Detrick, Ms.: U.S. Army Medical Research and Materiel Command, May 12–16, 1996, p. 1284.

Marks, M., and A. Collins, "Effects of Chronic Nicotine Infusion on Tolerance Development and Nicotine Receptors," *J Pharmacol Exp Therapeutics,* 226(3), 1983, pp. 283–291.

Marks, M., J. Pauly, et al., "Nicotine Binding and Nicotinic Receptor Subunit RNA After Chronic Nicotine Treatment," *J Neuroscience,* 12(7), 1992, pp. 2765–2784.

Marks, M., J. Stitzel, et al., "Time-Course Study of the Effects of Chronic Nicotine Infusion on Drug Response and Brain Receptors," *J Pharmacol Exp Therapeutics,* 235(3), 1985, pp. 619–628.

Marks, M., L. Artman, et al., "Cholinergic Adaptations to Chronic Oxotremorine Infusion," *J Pharmacol Exp Therapeutics,* 218, 1981, pp. 337–343.

Marrs, T., "Organophosphate Poisoning," *Pharmacol Ther,* 58, 1993, pp. 51–66.

Marshall, G., L. Davis, and C. Sherbourne, *A Review of the Scientific Literature As It Pertains to Gulf War Illnesses, Vol. 4: Stress,* Santa Monica, Calif.: RAND, MR-1018/4, 1999.

Martin, G. R., "Pre-Clinical Pharmacology of Zolmitriptan (Zomig; formerly 311C90), a Centrally and Peripherally Acting 5HT1B/1D Agonist for Migraine," *Cephalgia,* Supplement 18, October 17, 1997, pp. 4–14.

Martin, H., and J. Standerwick, "The Effect of Pyridostigmine upon Exercise Ventilation and Cardiac Frequency in Healthy Men," Chemical Defence Establishment Technical Note 445, Porton Down, U.K., 1980.

Martin, R., "Bioinorganic Chemistry of Aluminum," in H. Sigel, ed., *Metal Ions in Biological Systems,* New York: Marcel Dekker, 1988, pp. 1–57.

Martyn, C., C. Osmond, et al., "Geographical Relations Between Alzheimer's Disease and Aluminium in Drinking Water," *Lancet,* 1, 1989, pp. 59–62.

Maselli, R., and C. Leung, "Analysis of Neuromuscular Transmission Failure Induced by Anticholinesterases," *Ann NY Acad Sci,* 1993a, pp. 402–404.

Maselli, R., and C. Leung, "Analysis of Anticholinesterase-Induced Neuromuscular Transmission Failure," *Muscle and Nerve,* 16, 1993b, pp. 548–553.

Mason, H., E. Waine, et al., "Aging and Spontaneous Reactivation of Human Plasma Cholinesterase Activity After Inhibition by Organophosphorus Pesticides," *Human and Experimental Toxicology,* 12, 1993, pp. 497–503.

Matters, D., "Disturbances of Liver Porphyrin Metabolism Caused by Drugs," *Pharmacological Reviews,* 19, 1967, p. 537.

Matthew, C. B., R. P. Francesconi, and R. W. Hubbard, "Physostigmine: Dose-Response Effects on Endurance and Thermoregulation During Exercise," *Life Sci,* 47(4), 1990, pp. 335–343.

Matthew, C. B., R. P. Francesconi, et al., "Chronic vs. Acute Carbamate Administration in Exercising Rats," *Life Sci,* 47(4), 1990, pp. 335–343.

Matthew, C., J. Glenn, et al., "Acute Subchronic Pyridostigmine Administration: Effects on the Anticholinergic Properties of Atropine," *Proceedings of the 1993 Medical Defense Bioscience Review,* 2, 1993, pp. 605–614.

Matthew, C., J. Glenn, et al., "Cholinergic Drug Interactions and Heat Tolerance," *Life Sci,* 54(17), 1994, pp. 1237–1245.

Matthew, C. B., R. W. Hubbard, and R. P. Francesconi, "A Heat-Stressed Rat Model to Determine Relative Anticholinergic and Anticholinesterase Drug Potency," *Aviat Space Environ Med,* 57(11), 1986, pp. 1061–1065.

Matthew, C. B., R. W. Hubbard, and R. P. Francesconi, "Atropine, Diazepam, and Physostigmine: Thermoregulatory Effects in the Heat-Stressed Rat," *Life Sci,* 44(25), 1989, pp. 1921–1927.

Matthew, C. B., R. W. Hubbard, et al., "Carbamate-Induced Performance and Thermoregulatory Decrements Restored with Diazepam and Atropine," *Aviat Space Environ Med,* 58(12), 1987, pp. 1183–1187.

Matthew, C. B., R. W. Hubbard, et al., "Carbamates, Atropine, and Diazepam: Effects on Performance in the Running Rat," *Life Sci,* 42(20), 1988, pp. 1925–1931.

Matyszak, M. K., and V. H. Perry, "Demyelination in the Central Nervous System Following a Delayed-Type Hypersensitivity Response to Bacillus Calmette-Guerin," *Neuroscience,* 64(4), 1995, pp. 967–977.

Maurissen, J., "Psychophysical Testing in Human Populations Exposed to Neurotoxicants," *Neurobehavioral Toxicology and Teratology,* 7, 1985, pp. 309–317.

Maxwell, D., K. Brecht, et al., "Comparison of Antidote Protection Against Soman by Pyridostigmine, HI-6 and Acetylcholinesterase," *J Pharmacol Exp Therapeutics,* 264(3), 1993, pp. 1085–1089.

Maycock, G., "Sleepiness and Driving: The Experience of UK Car Drivers," *J of Sleep Res* 5(4), 1996, pp. 229–237.

McCabe, W., J. Hammarsten, et al., "Elevations of Serum Cholesterol in Man in Association with Life Stress and Independent of Diet and Exercise," *Abstract, J. Lab & Clin Med,* 54, 1959, p. 922.

McCain, W. C., "Acute Oral Toxicity Study of Pyridostigmine Bromide, Permethrin, and DEET in the Laboratory Rat," *J Toxicol and Env Health,* 50, 1997, pp. 113–124.

McConnell, R., A. Fidler, et al., "Health Hazard Evaluation Determination Report," NIOSH, U.S. Department of Health and Human Services, 1986.

McConnell, R., M. Keifer, et al., "Elevated Tactile Vibration Threshold Among Workers Previously Poisoned with Methamidofos and Other Organophosphate Pesticides," *Am J Ind Med,* 25, 1994, pp. 325–334.

McEvoy, G., ed., *AHFS Drug Information,* Bethesda, Md.: American Society of Hospital Pharmacists, 1991.

McEwen, B., and R. Sapolsky, "Stress and Cognitive Function," *Curr Opin Neurobiol,* 5, 1995, pp. 205–216.

McGarrigle, R., N. Adams, et al., "The Effectiveness of a Carbamate in Prophylaxis Against Nerve Agent in Dogs and Monkeys," Aberdeen Proving Ground, Md.: Chemical Research Development and Engineering Center, 1976.

McGehee, D., M. Heath, et al., "Nicotine Enhancement of Fast Excitatory Synaptic Transmission in CNS by Presynaptic Receptors," *Science,* 269(5231), 1995, pp. 1692–1696.

McKee, W., and B. Wollcott, "Report on Exposures of Unprotected Men and Rabbits to Low Concentrations of Nerve Gas Vapour," Porton Technical Paper 143, 1949.

McNall, P., B. Wolfson, et al., "Use of Pyridostigmine for the Reversal of Neuromuscular Blockade," *Anesthesia and Analgesia . . . Current Researches,* 48(6), 1969, pp. 1026–1032.

McPhail, R., "Studies on the Flavor Aversions Induced by N-Substituted Carbamates and by Alkyl-Tin Compounds," *Toxicologist,* 1, 1981, p. 44.

McPhillips, J., "Altered Sensitivity to Drugs Following Repeated Injections of a Cholinesterase Inhibitor in Rats," *Toxicol Appl Pharmacol,* 14, 1969, pp. 67–73.

Medical Letter, "Prevention and Treatment of Nerve Gas Poisoning," *Medical Letter,* 32(831), 1990, pp. 103–104.

Medical Letter, "Treatment of Nerve Gas Poisoning," *Medical Letter*, 37(948), 1995, pp. 43–44.

Meggs, W., and C. Cleveland, "Rhinolaryngoscopic Examination of Patients with the Multiple Chemical Sensitivity Syndrome," *Arch Environ Health*, 48(1), 1993, pp. 14–18.

Melnick, J. L., E. Adam, et al., "Cytomegalovirus and Atherosclerosis," *Eur Heart J*, 14, 1993, Supplement K, pp. 30–38.

Melnick, S. L., E. Shahar, et al., "Past Infection by Chlamydia Pneumoniae Strain TWAR and Asymptomatic Carotid Atherosclerosis. Atherosclerosis Risk in Communities (ARIC) Study Investigators," *Am J Med*, 95(5), 1993, pp. 499–504.

Meltzer, H. Y., R. C. Arora, et al., "Serotonin Uptake in Blood Platelets of Psychiatric Patients," *Archives of General Psychiatry*, 38(12), 1981, pp. 1322–1326.

Merrill, J., and J. Weller, "Treatment of Bromism with the Artificial Kidney," *Ann Intern Med*, 37, 1952, pp. 186–190.

Meshul, C., A. Boyne, et al., "Comparison of the Ultrastructural Myopathy Induced by Anticholinesterase Agents at the End Plates of Rat Soleus and Extensor Muscles," *Experimental Neurology*, 89(1), 1985, pp. 96–114.

Metcalf, D., and J. Holmes, "EEG, Psychological and Neurological Alterations in Humans with Organophosphorus Exposure," *Ann NY Acad Sci*, 160, 1969, pp. 359–365.

Metcalf, J., statement made by Rep. Jack Metcalf (R-Wash.) to the Subcommittee on Human Resources, Government Reform Committee, 1997.

Miczek, K., and P. Donat, "Brain 5 HT Systems and Inhibition of Aggressive Behavior," in T. Archer, P. Bevan, and A. Cools, eds., *Behavioral Pharmacology of 5-HT*, Hillsdale, N.J.: Lawrence Erlbaum Associates, 1989.

Miczek, K., J. Mos, et al., "Brain 5-HT and Inhibition of Aggressive Behavior in Animals: 5-HIAA and Receptor Subtypes," *Psychopharmacol Bull*, 25, 1989, pp. 399–403.

Midtling, J. E., P. G. Barnett, et al., "Clinical Management of Field Worker Organophosphate Poisoning," *Western J Med*, 142(4), 1985, pp. 514–518.

Milatovic, D., and W.-D. Dettbarn, "Modification of Acetylcholinesterase During Adaptation to Chronic, Subacute Paraoxon Application in Rat," *Toxicol Appl Pharmacol*, 136, 1996, pp. 20–28.

Miller, C., "Possible Models for Multiple Chemical Sensitivity: Conceptual Issues and Role of the Limbic System," *Toxicol Ind Health*, 8(4), 1992, pp. 181–202.

Miller, C., "White Paper: Chemical Sensitivity: History and Phenomenology," *Toxicol Ind Health*, 10(4/5), 1994, pp. 253–276.

Miller, C., "Chemical Sensitivity: Symptom, Syndrome, or Mechanism for Disease?" *Toxicology*, 111, 1996a, pp. 69–86.

Miller, C., invited testimony, Committee on Government Reform and Oversight, Subcommittee on Human Resources and Intergovernmental Relations, U.S. House of Representatives, 1996b.

Miller, .C., invited presentation, Presidential Advisory Committee on Gulf War Veterans' Illnesses, 1996c.

Miller, C., "Toxicant-Induced Loss of Tolerance—An Emerging Theory of Disease?" *Environmental Health Perspectives*, 105, 1997, Supplement 2, pp. 445–453.

Miller, C., and H. Mitzel, "Chemical Sensitivity Attributed to Pesticide Exposure Versus Remodelling," *Archives of Environmental Health*, 50(2), 1995, pp. 119–129.

Miller, C., N. Ashford, et al., "Empirical Approaches for the Investigation of Toxicant-Induced Loss of Tolerance," *Environmental Health Perspectives*, 105, 1997, Supplement 2, pp. 515–519.

Miller, R., L. Van Nyhuis, et al., "Comparative Times to Peak Effect and Durations of Action of Neostigmine and Pyridostigmine," *Anesthesiology*, 41, 1974, pp. 27–33.

Milner, I. B., B. N. Axelrod, et al., "Is There a Gulf War Syndrome?" *JAMA*, 271(9), 1994, p. 661.

Mirakhur, R., "Spontaneous Recovery or Evoked Reversal of Neuromuscular Block," *Acta Anaesthesiol Scand*, 39, 1995, Supplement 106, pp. 62–63.

Misra, U., M. Prasad, et al., "A Study of Cognitive Functions and Event Related Potentials Following Organophosphate Exposure," *Electromyogr Clin Neurophysiol*, 34, 1994, pp. 197–203.

MMWR, "Neurological Findings Among Workers Exposed to Fenthion in a Veterinary Hospital—Georgia," *MMWR*, 34, 1985, pp. 402–403.

Modrow, H., and J. McDonough, "Effects of Soman and Pyridostigmine on Variable Interval Responding," *Neurobehav Toxicol Teratol*, 7, 1985, pp. 528–529.

Mohs, R., B. Davis, et al., "Cognitive Effects of Physostigmine and Choline Chloride in Normal Subjects," in K. Davis and P. Berger, eds., *Brain Acetylcholine and Neuropsychiatric Disease*, New York: Plenum Press, 1979, pp. 237–251.

Mohs, R., B. Davis, et al., "Oral Physostigmine Treatment of Patients with Alzheimer's Disease," *Am J Psychiatry,* 142, 1985, pp. 28–33.

Monroe, R., "Episodic Behavioral Disorders and Limbic Ictus," in B. Doane and K. Livingston, eds., *The Limbic System: Functional Organization and Clinical Disorders,* New York: Raven Press, Ltd., 1986, pp. 251–266.

Moretto, A., M. Bertolazzi, et al., "Phenylmethanesulfonyl Fluoride Elicits and Intensifies the Clinical Expression of Neuropathic Insults," *Arch Toxicol* 66(1), 1992, pp. 67–72.

Moretto, A., M. Bertolazzi, et al., "The Phosphorothioic Acid O-(2-chloro-2,3,3-trifluorocyclobutyl) O-Ethyl S-Propyl Ester Exacerbates Organophosphate Polyneuropathy Without Inhibition of Neuropathy Target Esterase," *Toxicol Appl Pharmacol,* 129(1), 1994, pp. 133–137.

Moretto, A., and M. Lotti, "Promotion of Peripheral Axonopathies by Certain Esterase Inhibitors," *Toxicol Ind Health,* 9(6), 1993, pp. 1037–1046.

Moretto, A., and M. Lotti, "Poisoning by Organophosphorus Insecticides and Sensory Neuropathy," *J Neurol Neurosurg Psychiatry,* 64(4), 1998, pp. 463–468.

Morgan, J., and E. Weaver, "Chronic Bromism Simulating Neurological Diseases," *Virginia Medical Monthly,* 96, 1969, pp. 262–264.

Moriearty, P., and R. Becker, "Inhibition of Human Brain and RBC Acetylcholinesterase (AChE) by Heptylphysostigmine (HPTL)," *Metho Find Exp Clin Pharmacol,* 14(8), 1992, pp. 615–621.

Morse, J., and J. Davis, "Regulation of Ischemic Hippocampal Damage in the Gerbil: Adrenalectomy Alters the Rate of CA1 Cell Disappearance," *Exp Neurol,* 110, 1990, p. 86.

Moser, V., "Comparisons of the Acute Effects of Cholinesterase Inhibitors Using a Neurobehavioral Screening Battery in Rats," *Toxicologist,* 14, 1994, p. 241.

Moss, J., "Synergism of Toxicity of N,N-Diethyl-m-Toluamide to German Cockroaches (Orthoptera: Blattellidae) by Hydrolytic Enzyme Inhibitors," *J Econ Entomol,* 89(5), 1996, pp. 1151–1155.

Mota, A., A. Bento, et al., "Role of the Serotonin Receptor Subtype 5-HT1D on Basal and Stimulated Growth Hormone Secretion," *J Clin Endocrinol and Metabol,* 80(6), 1995, pp. 1973–1977.

Moya-Quiles, M., E. Munoz-Delgado, et al., "Effect of Pyrethroid Insecticide Allethrin on Membrane Fluidity," *Biochemistry and Molecular Biology International,* 36(6), 1995, pp. 1299–1308.

Moylan-Jones, R., "A Trial of Pyridostigmine Pretreatment for Nerve Agent Poisoning in Man," Chemical Defence Establishment, Technical Note 217, Porton Down, U.K., 1975.

Moylan-Jones, R., D. Parkes, et al., "The Pharmacokinetics of Pyridostigmine in Humans. Part II. Multiple Dose Studies," Chemical Defence Establishment, Technical Paper 258, Porton Down, U.K., 1979.

Moylan-Jones, R., D. Parkes, et al., "Selected Clinical Biochemical Observations in Men Taking Pyridostigmine," Chemical Defence Establishment, Technical Note 476, Porton Down, U.K., August 1981.

Moylan-Jones, R., D. Parkes, et al., "The Effect of Standard Field ("Compo") Rations on the Absorption of Pyridostigmine from the Tablets NAPS L1A1 (U)," Chemical Defence Establishment, Porton Down, U.K., 1984.

Muhlestein, J. B., E. H. Hammond, et al., "Increased Incidence of Chlamydia Species Within the Coronary Arteries of Patients with Symptomatic Atherosclerotic Versus Other Forms of Cardiovascular Disease," *J Am Coll Cardiol*, 27(7), 1996, pp. 1555–1561.

Mukhopadhyay, S., and M. Poddar, "Caffeine-Induced Locomotor Activity: Possible Involvement of GABAergic-Dopaminergic-Adenosinergic Interaction," *Neurochemical Research*, 20(1), 1995, pp. 39–44.

Muldoon, M., E. Bachen, et al., "Acute Cholesterol Responses to Mental Stress and Change in Posture," *Arch Intern Med*, 152, 1992, pp. 775–780.

Mumford, S., Memorandum 30, Serial No. 33, Chemical Defence Establishment, Porton Down, U.K., 1950.

Murialdo, G., S. Fonzi, et al., "Effects of Pyridostigmine, Corticotropin-Releasing Hormone and Growth Hormone-Releasing Hormone on the Pituitary-Adrenal Axis and on Growth Hormone Secretion in Dementia," *Neuropsychobiology*, 28, 1993, pp. 177–183.

Murphy, F., H. Kang, et al., "Executive Summary: Cooperative Study #458, National Health Survey of Persian Gulf Veterans and Their Families," *VA Cooperative Studies Program*, 1998.

Murphy, M., D. Blick, et al., *Physiological and Performance Effects of Pyridostigmine Bromide in Rats and Monkeys*, Fifth Annual Chemical Defense and Bioscientific Review Abstract, Aberdeen Proving Ground, Md.: U.S. Army Medical Research Institute of Chemical Defense, 1985.

Murphy, M., D. Blick, et al., "Effects of Diazepam on Soman-Induced Lethality, Convulsions, and Performance Deficit," Systems Research Laboratories, a division of Arvin/Calspan, with Texas A&M Research Foundation, 1989.

Murphy, M., D. Blick, et al., "Diazepam as a Treatment for Nerve Agent Poisoning in Primates," *Aviat Space Environ Med*, 64, 1993, pp. 110–115.

Murphy, R., and F. Zemlan, "Differential Effects of Substance P on Serotonin-Modulated Spinal Nociceptive Reflexes," *Psychopharmacology (Berlin)*, 93, 1987, pp. 118–121.

Murray, C., and H. Fibiger, "Learning and Memory Deficits After Lesions of the Nucleus Basalis Magnocellularis: Reversal by Physostigmine," *Neuroscience*, 14, 1985, pp. 1025–1032.

Mutch, E., P. Blain, et al., "Interindividual Variations in Enzymes Controlling Organophosphate Toxicity in Man," *Human and Experimental Toxicology*, 11, 1992, pp. 109–116.

Nagayama, M., F. Akahori, et al., "Effects of Selected Organophosphate Insecticides on Serum Cholinesterase Isoenzyme Patterns in the Rat," *Vet Human Toxicol*, 38(3), 1996, pp. 196–199.

Narahashi, T., "Nerve Membrane Ionic Channels as the Primary Target of Pyrethroid," *Neurotoxicol*, 6, 1985, pp. 3–22.

Natelson, B., J. Ottenweller, et al., "Persisting Effects of Oral Pyridostigmine Bromide on the Behavior of Rats," *Society for Neuroscience*, 22, 1996, p. 95.3.

National Institutes of Health, "The Persian Gulf Experience and Health," 1994.

Nelson, J. D., N. L. Adams, "Intensive Care of the Soman Intoxicated Primate," *The Pharmacologist*, 24, 1982, p. 220.

"Nerve Agents: GA GB GD GF VX," http://chemdef.apgea.army.mil., accessed 1997.

Nethercott, J., L. Davidoff, et al., "Multiple Chemical Sensitivities Syndrome: Toward a Working Case Definition," *Archives of Environmental Health*, 48(1), 1993, pp. 19–26.

Newmark, J., and W. Clayton, "Persian Gulf Illnesses: Preliminary Neurological Impressions," *Military Medicine*, 160, pp. 505–507.

Nicolson, G. L., and N. L. Nicolson, "Chronic Fatigue Illness and Operation Desert Storm," *J Occup Environ Med*, 38, 1995, pp. 14–16.

Nicolson, G. L., and N. L. Nicolson, "The Eight Myths of Operation 'Desert Storm' and Gulf War Syndrome," *Med Conflict and Survival*, 13, 1997, pp. 140–146.

Nieto, F. J., E. Adam, et al., "Cohort Study of Cytomegalovirus Infection as a Risk Factor for Carotid Intimal-Medial Thickening, a Measure of Subclinical Atherosclerosis," *Circulation*, 94(5), 1996, pp. 922–927.

Nilsson, A., "Connection Between Smoking and Reduced Risk of Ulcerative Colitis. Does Nicotine Mediate a Protective Effect?" *Lakartidningen,* 92(50), 1995, pp. 4788–4792.

Nilsson-Haransson, L., Z. Lai, et al., "Tetrahydroaminoacridine Induces Opposite Changes in Muscarinic and Nicotinic Receptors in the Rat Brain," *Eur J Pharmacol,* 186, 1990, pp. 301–305.

Noble, D., "Back into the Storm: Reanalyzing Health Effects of the Gulf War," *Analytic Chemistry,* 66(15), 1994, pp. 805–808.

"Nonpsychotropic Drugs May Cause Sleep Disturbances," *Drugs and Therapy Perspectives*, 10(12), 1997, pp. 10–13.

Nordberg, A., G. Wahlstrom, et al., "Effect of Long-Term Nicotine Treatment on [3H]nicotine Binding Sites in the Rat's Brain," *Drug and Alcohol Dependence,* 16, 1985, pp. 9–17.

Nordgren, I., B. Karlen, et al., "Intoxications with Anticholinesterases: Effect of Different Combinations of Antidotes on the Dynamics of Acetylcholine in Mouse Brain," *Pharmacology and Toxicology,* 70, 1992, pp. 384–388.

Nose, T., and H. Takemoto, "Effect of Oxotremorine on Homovanillic Acid Concentration in Striatum of Rat," *Eur J Pharmacol,* 25, 1974, p. 51.

Obermeyer, W. H., and R. M. Benca, "Effects of Drugs on Sleep," *Neurol Clin,* 14(4), 1996, pp. 827–840.

Office of the Special Assistant to the Secretary of Defense for Gulf War Illnesses (OSAGWI), "Case Narrative: Khamisiyah," Washington, D.C., 1997.

Ohara, M., M. Hirohata, et al., "Family of a Patient with Serum Cholinesterase Deficiency," *Internal Medicine,* 31(3), 1992, pp. 397–399.

Ohno, M., M. Kobayashi, et al., "Working Memory Failure by Combined Blockade of Muscarinic and Beta-Adrenergic Transmission in the Rat Hippocampus," *Neuroreport,* 8(7), 1997, pp. 1571–1575.

Ohtawa, M., M. Seko, et al., "Effects of Aluminium Ingestion on Lipid Peroxidation in Rats," *Chem Pharm Bull,* 31, 1983, pp. 1415–1418.

O'Keane, V., K. Abel, et al., "Growth Hormone Responses to Pyridostigmine in Schizophrenia: Evidence for Cholinergic Dysfunction," *Biol Psychiatry,* 36, 1994, pp. 582–588.

O'Keane, V., and T. Dinan, "Sex Steroid Priming Effects on Growth Hormone Response to Pyridostigmine Throughout the Menstrual Cycle," *J Clin Endocrinology and Metabolism,* 75(1), 1992, pp. 11–14.

O'Keane, V., K. O'Flynn, et al., "Pyridostigmine-Induced Growth Hormone Responses in Healthy and Depressed Subjects: Evidence for Cholinergic Supersensitivity in Depression," *Psychological Medicine,* 22, 1992, pp. 55–60.

Okhawa, H., H. Oshita, et al., "Comparison of Inhibitory Activity of Various Organophosphorus Compounds Against Acetylcholinesterase and Neurotoxic Esterase of Hens with Respect to Delayed Neurotoxicity," *Biochem Pharmacol,* 29, 1980, pp. 2721–2727.

Olivier, B., J. Mos, et al., "Modulatory Action of Serotonin in Aggressive Behaviour," in T. Archer, P. Bevan, and A. Cools, eds., *Behavioral Pharmacology of 5-HT,* Hillsdale, N.J.: Lawrence Erlbaum Associates, 1989.

O'Neill, J., "Non-Cholinesterase Effects of Anticholinesterases," *Fundam Appl Toxicol,* 1, 1981, pp. 154–160.

Ortiz, D., L. Yanez, et al., "Acute Toxicological Effects in Rats Treated with a Mixture of Commercially Formulated Products Containing Methyl Parathion and Permethrin," *Ecotoxicol Environ Saf,* 32(2), 1995, pp. 154–158.

Osame, M., M. Kawabuchi, et al., "Experimental Nemaline Rods Induced by Anticholinesterase Drug (Neostigmine Methylsulfate)," *Proc Jpn Acad,* 51, 1975, pp. 598–603.

Osimitz, T. G., and R. H. Grothaus, "The Present Safety Assessment of DEET," *J Am Mosq Control Assoc,* 11(2 Pt 2), 1995, pp. 274–278.

Osimitz, T. G., and J. V. Murphy, "Neurological Effects Associated with Use of the Insect Repellent N,N-Diethyl-m-Toluamide (DEET)," *J Toxicol Clin Toxicol,* 35(5), 1997, pp. 435–441.

Ottenweller, J., personal communication, 1998.

Overstreet, D., L. Dilsaver, et al., "Effects of Light on Responsiveness to a Muscarinic Agonist in Rats Selectively Bred for Endogenously Increased Cholinergic Function," *Psychiatry Res,* 33, 1990, pp. 139–150.

Overstreet, D., D. Janowsky, et al., "Enhanced Elevation of Corticosterone Following Arecoline Administration to Rats Selectively Bred for Increased Cholinergic Function," *Psychopharmacology (Berl),* 88, 1986a, pp. 129–130.

Overstreet, D., D. Janowsky, et al., "Stress-Induced Immobility in Rats with Cholinergic Supersensitivity," *Biol Psychiatry,* 21, 1986b, pp. 657–664.

Overstreet, D., D. Janowsky, et al., "Alcoholism and Depressive Disorders: Is Cholinergic Sensitivity a Biological Marker?" *Alcohol Alcohol,* 24, 1989, pp. 253–255.

Overstreet, D., D. Janowsky, et al., "Swim Test Immobility Co-Segregates with Serotonergic but Not Cholinergic Sensitivity in Cross-Breeds of Flinders Line Rats," *Psychiatr Genet*, 4, 1994, pp. 101–107.

Overstreet, D., A. Rezvani, et al., "Impaired Active Avoidance Responding in Rats Selectively Bred for Increased Cholinergic Function," *Physiol Behav*, 47, 1990, pp. 787–788.

Overstreet, D., A. Rezvani, et al., "Genetic Animal Models of Depression and Ethanol Preference Provide Support for Cholinergic and Serotonergic Involvement in Depression and Alcoholism," *Biol Psychiatry*, 31, 1992, pp. 919–936.

Overstreet, D., R. Russell, et al., "Genetic and Pharmacological Models of Cholinergic Supersensitivity and Affective Disorders," *Experientia*, 44, 1988, pp. 465–472.

Owens, M., D. Overstreet, et al., "Alterations in the Hypothalamic Pituitary-Adrenal Axis in a Proposed Animal Model of Depression with Genetic Muscarinic Susceptibility," *Neuropsychopharmacology*, 4, 1991, pp. 87–93.

Padilla, S., "The Neurotoxicology of Cholinesterase-Inhibiting Insecticides: Past and Present Evidence Demonstrating Persistent Effects," *Inhalation Toxicology*, 7, 1995, pp. 903–907.

Pappata, S., B. Tavitian, et al., "In Vivo Imaging of Human Cerebral Acetylcholinesterase," *J Neurochem*, 67(2), 1996, pp. 876–879.

Park, K., D. Kim, et al., "Pyridostigmine Toxicity: Electrophysiological Study," *Electromyogr Clin Neurophysiol*, 33, 1993, pp. 323–328.

Parker, F., J. Barber, et al., "Laboratory Techniques for Determining the Effects of Pyridostigmine Bromide," USAF School of Aerospace Medicine, Brooks AFB, Tex., 1986.

Parker, F., J. Barber, et al., "Chemical Defense Pretreatment Drugs in the Aerospace Environment: An Overview of Biochemical Analyses from Pyridostigmine Bromide Studies Conducted for the USAF School of Aerospace Medicine," USAF School of Aerospace Medicine, Brooks AFB, Tex., 1989.

Pascuzzo, G., A. Akaike, et al., "The Nature of the Interactions of Pyridostigmine with the Nicotinic Acetylcholine Receptor-Ionic Channel Complex I. Agonist, Desensitizing, and Binding Properties," *Mol Pharmacol*, 25, 1984, pp. 92–101.

Patrick, J., personal communication, 1997.

Patrick, J., P. Sequela, et al., "Functional Diversity of Neuronal Nicotinic Acetylcholine Receptors," in A. Cuello, ed., *Progress in Brain Research*, 98, 1993, pp. 113–120.

Patterson, S., J. Gottdiener, et al., "Effects of Acute Mental Stress on Serum Lipids: Mediating Effects of Plasma Volume," *Psychosomatic Med*, 55, 1993, pp. 525–532.

Pauly, J., M. Marks, et al., "An Autoradiographic Analysis of Cholinergic Receptors in Mouse Brain After Chronic Nicotinic Treatment," *J Pharmacol Exp Therapeutics*, 258(3), 1991, pp. 1127–1136.

PB1 Internet Site, "Nerve Agents: GA GB GD GF VX," accessed 1997.

Peacock, M., M. Morris, et al., "Sleep Apnea-Hypopnea Syndrome in a Sample of Veterans of the Persian Gulf War," *Military Medicine*, 162(4), 1997, pp. 249–251.

Pelckmans, M., W. Verdickt, et al., "Bromism: Rare But Still Present," *Acta Clinica Belgica*, 38(6), 1983, pp. 397–400.

Pelligrini, G., and R. Santi, "Potentiation of Toxicity of Organophosphorus Compounds Containing Carboxylic Acid Functions Towards Warm-Blooded Animals by Some Organophosphorus Impurities," *J Agric Food Chem*, 20, 1972, pp. 944–950.

Penman, A., R. Tarver, et al., "No Evidence of Increase in Birth Defects and Health Problems Among Children Born to Persian Gulf War Veterans in Mississippi," *Milit Med*, 161, 1996, pp. 1–6.

Pennisi, E., "Chemicals Behind Gulf War Syndrome?" *Science*, 272, 1996, pp. 479–480.

Perrotta, D., "Long-Term Health Effects Associated with Sub-Clinical Exposures to GB and Mustard," Environmental Committee Armed Forces Epidemiological Board, 1996.

Persian Gulf Veterans Coordinating Board, "Unexplained Illnesses Among Desert Storm Veterans," *Arch of Intern Med*, 155, 1995, pp. 262–268.

Persian Gulf War (PGW) Illnesses Task Force, "Khamisiyah: A Historical Perspective on Related Intelligence," 1997, pp. 1–24.

Peters, B., and H. Levin, "Memory Enhancement After Physostigmine in the Amnesic Syndrome," *Arch Neurol*, 34, 1977, p. 215.

Petersdorf, R., W. Page, et al., eds., *Interactions of Drugs, Biologics, and Chemicals in US Military Forces (Institute of Medicine)*, Washington, D.C.: National Academy Press, 1996.

Peterson, R., "Scopolamine Induced Learning Failures in Man," *Psychopharmacology*, 52, 1977, p. 283.

Petrali, J., *A Study of the Effect of Soman on the Rat Blood-Brain Barrier*, 4th Annual Chemical Defense Bioscience Review, Aberdeen Proving Ground, Md.: U.S. Army Medical Research Institute of Chemical Defense, 1984.

Phillips, L. H., and J. C. Torner, "Epidemiologic Evidence for a Changing Natural History of Myasthenia Gravis," *Neurology,* 47(5), 1996, pp. 1233–1238.

Picciotto, M., M. Zoli, et al., "Acetylcholine Receptors Containing the ß2 Subunit Are Involved in the Reinforcing Properties of Nicotine," *Nature,* 391, 1998, pp. 173–177.

Piesner, A., P. Arlien-Soborg, et al., "Neurological Complications and Japanese Encephalitis Vaccination," *Lancet,* 348, 1996, pp. 202–203.

Ploeckinger, B., K. Dantendorfer, et al., "Rapid Decrease of Serum Cholesterol and Postpartum Depression," *BMJ,* 313, 1996, pp. 664–679.

Pollay, M., "The Processes Affecting the Distribution of Bromide in Blood, Brain, and CSF," *Exp Neurol,* 17, 1967, pp. 74–85.

Pool, W., and D. Hane, "Acute Toxicity of Pyridostigmine Bromide (Mestinon) in Adult and Neonatal Rats," Nutley, N.J., Roche Laboratories (internal report), 1972.

Pope, C., "Pyridostigmine, Organophosphates and Gulf War Illnesses: Background Material and Preliminary Assessments," prepared for Investigation and Analysis Directorate, OSAGWI, 1997.

Pope, C., T. Chakraborti, et al., "Long-Term Neurochemical and Behavioral Effects Induced by Acute Chlorpyrifos Treatment," *Pharmacol Biochem Behav,* 42, 1992, pp. 251–256.

Pope, C. N., and S. Padilla, "Promotion of Organophosphate-Induced Delayed Polyneuropathy by Phenylmethanesulfonyl Fluoride," *Toxicol Appl Pharmacol,* 110(1), 1991, pp. 179–180.

Pope, C. N., D. Tanaka, Jr., and S. Padilla, "The Role of Neurotoxic Esterase (NTE) in the Prevention and Potentiation of Organophosphorous-Induced Delayed Neurotoxicity," *Chemico-Biological Interactions,* 87(1-3), 1993, pp. 395–406.

Prendergast, M., statement by Deputy Commissioner and Senior Advisor to the Commissioner, Food and Drug Administration, Department of Health and Human Services, before the Presidential Advisory Committee on Gulf War Veterans' Illnesses, 1997.

Preston, K., and C. Schuster, "Conditioned Gustatory Avoidance Induced by Cholinergic Agents," *Pharmacol Biochem Behav,* 15, 1981, pp. 827–828.

Preusser, H.-J., "Die Ultrastruktur der motorischen Endplatte im Zwerchfell der Ratte und Veranderungen nach Inhibierung der Acetylcholinesterase," *Zellforsch*, 80, 1967, pp. 436–457.

Prioux-Guyonneau, M., C. Coudray-Lucas, et al., "Modification of Rat Brain 5-Hydroxytryptamine Metabolism by Sublethal Doses of Organophosphate Agents," *Acta Pharmacologica et Toxicologica*, 51(4), 1982, pp. 278–284.

Procopio, M., C. Invitti, et al., "Effect of Arginine and Pyridostigmine on the GHRH-Induced GH Rise in Obesity and Cushing's Syndrome," *International J of Obesity*, 19, 1995, pp. 108–112.

Prusaczyk, W., and M. Sawka, "Effects of Pyridostigmine Bromide on Human Thermoregulation During Cold Water Immersion," *J Appl Physiol*, 71, 1991, pp. 432–437.

Pscheidt, G. R., Z. Votava, and H. E. Himwich, "Effect of Physostigmine on the Level of Brain Biogenic Amines in Rats and Rabbits," *Biochem Pharmacol*, 16(6), 1967, pp. 1132–1134.

Pucilowski, O., B. Eichelman, et al., "Enhanced Affective Aggression in Genetically Bred Hypercholinergic Rats," *Neuropsychobiology*, 24, 1990, pp. 37–41.

Pullan, R. D., "Colonic Mucus, Smoking and Ulcerative Colitis," *Ann R Coll Surg Engl*, 78(2), 1996, pp. 85–91.

Pullan, R. D., J. Rhodes, et al., "Transdermal Nicotine for Active Ulcerative Colitis," *New Engl J Med*, 330(12), 1994, pp. 811–815.

Puolakkainen, M., C. C. Kuo, et al., "Serological Response to Chlamydia Pneumoniae in Adults with Coronary Arterial Fatty Streaks and Fibrolipid Plaques," *J Clin Microbiol*, 31(8), 1993, pp. 2212–2214.

Puttfarcken, P. S., A. M. Manelli, et al., "Evidence for Nicotinic Receptors Potentially Modulating Nociceptive Transmission at the Level of the Primary Sensory Neuron: Studies with F11 Cells," *J Neurochem*, 69(3), 1997, pp. 930–938.

Pyridostigmine Bromide New Drug Application (pending), filed May 1996.

Radcliffe, M., P. Ashurst, et al., "Unexplained Illness: The Mind Versus the Environment," *J Royal Society of Medicine*, 88, 1995, pp. 678–679.

Ram, Z., M. Molcho, et al., "The Effect of Pyridostigmine on Respiratory Function in Healthy and Asthmatic Volunteers," *Isr J Med Sci*, 27, 1991, pp. 664–668.

Rama, D., "Biological Monitoring for Organophosphate/Carbamate Pesticides—the Cholinesterase Assay," *SAMJ*, 84, 1994, pp. 298–299.

Rao, T. S., L. D. Correa, et al., "Evaluation of Anti-Nociceptive Effects of Neuronal Nicotinic Acetylcholine Receptor (NAChR) Ligands in the Rat Tail-Flick Assay," *Neuropharmacology*, 35(4), 1996, pp. 393–405.

Rapaport, M., S. C. Risch, et al., "The Effects of Physostigmine Infusion on Patients with Panic Disorder," *Biol Psychiatry*, 29(7), 1991, pp. 658–664.

Rapoport, S., *Blood-Brain Barrier in Physiology and Medicine*, New York: Raven Press, 1976.

Raskind, M., E. Peskind, et al., "Neuroendocrine Response to Physostigmine in Alzheimer's Disease," 46, 1989, pp. 535–540.

Rausch, J. L., D. S. Janowsky, et al., Physostigmine Effects on Serotonin Uptake in Human Blood Platelets," *Eur J Pharmacol*, 109(1), 1985, pp. 91–96.

Rausch, J. L., N. S. Shah, et al., "Platelet Serotonin Uptake in Depressed Patients: Circadian Effect," *Biol Psychiatry*, 17(1), 1982, pp. 121–123.

Ray, S., and M. Poddar, "Central Cholinergic-Dopaminergic Interaction in Carbaryl-Induced Tremor," *Eur J Pharmacol*, 119, 1986, pp. 251–253.

Redhead, K., G. Quinlan, et al., "Aluminium-Adjuvanted Vaccines Transiently Increase Aluminium Levels in Murine Brain Tissue," *Pharmacology and Toxicology*, 70, 1992, pp. 278–280.

Rest, K., "Advancing the Understanding of Multiple Chemical Sensitivity (MCS): Overview and Recommendations from an AOEC Workshop," *Toxicol Ind Health*, 8, 1992, pp. 1–13.

Rettig, R. A., *Military Use of Drugs Not Approved by the FDA for CW/BW Defense: Lessons from the Gulf War*, Santa Monica, Calif.: RAND, MR-1018/9, 1999.

Revell, T., "The Gulf War Syndrome" (letter) (see comments), *BMJ* (Clinical Research Edition), 310(6986), 1995, p. 1073.

Rhodes, J., and G. Thomas, "Nicotine Treatment in Ulcerative Colitis. Current Status," *Drugs*, 49(2), 1995, pp. 157–160.

Richelson, E., "Desensitization of Muscarinic Receptor-Mediated Cyclic GMP Formation by Cultured Nerve Cells," *Nature (London)*, 272, 1978, pp. 366–368.

Richter, E., P. Chuwers, et al., "Health Effects from Exposure to Organophosphate Pesticides in Workers and Residents in Israel," *Isr J Med Sci*, 28, 1992, pp. 584–597.

Rider, J., L. Ellinwood, et al., "Production of Tolerance in the Rat to Octamethyl Pyriophosphormaide (OMPA)," *Proc Soc Exp Biol Med*, 81, 1952, pp. 455–459.

Risch, S. C., P. Cohen, et al., "Physostigmine Induction of Depressive Symptomatology in Normal Human Subjects," *Psychiatry Res*, 4, 1981, pp. 89–94.

Risch, S. C., D. Janowsky, et al., "Muscarinic Supersensitivity of Anterior Pituitary ACTH and Beta Endorphin Release in Major Depressive Illness," *Peptides*, 9, 1981, pp. 789–792.

Risch, S. C., D. Janowsky, et al., "Cholinomimetic-Induced Co-Release of Prolactin and Beta-Endorphin in Man," *Psychopharmacol Bull*, 18, 1982a, pp. 21–25.

Risch, S. C., D. Janowsky, et al., "Correlated Cholinomimetic-Stimulated Beta-Endorphin and Prolactin Release in Humans," *Peptides*, 3, 1982b, pp. 319–322.

Risch, S. C., N. Kalin, et al., "Cholinergic Challenges in Affective Illness: Behavioral and Neuroendocrine Correlates," *J Clin Psychopharmacol*, 1, 1981, pp. 186–192.

Risch, S. C., N. Kalin, et al., "Co-Release of ACTH and Beta-Endorphin Immunoreactivity in Human Subjects in Response to Central Cholinergic Stimulation," *Science*, 222, 1983, p. 77.

Roach, J., A. Eliasson, et al., "The Effect of Pyridostigmine on Bronchial Hyperreactivity," Army ACP Meeting, abstract, 1991, p. 451.

Robbins, T. W., G. McAlonan, et al., "Cognitive Enhancers in Theory and Practice: Studies of the Cholinergic Hypothesis of Cognitive Deficits in Alzheimer's Disease," *Behav Brain Res*, 83(1–2), 1997, pp. 15–23.

Roberts, D., "EMG Voltage and Motor Nerve Conduction Velocity in Organophosphorus Pesticide Factory Workers," *Int Arch Occup Environ Hlth*, 1974, pp. 267–274.

Roberts, D., and S. Thesleff, "Acetylcholine Release from Motor-Nerve Endings in Rats Treated with Neostigmine," *Eur J Pharmacol*, 6, 1969, pp. 281–285.

Roberts, D. E., M. N. Sawka, et al., "Pyridostigmine Bromide Does Not Alter Thermoregulation During Exercise in Cold Air," *Can J Physiol Pharmacol*, 72, 1994, pp. 788–793.

Robinson, D., and R. McGee, "Agonist-Induced Regulation of Neuronal Nicotinic Acetylcholine Receptor of PC12 Cells," *Mol Pharmacol*, 27, 1985, pp. 409–417.

Robinson, T., and J. Becker, "Enduring Changes in Brain and Behavior Produced by Chronic Amphetamine Administration: A Review and Evaluation of Animal Models of Amphetamine Psychosis," *Brain Res Rev*, 11, 1986, pp. 157–198.

Robinson, T., J. Becker, et al., "Long-Term Facilitation of Amphetamine-Induced Rotational Behavior and Striatal Dopamine Release Produced by a Single Exposure to Amphetamine: Sex Differences," *Brain Res.* 253, 1982, pp. 231–241.

Rockefeller Report, "Investigational Drugs Used in the Persian Gulf War," 1997.

Rodnitzky, R., H. Levin, et al., "Occupational Exposure to Organophosphate Pesticides: Neurobehavioral Study," *Arch Environ Health*, 30, 1975, pp. 98–103.

Roland, E., J. Jan, et al., "Toxic Encephalopathy in a Child After Brief Exposure to Insect Repellents," *Can Med Assoc J*, 132, 1985, pp. 155–156.

Role, L., and D. Berg, "Nicotinic Receptors in the Development and Modulation of CNS Synapses," *Neuron*, 16(6), 1996, pp. 1077–1085.

Romano, J., and J. King, "Conditioned Taste Aversion and Cholinergic Drugs: Pharmacological Antagonism," *Pharmacology Biochemistry and Behavior*, 27, 1987, pp. 81–85.

Romano, J., and M. Landauer, "Effects of the Organophosphorus Compound, O-Ethyl-N-Dimethyl-Phosphoramidocyanidate (Tabun) on Flavor Aversions, Locomotor Activity, and Rotarod Performance in Rats," *Fundam Appl Toxicol*, 6, 1986, pp. 62–68.

Romano, J., J. King, et al., "A Comparison of Physostigmine and Soman Using Taste Aversion and Nociception," *Neurobehav Toxicol Teratol*, 7, 1985, pp. 243–249.

Rose, G., and A. Dewar, "Intoxication with Four Synthetic Pyrethroids Fails to Show Any Correlation Between Neuromuscular Dysfunction and Neurochemical Abnormalities in Rats," *Arch Toxicol*, 53, 1983, pp. 297–316.

Rosenstock, H. A., "Sertraline Withdrawal in Two Brothers: A Case Report," *International Clin Psychopharmacology*, 11(1), 1996, pp. 58–59.

Rosenstock, L., M. Keifer, et al., "Chronic Central Nervous System Effects of Acute Organophosphate Pesticide Intoxication," *Lancet*, 338, 1991, pp. 223–227.

Roskams, A., and J. Connor, "Aluminium Access to the Brain: A Role for Transferring and Its Receptor," *Proc Natl Acad Sci*, 87, 1990, pp. 9024–9027.

Rostker, Bernard, letter to Gulf War veterans, July 24, 1997, http://www.mendonet.com/588th/letter.htm, (http://www.gulfweb.org/).

Rothenberg, D., A. Berns, et al., "Bromide Intoxication with Carbromal Preparations," *J Toxicol Clin Toxicol*, 23, 1990, pp. 341–346.

Rothrock, J., "Making Sense of the New Migraine Drugs," UCSD Department of Medicine, Grand Rounds, La Jolla, Calif., January 12, 1999.

Rotman, A., "Blood Platelets in Psychopharmacological Research," *Progress in Neuro-Psychopharmacol and Biol Psychiatry,* 7(2-3), 1983, pp. 135–151.

Roy, M., P. Koslowe, et al., "Signs, Symptoms and Ill-Defined Conditions in Persian Gulf War Veterans: Findings from the Comprehensive Clinical Evaluation Program," *Psychosomatic Medicine,* 60, 1998, pp. 663–668.

Rubin, L., and M. Goldberg, "Effect of Sarin on Dark Adaptation in Man: Threshold Changes," *J Appl Physiol,* II(3), 1957, pp. 439–444.

Rubin, L., and M. Goldberg, "Effect of Sarin on Dark Adaptation in Man: Mechanisms of Action," *J Appl Physiol,* II(3), 1957, pp. 445–449.

Rupniak, N. M., S. Patel, et al., "Antinociceptive and Toxic Effects of (+)-Epibatidine Oxalate Attributable to Nicotinic Agonist Activity," *Br J Pharmacol,* 113(4), 1994, pp. 1487–1493.

Russ, C., J. Powell, et al., "K Variant of Butyryl Cholinesterase and Late-Onset Alzheimer's Disease," *Lancet,* 351, 1998, p. 881.

Russell, R., R. Booth, et al., "Behavioral, Neurochemical and Physiological Effects of Repeated Exposures to Subsymptomatic Levels of the Anticholinesterase, Soman," *Neurobehav Toxicol Teratol,* 8, 1986, pp. 675–685.

Russell, R. W., R. A. Booth, et al., "Roles of Neurotransmitter Receptors in Behavior: Recovery of Function Following Decreases in Muscarinic Receptor Density Induced by Cholinesterase Inhibition," *Behav Neurosci,* 103(4), 1989, pp. 881–892.

Russell, R., D. Overstreet, et al., "Experimental Tests of Hypothesis About Neurochemical Mechanisms Underlying Behavioral Tolerance to the Anticholinesterase, Diisopropyl Fluorophosphate," *J Pharmacol Exp Therapeutics,* 192, 1975, pp. 73–85.

Rustam, H., R. Von Burg, et al., "Evidence for a Neuromuscular Disorder in Methylmercury Poisoning," *Arch Environ Health,* 30, 1975, pp. 190–195.

Ryan, C., L. Morrow, et al., "Cacosmia and Neurobehavioral Dysfunction Associated with Occupational Exposure to Mixtures of Organic Solvents," *Am J Psychiatry,* 145(11), 1988, pp. 1442–1445.

Ryder, R., T. Hayes, et al., "How Soon After Myocardial Infarction Should Plasma Lipid Values Be Assessed?" *BMJ,* 289, 1984, pp. 1651–1653.

Safer, D., and R. Allen, "The Central Effects of Scopolamine in Man," *Biol Psychiatry,* 3, 1971, p. 347.

Saikku, P., "Chlamydia Pneumoniae and Atherosclerosis—An Update," *Scand J Infect Dis Suppl,* 104, 1997, pp. 53–56.

Saleh, M., M. Zied, et al., "Gamma Aminobutyric Acid Radioreceptor-Assay: A Possible Biomarker for Human Exposure to Certain Agrochemicals," *J Environ Sci Health,* B28(6), 1993, pp. 687–699.

Salpeter, M., H. Kasprzak, et al., "Endplates After Esterase Inactivation in Vivo: Correlation Between Esterase Concentration, Functional Response and Fine Structure," *J Neurocytol,* 8, 1979, pp. 96–115.

Sanchez-Arroyos, R., J. Gaztelu, et al., "Hippocampal and Entorhinal Glucose Metabolism in Relation to Cholinergic Theta Rhythm," *Brain Res Bull,* 32, 1993, pp. 171–178.

Sandborn, W. J., W. J. Tremaine, et al., "Transdermal Nicotine for Mildly to Moderately Active Ulcerative Colitis. A Randomized, Double-Blind, Placebo-Controlled Trial," *Ann Intern Med,* 126(5), 1997, pp. 364–371.

Sandyk, R., and G. I. Awerbuch, "The Co-Occurrence of Multiple Sclerosis and Migraine Headache: the Serotoninergic Link," *Int J Neurosci,* 76(3-4), 1994, pp. 249–257.

Sangster, B., J. Blom, et al., "The Influence of Sodium Bromide in Man: A Study in Human Volunteers with Special Emphasis on the Endocrine and the Central Nervous System," *Food Chem Toxicol,* 21, 1983, pp. 409–419.

Santolucito, J. A., and G. Morrison, "EEG of Rhesus Monkeys Following Low-Level Feeding of Pesticides," *Toxicol Appl Pharmacol,* 19, 1971, pp. 147–154.

Sapolsky, R., *Stress, the Aging Brain, and the Mechanisms of Neuronal Death.* Cambridge, Mass.: MIT Press, 1992.

Sapolsky, R., and W. Pulsinelli, "Glucocorticoids Potentiate Ischemic Injury to Neurons: Therapeutic Implications," *Science,* 121, 1985, p. 1605.

Sargin, H., S. Cirak, et al., "A Case of Porphyria Due to Carbaryl Intoxication," *Human and Experimental Toxicology,* 11, 1992, p. 373.

Sarno, A., "More on Desert Storm (letter)," *JAMA,* 266(23), 1991, p. 3282.

Sarter, M., and J. P. Bruno, "Cognitive Functions of Cortical Acetylcholine: Toward a Unifying Hypothesis," *Brain Res Rev,* 23(1-2), 1997, pp. 28–46.

Saskin, P., H. Moldofsy, et al., "Sleep and Posttraumatic Rheumatic Pain Modulation Disorder (Fibrositis Syndrome)," *Psychosomatic Medicine,* 48(5), 1986, pp. 319–323.

Sastry, B., and C. Sadavongvivad, "Cholinergic Systems in Non-Nervous Tissues," *Pharmacological Reviews,* 30(1), 1979, pp. 65–132.

Sato, M., R. Racine, et al., "Kindling: Basic Mechanisms and Clinical Validity," *Electroencephalogr Clin Neurophysiol*, 76, 1990, pp. 459–472.

Savage, E., R. Keefe, et al., "Chronic Neurologic Sequelae of Acute Organophosphate Pesticide Poisoning," *Archives of Environmental Health*, 43(1), 1988, pp. 38–45.

Sayed, A., "Mania and Bromism," *Am J Psychiatry*, 133, 1976, p. 228.

Scadding, G., C. Havard, et al., "The Long Term Experience of Thymectomy for Myasthenia Gravis," *J Neurol Neurosurg Psychiatry*, 48, 1985, pp. 401–406.

Schachter, S., American Epilepsy Society meeting, Boston, Mass., 1997.

Schiller, G., "Reduced Binding of (3H) Quinuclidinyl Benzilate Associated with Chronically Low Acetylcholinesterase Activity," *Life Sci*, 24, 1979, pp. 1159–1164.

Schmitz, E. B., J. Moriarty, et al., "Psychiatric Profiles and Patterns of Cerebral Blood Flow in Focal Epilepsy: Interactions Between Depression, Obsessionality, and Perfusion Related to the Laterality of the Epilepsy," *J Neurol Neurosurg Psychiatry*, 62(5), 1997, pp. 458–463.

Schoenig, G. P., R. E. Hartnagel, Jr., et al., "Absorption, Distribution, Metabolism, and Excretion of N,N-Diethyl-M-Toluamide in the Rat," *Drug Metab Dispos*, 24(2), 1996, pp. 156–163.

Schoenig, G., R. Hartnagel, et al., "Neurotoxicity Evaluation of N, N-Diethyl-*m*-Toluamide (DEET) in Rats," *Fundam Appl Toxicol*, 21, 1993, pp. 355–365.

Schon, F., M. Drayson, et al., "Myasthenia Gravis and Elderly People," *Age Ageing*, 25(1), 1996, pp. 56–58.

Schottenfeld, R. S., "Workers with Multiple Chemical Sensitivities: A Psychiatric Approach to Diagnosis and Treatment," *Occup Med: State Art Rev*, 2(4), 1987, pp. 739–754.

Schrand, J. R., "Is Sleep Apnea a Predisposing Factor for Tobacco Use?" *Med Hypotheses*, 47(6), 1996, pp. 443–448.

Schulman, H., "Calcium Dependent Protein Kinases and Neuronal Function," *TIPS*, 5, 1984, pp. 188–192.

Schuschereba, S., P. Bowman, et al., "Myopathic Alterations in Extraocular Muscle of Rats Subchronically Fed Pyridostigmine Bromide," *Toxicologic Pathology*, 18(3), 1990, pp. 387–395.

Schwab, B., and S. Murphy, "Induction of Anticholinesterase Tolerance in Rats Using Doses of Disulfoton Which Produce No Cholinergic Signs," *J Toxicol Environ Health*, 8, 1981, pp. 199–204.

Schwab, B., H. Hand, et al., "Reduced Muscarinic Receptor Biding in Tissues of Rats Tolerant to the Insecticide Disulfoton," *Neurotoxicology*, 2, 1981, pp. 635–648.

Schwab, B., L. Costa, et al., "Muscarinic Receptor Alterations as a Mechanism of Anticholinesterase Tolerance," *Toxicol Appl Pharmacol*, 71, 1983, pp. 14–23.

Schwartz, R., and K. Kellar, "Cholinergic Receptor Binding Sites in Brain: Regulation in Vivo," *Science*, 220, 1983, pp. 214–216.

Schwartz, R., and K. Kellar, "In Vivo Regulation of [3H] Acetylcholine Recognition Sites in Brain by Nicotinic Cholinergic Drugs," *J Neurochemistry*, 45, 1985, pp. 427–433.

Schwartz, R. B., A. L. Komaroff, et al., "SPECT Imaging of the Brain: Comparison of Findings in Patients with Chronic Fatigue Syndrome, AIDS Dementia Complex, and Major Unipolar Depression," *AJR Am J Roentgenol*, 162(4), 1994, pp. 943–951.

Schwarz, M., D. Glick, et al., "Engineering of Human Cholinesterases Explains and Predicts Diverse Consequences of Administration of Various Drugs and Poisons," *Pharmacol Ther*, 67(2), 1995, pp. 283–322.

Schwarz, M., Y. Loewenstein-Lichtenstein, et al., "Successive Organophosphate Inhibition and Oxime Reactivation Reveals Distinct Responses of Recombinant Human Cholinesterase Variants," *Molecular Brain Res*, 31(2), 1995, pp. 101–110.

Scott, M. H. W. Reading, and J. B. Loudon, "Studies on Human Platelets in Affective Disorder," *Psychopharmacol*, 60(2), 1979, pp. 131–135.

Scremin, O., K. Allen, et al., "Physostigmine Enhances Blood Flow-Metabolism Ratio in Neocortex," *Neuropsychopharmacology*, 1, 1988, pp. 297–303.

Segal, M., and J. M. Auerbach, "Muscarinic Receptors Involved in Hippocampal Plasticity," *Life Sci*, 60(13-14), 1997, pp. 1085–1091.

Sejnowski, T., personal communication, 1997.

Senanayake, N., "Polyneuropathy Following Insecticide Poisoning," *J Neurol*, 232, 1985, p. 203.

Senanayake, N., and L. Karielledde, "Neurotoxic Effects of Organophosphorus Insecticides. An Intermediate Syndrome," *New Engl J Med*, 316, 1987, pp. 761–763.

Shale, D., D. Lane, et al., "Air-Flow Limitation in Myasthenia Gravis: The Effect of Acetylcholinesterase Inhibitor Therapy on Air-Flow Limitation," *Am Rev Respir Dis*, 128, 1983, pp. 618–621.

Sharabi, Y., Y. L. Danon, et al., "Survey of Symptoms Following Intake of Pyrido-stigmine During the Persian Gulf War," *Isr J Med Sci*, 27, 1991, pp. 656–658.

Sharma, H., F. Nyberg, et al., "Histamine Modulates Heat Stress-Induced Changes in Blood-Brain Barrier Permeability, Cerebral Blood Flow, Brain Oedema and Serotonin Levels: An Experimental Study in the Young Rat," *Neuroscience*, 50, 1992, pp. 445–454.

Sharp, B., H. Beyer, et al., "Attenuation of the Plasma Prolactin Response to Restraint Stress After Acute and Chronic Administration of Nicotine to Rats," *J Pharmacol Exp Therapeutics*, 241(2), 1987, pp. 438–442.

Shaw, K.-P., Y. Aracava, et al., "The Reversible Cholinesterase Inhibitor Physostigmine Has Channel-Blocking and Agonist Effects on the Acetyl-choline Receptor-Ion Channel Complex," *Mol Pharmacol*, 28(6), 1985, pp. 527–538.

Shays, C., statement, Subcommittee on Human Resources, House Committee on Government Reform and Oversight, 1997.

Sherby, S., A. Eldefrawi, et al., "Comparison of Actions of Carbamate Anti-cholinesterases on the Nicotinic Acetylcholine Receptor," *Mol Pharmacol*, 27, 1985, pp. 343–348.

Shih, T., "Time-Course Effects of Soman on Acetylcholine and Choline Levels in Six Discrete Areas of the Rat Brain," *Psychopharmacology*, 78, 1982, pp. 170–175.

Shiloff, J., and J. Clement, "Effects of Subchronic Pyridostigmine Pretreatment on the Toxicity of Soman," *Can J Physiol Pharmacol*, 64, 1986, pp. 1047–1049.

Shipley, M., "Transport of Molecules from Nose to Brain: Transneuronal Ante-grade and Retrograde Labeling in the Rat Olfactory System by Wheat Germ Agglutinin-Horseradish Peroxidase Applied to the Nasal Epithelium," *Brain Res Bull*, 15, 1985, pp. 129–142.

Shytle, R., A. Silver, et al., "Transdermal Nicotine for Tourette's Syndrome," *Drug Dev Res*, 38, 1996, pp. 290–298.

Sidell, F., clinical notes on chemical casualty care: pyridostigmine, Aberdeen Proving Ground, Md.: U.S. Army Medical Research Institute of Chemical Defense, Department of the Army, 1990.

Sidell, F. R., and J. Borak, "Chemical Warfare Agents: II Nerve Agents," *Ann Emergency Med*, 21(7), 1992, pp. 865–871.

Sidell, F., and W. Groff, "The Reactivatability of Cholinesterase Inhibited by VX and Sarin in Man," *Toxicol Appl Pharm*, 27, 1974, pp. 241–252.

Sillanpaa, M. C., L. M. Agar, et al., "Gulf War Veterans: A Neuropsychological Examination," *J Clin Exp Neuropsychol,* 19(2), 1997, pp. 211–219.

Silver, W., and J. Maruniak, "Trigeminal Chemoreception in the Nasal and Oral cavities," *Chemical Senses,* 6(4), 1981, pp. 295–305.

Silverstein, M. D., B. A. Lashner, and S. B. Hanauer, "Cigarette Smoking and Ulcerative Colitis: A Case-Control Study," *Mayo Clin Proc,* 69(5), 1994, pp. 425–429.

Simasko, S., J. Soares, et al., "Two Components of Carbamylcholine-Induced Loss of Nicotinic Acetylcholine Receptor Function in the Neuronal Cell Line PC12," *Mol Pharmacol,* 30, 1986, pp. 6–12.

Simon, G., W. Daniell, et al., "Immunologic, Psychological, and Neuropsychological Factors in Multiple Chemical Sensitivity," *Annals of Internal Medicine,* 19(2), 1993, pp. 97–103.

Simon, T., D. Hickey, et al., "Single Photon Emission Computed Tomography of the Brain in Patients with Chemical Sensitivities," *Toxicol Ind Health,* 10(4/5), 1994, pp. 573–577.

Sitaram, N., and J. Gillin, "Acetylcholine: Possible Involvement in Sleep and Analgesia," in K. L. Davis and P. A. Berger, eds., *Brain Acetylcholine and Neuropsychiatric Disease,* New York: Plenum Press, 1979, pp. 311–343.

Sitaram, N., and J. Gillin, "Development and Use of Pharmacological Probes of the CNS in Man: Evidence of Cholinergic Abnormality in Primary Affective Illness," *Biological Psychiatry,* 15(6), 1980, pp. 925–955.

Sitaram, N., D. Jones, et al., "Supersensitive ACh REM Induction as a Genetic Vulnerability Marker," *Int J Neurosci,* 32, 1985, pp. 777–778.

Sitaram, N., D. Jones, et al., "The Association of Supersensitivie Cholinergic REM Induction and Affective Illness Within Pedigrees," *J Psychiatr Res,* 21, 1987, pp. 487–497.

Sitaram, N., J. Nurnberger, et al., "Cholinergic Regulation of Mood and REM Sleep. A Potential Model and Marker for Vulnerability to Depression," *Am J Psychiatry,* 139, 1982, pp. 571–576.

Smit, M., F. Ehlert, et al., "Decreased Agonist and Antagonist Binding to the Muscarinic Cholinergic Receptor Following Chronic Cholinesterase Inhibition," *Fed Proc,* 39, 1980a, p. 388.

Smit, M., F. Ehlert, et al., "Differential Regulation of Muscarinic Agonist Binding Sites Following Chronic Cholinesterase Inhibition," *Eur J Pharmacol* 66, 1980b, pp. 379–380.

Smith, A. P., "The Reversal by Pyridostigmine of Soman-Induced Neuromuscular Blockade in Primate Respiratory Muscle," Chemical Defence Establishment Technical Paper 302, Porton Down, U. K., 1981.

Smith, D., W. Stavinoha, et al., "Cholinesterase Inhibition in Relation to Fitness to Fly," *Aerospace Med*, 39, 1968, pp. 754–758.

Sneddon, J. M., "Blood Platelets as a Model for Monoamine-Containing Neurones," *Prog Neurobiol*, 1(2), 1973, pp. 151–198.

Snodgrass, H., "Permethrin Transfer from Treated Cloth to the Skin Surface: Potential for Exposure in Humans," *J Toxicol Env Health*, 35, 1992, pp. 91–105.

Snodgrass, H., D. Nelson, et al., "Dermal Penetration and Potential for Placental Transfer of the Insect Repellent, *N,N*-Diethyl-*m*-Toluamide," *Am Ind Hyg Assoc J*, 43, 1982, pp. 747–753.

Socci, D. J., P. R. Sanberg, and G. W. Arendash, "Nicotine Enhances Morris Water Maze Performance of Young and Aged Rats," *Neurobiol of Aging*, 16(5), 1995, pp. 857–860.

Soliman, S., "Comparative Studies in the Neurotoxicity of Organophosphorus Compounds in Different Animal Species," *Neurotoxicology*, 4(4), 1983, pp. 107–116.

Somani, S., "Binding of Quaternary Amines to Subcellular Constituents (Abstract)," *Ind J Pharmacol*, 1977.

Somani, S., "Metabolism and Pharmacokinetics of Pyridostigmine in Rat After Multiple Dosing," *Pharmacologist*, 25, 1983, p. 97.

Somani, S., "Gulf War Syndrome: Potential Effects of Low-Level Exposure to Sarin and/or Pyridostigmine Under Conditions of Physical Stress," testimony, Subcommittee on Human Resources, U.S. House of Representatives, 1997.

Somani, S. M., J. B. Roberts, et al., "Pyridostigmine Metabolism in Man," *Clin Pharmacol Ther*, 13, 1972, pp. 393–399.

Somnier, F. E., "Myasthenia Gravis," *Dan Med Bull*, 43(1), 1996, pp. 1–10.

Soreq, H., "Mutations and Impaired Expression in the AChE and BChE Genes: Neurological Implications," *Biomed and Pharmacother*, 48, 1994, pp. 253–259.

Soreq, H., "Cholinergic Symptoms and Gulf War Syndrome," *Nature Medicine*, 1(12), 1995, p. 1226.

Soreq, H., "Acetylcholinesterase: The Problem or the Solution?" (abstract), CDC Conference on The Health Impact of Chemical Exposures During the Gulf War, Atlanta, Ga., February 28–March 2, 1999.

Soreq, H., G. Ehrlich, et al., "Mutations and Impaired Expression in the AChE and BChE Genes: Neurological Implications," *Biomed and Pharmacother,* 48, 1994, pp. 253–259.

Sorlie, P. D., E. Adam, et al., "Cytomegalovirus/Herpesvirus and Carotid Atherosclerosis: The ARIC Study," *J Med Virol,* 42(1), 1994, pp. 33–37.

Sparks, P., W. Daniell, et al., "Multiple Chemical Sensitivity Syndrome: A Clinical Perspective I. Case Definition, Theories of Pathogenesis, and Research Needs," *JOM,* 36(7), 1994, pp. 718–737.

Spencer, T., J. Hill, et al., "Evaporation of Diethyltoluamide from Human Skin in Vivo and in Vitro," *J Invest Dermatol,* 72, 1979, pp. 317–319.

Sprague, G., L. Sandvik, et al., "Time-Course for Neurotoxic Esterase Inhibition in Hens Given Multiple Diisopropyl Fluorophosphate Injections," *Neurotoxicology,* 2, 1981, pp. 523–532.

Stallcup, W., and J. Patrick, "Substance P Enhances Cholinergic Receptor Desensitization in a Clonal Nerve Cell Line," *Proc Natl Acad Sci USA,* 77(1), 1980, pp. 634–638.

Stanton, M., W. Mundy, et al., "Time-Dependent Effects of Acute Chlorpyrifos Administration on Spatial Delayed Alternation and Cholinergic Neurochemistry in Weanling Rats," *NeuroToxicology,* 15(1), 1994, pp. 201–208.

Staudenmayer, H., and J. Selner, "Neuropsychology During Relaxation in Generalized, Universal 'Allergic' Reactivity to the Environment: A Comparison Study," *J Psychosom Res,* 34(3), 1990.

Staudenmayer, H., J. Selner, et al., "Double-Blind Provocation Chamber Challenges in 20 Patients Presenting with 'Multiple Chemical Sensitivity,'" *Regulatory Toxicology and Pharmacology,* 18(3), 1993, pp. 44–53.

Steenland, K., "Chronic Neurological Effect of Organophosphate Pesticides," *BMJ,* 312, 1996, pp. 1312–1313.

Steinberg, B., S. Weston, et al., "Affective Instability in Personality Disordered Patients Correlates with Mood Response to Physostigmine Challenge," *Biol Psychiatry,* 33, 1993, p. 86.

Stephens, R., A. Spurgeon, et al., "Organophosphates: The Relationship Between Chronic and Acute Exposure Effects," *Neurotoxicology and Teratology,* 18(4), 1996, pp. 449–453.

Stephenson, L., and M. Kolka, "Acetylcholinesterase Inhibitor, Pyridostigmine Bromide, Reduces Skin Blood Flow in Humans," U.S. Army Research Institute of Environmental Medicine, 1989.

Stephenson, L., and M. Kolka, "Acetylcholinesterase Inhibitor, Pyridostigmine Bromide, Reduces Skin Blood Flow in Humans," *Am J Physiol*, 71, 1990, pp. 432–437.

Stern, K., and M. McClintock, "Regulation of Ovulation by Human Pheromones," *Nature*, 392, 1998, pp. 177–179.

Sterri, S., S. Lyngas, et al., "Toxicity of Soman After Repetitive Injection of Sublethal Doses in the Rat," *Acta Pharmacol Toxicol*, 46, 1980, pp. 1–7.

Stewart, J., and I. Koplovitz, "The Effect of Pyridostigmine Pretreatment on the Efficacy of Atropine and Oxime Treatment of Cyclohexylmethylphosphonofluroidate (CMFF) Poisoning in Rodents," Aberdeen Proving Ground, Md., U.S. Army Medical Research Institute of Chemical Defense, 1993.

Stokes, L., A. Stark, et al., "Neurotoxicity Among Pesticide Applicators Exposed to Organophosphates," *Occupational and Environmental Medicine*, 52, 1995, pp. 648–653.

Stoller, A., J. Krupinski, et al., "Organophosphorous Insecticides and Major Mental Illness: An Epidemiological Investigation," *Lancet*, i, 1965, pp. 1387–1388.

Stoohs, R., C. Guilleminault, et al., "Traffic Accidents in Commercial Long-Haul Drivers: The Influence of Sleep-Disordered Breathing and Obesity," *Sleep*, 17(7), 1994, pp. 619–623.

Storzbach, D., L. Binder, et al., *Objective Cognitive Performance of Persian Gulf War Veterans with High Scores on Measures of Post-Traumatic Stress Symptoms*, Conference on Federally Sponsored Gulf War Veterans' Illnesses Research, June 17–19, 1998, Pentagon City, Va.

Stretch, R., P. Bliese, et al., "Physical Health Symptomatology of Gulf War-Era Service Personnel from the States of Pennsylvania and Hawaii," *Milit Medicine*, 160, 1995, pp. 131–136.

Stretch, R., P. Bliese, et al., "Post-Traumatic Stress Disorder Symptoms Among Gulf War Veterans," *Milit Medicine*, 161, 1996a, pp. 407–410.

Stretch, R., P. Bliese, et al., "Psychological Health of Gulf War-Era Military Personnel," *Milit Medicine*, 161, 1996b, pp. 257–261.

Streufert, S., R. Pogash, et al., "Effects of Caffeine Deprivation on Complex Human Functioning," *Psychopharmacol*, 118(4), 1995a, pp. 377–384.

Streufert, S., R. Pogash, et al., "Alcohol Hangover and Managerial Effectiveness," *Alcohol, Clin and Experimental Res*, 19(5), 1995b, pp. 1141–1146.

Streufert, S., U. Satish, et al., "Excess Coffee Consumption in Simulated Complex Work Settings: Detriment or Facilitation of Performance?" *J Appl Psychology*, 82(5), 1997, pp. 774–782.

Subcommittee on Human Resources, "Gulf War Veterans' Illnesses: VA, DoD Continue to Resist Strong Evidence Linking Toxic Causes to Chronic Health Effects," House Committee on Government Reform and Oversight, 1997.

Subcommittee on Human Resources, "Status of Efforts to Identify Persian Gulf War Syndrome," House Committee on Government Reform and Oversight. 1997.

Sugiyama, S., T. Kato, et al., "Deterioration of Mitochondrial Function in Heart Muscles of Rats with Hypothyroidism," *J Clin Biochem Nutr*, 11, 1991, pp. 199–204.

Sultan, W., and W. Lennox, "Comparison of the Efficacy of Various Therapeutic Regimens, with and Without Pyridostigmine Prophylaxis, for Soman (GD) Poisoning in Mice and Rabbits," Aberdeen Proving Ground, Md.: U.S. Army Chemical Systems Laboratory, 1983.

Sumpter-Loebig, S., prepared statement of Sgt. Susan Sumpter-Loebig, U.S. Army (Ret.), Subcommittee on Human Resources, House Committee on Government Reform and Oversight, 1997.

Sutker, P. B., M. Uddo, et al., "Psychopathology in War-Zone Deployed and Nondeployed Operation Desert Storm Troops Assigned Graves Registration Duties," *J Abnorm Psychol*, 103(2), 1994, pp. 383–390.

Swamy, K. V., R. Ravikumar, and P. M. Mohan, "Changes in Cholinesterase System in Different Brain Areas During the Development of Behavioral Tolerance to Monocrotophos Toxicity in Male Albino Rats," *Biochem Int*, 27(4), 1992, pp. 661–669.

Tabershaw, I., and W. Cooper, "Sequelae of Acute Organic Phosphate Poisoning," *J Occup Med*, 8, 1966, pp. 5–20.

Talbot, B., D. Anderson, et al., "A Comparison of in Vivo and in Vitro Rates of Aging of Soman-Inhibited Erythrocyte Acetylcholinesterase in Different Animal Species," *Drug Chem Toxicol*, 11, 1988, pp. 289–305.

Tammings, C., R. Smith, et al., "Depression Associated with Oral Choline," *Lancet*, 2, 1976, p. 905.

Tandon, P., S. Padilla, et al., "Fenthion Produces a Persistent Decrease in Muscarinic Receptor Function in the Adult Rat Retina," *Toxicol Appl Pharmacol*, 125, 1994, pp. 271–280.

Tandon, P., S. Willig, et al., "Dose-Response Study of the Tissue-Specific Effects of Fenthion on Receptor Function in Rat CNS," *Toxicologist,* 14, 1994, p. 257.

Tankersley, M., K. Smith, et al., "Petition to Repeal the Interim Rule," 1996, pp. 1–27.

Tavitian, B., S. Pappata, et al., "In Vivo Visualization of Acetylcholinesterase with Positron Emission Tomography," *Neuroreport,* 4, 1993, pp. 535–538.

Tavitian, B., S. Pappata, et al., "Binding Characteristics of [11C]physostigmine, a PET Tracer for Acetylcholinesterase (abstract)," *J Cereb Blood Flow Metab,* 15(Suppl), 1995, p. S122.

Taylor, P., and J. Brown, "Acetylcholine," in G. Siegel, B. Agranoff, R. Albers, and P. Molinoff, eds., *Basic Neurochemistry,* New York: Raven Press, 1994, Chapter 11, pp. 231–260.

Taylor, J., E. El-Fakahany, et al., "Long-Term Regulation of Muscarinic Receptors on Cultured Nerve Cells," *Life Sci,* 25, 1979, pp. 2181–2187.

Teichman, S., A. Ferrick, et al., "Disopyramide-Pyridostigmine Interaction: Selection Reversal of Anticholinergic Symptoms with Preservation of Antiarrhythmic Effect," *JACC,* 10, 1987, pp. 633–641.

Thakore, J., and T. Dinan, "Loss of the Diurnal Variation of Pyridostigmine-Induced Growth Hormone Responses in Depression: The Effect of Cortisol," *International Clin Psychopharmacology,* 10, 1995, pp. 107–110.

Thomas, G. A., J. Rhodes, et al., "Nicotine and Gastrointestinal Disease," *QJM,* 89(7), 1996, pp. 485–488.

Thomas, G. A., J. Rhodes, et al., "Inflammatory Bowel Disease and Smoking—A Review," *Am J Gastroenterol,* 93(2), 1998, pp. 144–149.

Thomas, G. A., J. Rhodes, et al., "Transdermal Nicotine as Maintenance Therapy for Ulcerative Colitis," *New Engl J Med,* 332(15), 1995, pp. 988–992.

Thompson, M., "The Silent Treatment," *Nation,* 148(28), 1996.

Thomsen, T., H. Kewitz, and O. Pleul, "Estimation of Cholinesterase Activity in Undiluted Plasma and Erythrocytes as a Tool for Measuring in Vivo Effect of Reversible Inhibitors," *J Clin Chem Clin Biochem,* 26(7), 1988, pp. 469–475.

Tiedt, T., Gulf War Syndrome testimony, Human Resources Subcommittee, House Government Reform and Oversight Committee, 1994.

Tiedt, T., E. Albuquerque, et al., "Neostigmine-Induced Alterations at the Mammalian Neuromuscular Junction I. Muscle Contraction and Electrophysiology," *J Pharmacol Exp Therapeutics,* 205(2), 1978, pp. 326–339.

Tiersky, L., B. Natelson, et al., "Functional Status and Mood in Gulf War Veterans (GWVs) with Fatiguing Illness," conference on Federally Sponsored Gulf War Veterans' Illnesses Research, Arlington, Va., June 17–19, 1998.

Tizabi, Y., D. H. Overstreet, et al., "Antidepressant Effects of Nicotine in an Animal Model of Depression," *Psychopharmacol,* 142(2), 1999, pp. 193–199.

Toth, L., S. Karcsu, et al., "Histochemical Evidence for the Role of Ca2+ and Neutral Protease in the Development of the Subacute Myopathy Induced by Organophosphorous Compounds," *Acta Histochem,* 72, 1983, pp. 71–75.

Trainer, P., J. Kirk, et al., "Pyridostigmine Partially Reverses Dexamethasone-Induced Inhibition of the Growth Hormone Response to Growth Hormone-Releasing Hormone," *J Endocrinology,* 134, 1991, pp. 513–517.

Trasforini, G., A. Margutti, et al., "Evidence that Enhancement of Cholinergic Tone Increases Basal Plasma Levels of Calcitonin Gene-Related Peptide in Normal Man," *J Clin Endocrinology and Metabolism,* 78(3), 1994, pp. 763–766.

Trojan, D., and N. Cashman, "Anticholinesterases in Post-Poliomyelitis Syndrome," *Ann NY Acad Sci,* 753, 1995, pp. 285–295.

Trojan, D., and N. Cashman, "An Open Trial of Pyridostigmine in Post-Poliomyelitis Syndrome," *Canadian J of Neurological Sciences,* 22(3), 1995, pp. 223–227.

Tuitte, J. I., "Second Staff Report on US Chemical and Biological Warfare-Related Dual-Use Exports to Iraq and the Possible Impact on the Health Consequences of the War (Updated April 25, 1997)," 1997.

Tuomisto, J. E. Tukiainen, and U. G. Ahlfors, "Decreased Uptake of 5-Hydroxytryptamine in Blood Platelets from Patients with Endogenous Depression," *Psychopharmacol,* 65(2), 1979, pp. 141–147.

Uchida, S., K. Takeyasu, et al., "Changes in Muscarinic Acetylcholine Receptors of Mice by Chronic Administration of Diisopropylfluorophosphate and Papaverine," *Life Sci,* 24, 1979, pp. 1805–1812.

"UN Inspectors in Iraq Found VX Nerve Gas Production," http://cthesis.com/politics/0698/p_24_1.html, posted June 24, 1998.

Unwin, C., N. Blatchley, et al., "Health of UK Servicemen Who Served in the Persian Gulf War," *Lancet,* 353, 1999, pp. 169–178.

U.S. Army Medical Research Institute of Chemical Defense, "219. Pretreatment," *Medical Management of Chemical Casualties Handbook,* accessed from Internet, 1997.

U.S. Department of Defense, "Immunizations and Chemoprophylaxis," 1995.

U.S. Environmental Protection Agency, "Technical Support Document on Risk Assessment of Chemical Mixtures," 1988.

Uyama, O., et al., "Quantitative Evaluation of Vascular Permeability in the Gerbil Brain After Transient Ischemia Using Evans Blue Fluorescence," *J Cerebral Blood Flow Metab.* 8, 1988, pp. 282–284.

Vaerøy, H., R. Helle, et al., "Cerebrospinal Fluid Levels of ß-Endorphin in Patients with Fibromyalgia (Fibrositis Syndrome)," *J Rheumatol*, 15(12), 1988, pp. 1804–1806.

Vaerøy, H., R. Helle, et al., "Elevated CSF Levels of Substance P and High Incidence of Raynaud Phenomenon in Patients with Fibromyalgia: New Features for Diagnosis," *Pain*, 32(1), 1988, pp. 21–26.

Vaiseman, N., G. Koren, et al., "Pharmacokinetics of Oral and Intravenous Bromide in Normal Volunteers," *Clinical Toxicology*, 24(5), 1986, pp. 403–413.

Valcavi, R., M. Zini, et al., "The Late Growth Hormone Rise Induced by Oral Glucose Is Enhanced by Cholinergic Stimulation with Pyridostigmine in Normal Subjects," *Clinical Endocrinology*, 37, 1992, pp. 360–364.

Valcavi, R., O. Gaddi, et al., "Cardiac Performance and Mass in Adults with Hypopituitarism: Effects of One Year of Growth Hormone Treatment," *J Clin Endocrinology and Metabolism*, 80(2), 1995, pp. 659–666.

Vannucchi, M. G., C. Scali, et al., "Selective Muscarinic Antagonists Differentially Affect In Vivo Acetylcholine Release and Memory Performances of Young and Aged Rats," *Neuroscience*, 79(3), 1997, pp. 837–846.

Vasterling, J. J., K. Brailey, et al., "Attention and Memory Dysfunction in Posttraumatic Stress Disorder," *Neuropsychology*, 12(1), 1998, pp. 125–133.

Velicky, J., M. Titlbach, et al., "Potassium Bromide and the Thyroid Gland of the Rat: Morphology and Immunohistochemistry, RIA and INAA analysis," *Anat Anz*, 179(5), 1997, pp. 421–431.

Velicky, J., M. Titlbach, et al., "Long-Term Action of Potassium Bromide on the Rat Thyroid Gland," *Acta Histochem*, 100(1), 1988, pp. 11–23.

Velicky, J., M. Titlbach, et al., "Expression of the Proliferating Cell Nuclear Antigen (PCNA) in the Rat Thyroid Gland After Exposure to Bromide," *Acta Histochem*, 99(4), 1997, pp. 391–399.

Verschoyle, R., A. Brown, et al., "A Comparison of the Acute Toxicity, Neuropathology, and Electrophysiology of *N, N*-Diethyl-*m*-Toluamine and *N, N*-Dimethyl-2,2-Diphenylacetamide in Rats," *Fundam Appl Toxicol*, 18, 1990, pp. 79–88.

Viby-Mogensen, J., "Succinylcholine Neuromuscular Blockade in Subjects Heterozygous for Abnormal Plasma Cholinesterase," *Anesthesiology,* 55, 1981, p. 235.

Visseren, F. L., K. P. Bouter, et al., "Patients with Diabetes Mellitus and Atherosclerosis; A Role for Cytomegalovirus?" *Diabetes Res Clin Pract,* 36(1), 1997, pp. 49–55.

Vizi, E. S., L. G. Harsing, Jr., and G. Zsilla, "Evidence of the Modulatory Role of Serotonin in Acetylcholine Release from Striatal Interneurons," *Brain Res,* 212(1), 1981, pp. 89–99.

Vobecky, M., and A. Babicky, "Effect of Enhanced Bromide Intake on the Concentration Ratio I/Br in the Rat Thyroid Gland," *Biol Trace Elem Res,* 43(45), 1994, pp. 509–516.

Vobecky, M., A. Babicky, et al., "Effect of Increased Bromide Intake on Iodine Excretion in Rats," *Biol Trace Elem Res,* 55(3), 1996, pp. 215–219.

Vobecky, M., A. Babicky, et al., "Interaction of Bromine with Iodine in the Rat Thyroid Gland at Enhanced Bromide Intake," *Biol Trace Elem Res,* 54(3), 1996, pp. 207–212.

von Bredow, J., J. Jaxx, et al., "Estimate of the Lowest Dose of Diazepam Required to Treat Soman-Induced Convulsions in Pyridostigmine Pretreated, Atropine, Pralidoxime Chloride and Diazepam Treated Rhesus Monkeys," Aberdeen Proving Ground, Md.: U.S. Army Medical Research Institute of Chemical Defense, 1988.

von Bredow, J. D., N. L. Adams, et al., "Effectiveness of Oral Pyridostigmine Pretreatment and Cholinolytic-Oxime Therapy Against Soman Intoxication in Nonhuman Primates," *Fundam Appl Toxicol,* 17, 1991, pp. 761–770.

von Bredow, J., R. McGarrigle, et al., "Carbamate and Anticholinergic Prophylaxis Against Multilethal Concentrations of Soman in Primates," *Pharmacologist,* 24, 1982, p. 220.

von Mayersbach, H., "Circadian Liver Detoxification and Acetylcholinesterase Rhythmicity: Two Limiting Factors in Circadian E600 Toxicity," in L. Scheving, F. Halberg, and J. Pauly, eds., *Chronobiology,* Tokyo: Igaku Shoin, Ltd., 1974.

Wacks, I., J. Oster, et al., "Spurious Hyperchloremia and Hyperbicarbonatemia in a Patient Receiving Pyridostigmine Bromide Therapy for Myasthenia Gravis," *Am J Kidney Diseases,* XVI(1), 1990, pp. 76–79.

Wada, K., M. Ballivet, et al., "Functional Expression of a New Pharmacological Subtype of Brain Nicotinic Acetylcholine Receptor," *Science,* 240, 1987, pp. 330–334.

Wada, E., K. Wada, et al., "Distribution of Alpha2, Alpha3, Alpha4, and Beta2 Neuronal Nicotinic Receptor Subunit mRNAs in the Central Nervous System: A Hybridization Histochemical Study in the Rat," *J Comparative Neurology,* 284, 1989, pp. 314–335.

Wada, K., D. McKinnon, et al., "The Distribution of mRNA Encoded by a New Member of the Neuronal Nicotinic Acetylcholine Receptor Gene Family (Alpha5) in the Rat Central Nervous System," *Brain Res,* 526, 1990, pp. 45–53.

Wali, S. O., and M. H. Kryger, "Medical Treatment of Sleep Apnea," *Curr Opin Pulm Med,* 1(6), 1995, pp. 498–503.

Walsh, T., and D. Emerich, "The Hippocampus as a Common Target of Neurotoxic Agents," *Toxicol,* 49, 1988, pp. 137–140.

Wannarka, G., "Status of the Pyridostigmine Development Effort," *4th Annual Defense Bioscience Review,* 1984, pp. 107–120.

Watanabe, K., and H. Kang, "Military Service in Vietnam and the Risk of Death from Trauma and Selected Cancers," *AEP,* 5(5), 1995, pp. 407–412.

Watson, J. P., and R. A. Lewi, "Ulcerative Colitis Responsive to Smoking and to Nicotine Chewing Gum in a Patient with Alpha 1 Anti-Trypsin Deficiency," *Respir Med* 89(9), 1995, pp. 635–636.

Wecker, L., and W.-D. Dettbarn, "Paraoxon-Induced Myopathy: Muscle Specificity and Acetylcholine Involvement," *Experimental Neurology,* 51, 1976, pp. 281–291.

Wehrenberg, W., S. Wiviott, et al., "Pyridostigmine-Mediated Growth Hormone Release: Evidence for Somatostatin Involvement," *Endocrinology,* 130(3), 1992, pp. 1445–1450.

Wenger, B., M. D. Quigley, et al., "Seven-Day Pyridostigmine Administration and Thermoregulation During Rest and Exercise in Dry Heat," *Aviat Space Environ Med,* October 1993, pp. 905–911.

Wenger, C., and W. Latzka, "Effects of Pyridostigmine Bromide on Physiological Response to Heat, Exercise, and Hypohydration," *Aviat Space Environ Med,* 63(1), 1992, pp. 37–45.

Wertlake, P., A. Wilcox, et al., "Relationship of Mental and Emotional Stress to Serum Cholesterol Levels," *Proc Soc Exper Biol & Med,* 97, 1958, p. 163.

Westbrook, G., *Regulation of Glutamate Channels at Central Synapses,* International Symposium on the Cholinergic Synapse: Structure, Function and Regulation (3rd), University of Maryland, Baltimore, 1994.

Westernick, B., and J. Korf, "Influence of Drugs on Striatal and Limbic Homovanillic Acid Concentration in the Rat Brain," *Eur J Pharmacol*, 33, 1975, p. 31.

Westfall, T. C., H. Grant, and H. Perry, ""Release of Dopamine and 5-Hydroxytryptamine from Rat Striatal Slices Following Activation of Nicotinic Cholinergic Receptors," *General Pharmacol*, 14(3), 1983, pp. 321–325.

Wetherell, A., "Car Driver Behaviour Following Pyridostigmine Bromide Administration," Chemical Defence Establishment, Porton Down, U.K., 1988.

Wetherell, A., "Cognitive and Psychomotor Effects of Nerve Agent Immediate Treatments Containing 10 and 15 mg TL4914 Preceded by Two Days' Pretreatment with Pyridostigmine Bromide," Chemical Defence Establishment, Porton Down, U.K., 1988.

Wetherell, A., "Cognitive and Psychomotor Performance Tests and Experiment Design in Multiple Chemical Sensitivity," *Environ Health Perspect*, 105, Supplement 2, 1997, pp. 495–503.

Wetherell, A., "A Comparison of the Effects on Human Behaviour of Nerve Agent Immediate Treatment Containing 5 mg Diazepam with That Containing 15 mg TL4914," Chemical Defence Establishment, Porton Down, U.K., 1984.

Wetherell, A., "Effects of 5mg Diazepam and 15 and 30 mg TL4914 on Human Cognitive and Psychomotor Performance," Chemical Defence Establishment, Porton Down, U.K., 1984.

Wetherell, A., and J. Wainwright, "Comparative Effects on Human Behaviour of the Current Nerve Agent Immediate Treatment Incorporating 5mg Diazepam and the Proposed Treatment Incorporating 10mg TL4914," Chemical Defence Establishment, Porton Down, U.K., 1985.

Wetherell, J., "The Development of Pyridostigmine as a Nerve Agent Pretreatment," Technical Note 1296, Chemical Defence Establishment, Porton Down, U.K., 1992.

Wetherell, J., and M. French, "The Hydrolysis of Succinyuldithiocholine and Related Thiocholine Esters by Human Plasma and Purified Cholinesterase," *Biochem Pharmacol*, 35(6), 1986, pp. 939–945.

Wetherell, J., and M. French, "A Comparison of the Decarbamoylation Rates of Physostigmine-Inhibited Plasma and Red Cell Cholinesterases of Man with Other Species," *Biochem Pharmacol* 42, 1991, pp. 515–520.

Whetsell, W., "Current Concepts of Excitotoxicity," *J of Neuropathology and Experimental Neurology*, 55(1), 1996, pp. 1–13.

Whinnery, J., "Pyridostigmine Bromide: A Pre-Exposure Antidote for Specific Chemical Warfare Nerve Agents: A Condensed Review for the Aeromedical Specialist," USAF School of Aerospace Medicine, Brooks AFB, Tex., 1984.

White, R. F., M. Krengel, et al., "Neuropsychological Findings Among Persian Gulf War Veterans" (abstract), conference on Federally Sponsored Gulf War Veterans' Illnesses Research, June 17–19, 1998, p. 76.

Whybrow, P., and J. Ewing, "Self Perpetuation of Bromism," *Brit Med J,* 2, 1966, p. 886.

Wiley, R., J. Kotulak, et al., "The Effects of Pyridostigmine Bromide on Visual Performance," *Aviat Space Environ Med,* 63, 1992, pp. 1054–1059.

Williams, F., "Clinical Significance of Esterase in Man," *Clin Pharmacokinet,* 10, 1987, pp. 392–405.

Williams, J., "Human Response to Pyridostigmine Bromide," Air Force Aerospace Medical Research Laboratory, Dayton, Ohio, 1984.

Wills, J., "Pharmacological Antagonists of the Anticholinesterase Agents," in G. Koelle, ed., *Cholinesterases and Anticholinesterase Agents,* Berlin: Springer-Verlag, 1963, p. 896.

Wills, M., and J. Savory, "Aluminium Poisoning: Dialysis Encephalopathy, Osteomalacia, and Anaemia," *Lancet,* 2, 1983, pp. 29–33.

Wilson, J., E. Braunwald, et al., eds., *Harrison's Principles of Internal Medicine,* New York: McGraw-Hill, 1991.

Wimmer, M. L., R. Sandmann-Strupp, et al., "Association of Chlamydial Infection with Cerebrovascular Disease," *Stroke,* 27(12), 1996, pp. 2207–2210.

Winbladh, B., "Choroid Plexus Uptake of Acetylcholine," *Acta Physiol Scand,* 92, 1974, pp. 156–164.

Windheuser, J., J. Haslam, et al., "The Use of *N,N-* Diethyl-m-Toluamide to Enhance the Dermal and Transdermal Delivery of Drugs," *J Pharmacol Sci,* 71, 1982, pp. 1211–1213.

Wirth, J. A., "Organic Psychosyndrome and Sleep Apnea. Transdermal Nicotine—a New Therapy Concept?" *Pneumologie,* 49, 1995, Supplement 1, pp. 183–184.

Wolfe, A., D. Blick, et al., "Use of Cholinesterases as Pretreatment Drugs for the Protection of Rhesus Monkeys Against Soman Toxicity," *Toxicol Appl Pharmacol,* 117, 1992, pp. 189–193.

Wolfe, J., S. Proctor, et al., *Relationship of PTSD and Depression to Persian Gulf Health Problems,* Conference on Federally Sponsored Gulf War Veterans' Illnesses Research, June 17–19, 1998a, Pentagon City, Va.

Wolfe, J., S. Proctor, et al., "Re: 'Is Gulf War Syndrome Due to Stress? The Evidence Reexamined' (letter)," *Am J Epidem* 148(4), 1998b, p. 402.

Wolfe, J., S. Proctor, et al., "Health Symptoms Reported by Persian Gulf War Veterans Two Years After Return," *Amer J Ind Med*, 33, 1998c, pp. 104–113.

Wolthius, O., B. Groen, et al., "Effects of Low Doses of Cholinesterase Inhibitors on Behavioral Performance of Robot-Tested Marmosets," *Pharmacol Biochem Behav*, 51(2/3), 1995, pp. 443–456.

Wonnacott, S., D. Marshal, et al., *Presynaptic Nicotinic Receptor Modulation of Dopamine Release in Rat Brain*, International Symposium on the Cholinergic Synapse: Structure, Function and Regulation (3rd), University of Maryland, Baltimore, 1994.

Worek, F., and L. Szinicz, "Cardiorespiratory Function in Nerve Agent Poisoned and Oxime+Atropine Treated Guinea-Pigs: Effect of Pyridostigmine Pretreatment," *Arch Toxicol*, 69(5), 1995, pp. 322–329.

Worek, F., A. Kleine, et al., "Effect of Pyridostigmine Pretreatment on Cardiorespiratory Function in Tabun Poisoning," *Human and Experimental Toxicology*, 14, 1995, pp. 634–642.

Writer, J., R. De Fraites, et al., "Comparative Mortality Among U.S. Military Personnel in the Persian Gulf Region and Worldwide During Operations Desert Shield and Desert Storm," *JAMA*, 275, pp. 118–121.

Yamaguchi, M., R. Robson, et al., "Properties of Soleus Muscle Z-Lines and Induced Z-Line Analogs Revealed by Dissection with Ca2+-Activated Neutral Protease," *Anat Rec*, 206, 1983, pp. 345–362.

Yamamoto, K., Y. Sawada, et al., "Comparative Pharmacokinetics of Four Cholinesterase Inhibitors in Rats," *Biol Pharm Bull*, 18(9), 1995, pp. 1292–1295.

Yamamura, H., and S. Snyder, "Muscarinic Cholinergic Binding in Rat Brain," *Proc Nat Acad Sci USA*, 71(5), 1974, pp. 1725–1729.

Yanaura, M., M. Nakashima, et al., "Characterization of Slow Presynaptic Current of Apyslia LUQ Neurons in Culture," *Brain Res*, 629(1), 1993, pp. 88–94.

Yang, I., J. Woo, et al., "Combined Pyridostigmine-Thyrotrophin-Releasing Hormone Test for the Evaluation of Hypothalamic Somatostatinergic Activity in Healthy Normal Men," *Eur J Endocrinology*, 133, 1995, pp. 457–462.

Yonemitsu, Y., Y. Kaneda, et al., "The Immediate Early Gene of Human Cytomegalovirus Stimulates Vascular Smooth Muscle Cell Proliferation in Vitro and in Vivo," *Biochem Biophys Res Commun*, 231(2), 1997, pp. 447–451.

Young, G. D., "Pyridostigmine Bromide Interactive Studies: A Synopsis of Past, Current, and Future Studies," Directorate of Toxicology, USACHPPM, undated.

Young, J., "Desensitization and Agonist Binding to Cholinergic Receptors in Intestinal Smooth Muscle," *FEBS Lett,* 46, 1974, pp. 354–356.

Young, R., R. Rachal, and J. W. Huguley III, "Environmental Health Concerns of the Persian Gulf War," *J National Med Assoc,* 84(5), 1992, pp. 417–424.

Zadikoff, C., "Toxic Encephalopathy Associated with Use of Insect Repellent," *J Pediatr,* 95, 1979, pp. 140–142.

Zarrindast, M. R., M. Sadegh, and B. Shafaghi, "Effects of Nicotine on Memory Retrieval in Mice," *Eur J Pharmacol,* 295(1), 1996, pp. 1–6.

Zeller, M., prepared statement of SSgt. Mark J. Zeller before the Subcommittee on Human Resources, House Committee on Government Reform and Oversight, 1997.

Zhou, Y. F., E. Guetta, et al., "Human Cytomegalovirus Increases Modified Low Density Lipoprotein Uptake and Scavenger Receptor mRNA Expression in Vascular Smooth Muscle Cells," *J Clin Invest,* 98(9), 1996, pp. 2129–2138.

Ziem, G., "Multiple Chemical Sensitivity: Treatment and Followup with Avoidance and Control of Chemical Exposures," *Toxicol Ind Health,* 8, 1992, pp. 73–86.

Ziem, G., and J. McTamney, "Profile of Patients with Chemical Injury and Sensitivity," *Environmental Health Perspectives,* 105, 1997, Supplement 2, pp. 417–436.

Zoler, M., "Vagal Nerve Stimulation Needs Tweaking," *Internal Medicine News,* 1998, p. 21.

Zuckerman, D., P. Olson, et al., "Is Military Research Hazardous to Veterans' Health? Lessons from the Persian Gulf," accessed from the Internet, 1994.